T0345182

Introduction to Statistical Methods for Biosurveillance

Bioterrorism is not a new threat but, in an increasingly interconnected world, the potential for catastrophic outcomes is greater today than ever. The medical and public health communities are establishing biosurveillance systems designed to proactively monitor populations for possible disease outbreaks as a first line of defense.

The ideal biosurveillance system should identify trends not visible to individual physicians and clinicians in near-real time. Many of these systems use statistical algorithms to look for anomalies and to trigger epidemiologic investigation, quantification, localization, and outbreak management.

This book is focused on the design and evaluation of statistical methods for effective biosurveillance. Weaving public health and statistics together, it presents both basic and more advanced methods, all with a focus on empirically demonstrating added value. Although the emphasis is on epidemiologic surveillance and syndromic surveillance, the statistical methods can also be applied to a broad class of public health surveillance problems.

Ronald D. Fricker, Jr. is an Associate Professor of Operations Research at the Naval Postgraduate School (NPS). He holds a Ph.D. in statistics from Yale University. Prior to joining NPS, Dr. Fricker was a Senior Statistician at the RAND Corporation and the Associate Director of the National Security Research Division. Published widely in leading professional journals, he is a Fellow of the American Statistical Association, an Elected Member of the International Statistical Institute, and a former chair of the ASA Section on Statistics in Defense and National Security. He is a contributing editor to *Interfaces* and is on the editorial boards of *Statistics, Politics, and Policy* and the *International Journal of Quality Engineering and Technology*. Fricker's current research is focused on studying the performance of various statistical methods for use in biosurveillance, particularly syndromic surveillance, and statistical process control methodologies more generally.

Introduction to Statistical Methods for Biosurveillance

With an Emphasis on Syndromic Surveillance

RONALD D. FRICKER, JR.

Naval Postgraduate School

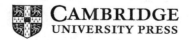

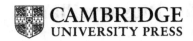

CAMBRIDGE
UNIVERSITY PRESS

Shaftesbury Road, Cambridge CB2 8EA, United Kingdom

One Liberty Plaza, 20th Floor, New York, NY 10006, USA

477 Williamstown Road, Port Melbourne, VIC 3207, Australia

314–321, 3rd Floor, Plot 3, Splendor Forum, Jasola District Centre, New Delhi – 110025, India

103 Penang Road, #05–06/07, Visioncrest Commercial, Singapore 238467

Cambridge University Press is part of Cambridge University Press & Assessment,
a department of the University of Cambridge.

We share the University's mission to contribute to society through the pursuit of
education, learning and research at the highest international levels of excellence.

www.cambridge.org
Information on this title: www.cambridge.org/9780521191340

First published 2013

A catalogue record for this publication is available from the British Library

Library of Congress Cataloging-in-Publication data
Fricker, Ronald D., 1960–
Introduction to statistical methods for biosurveillance : with an emphasis on syndromic
surveillance / Ronald D. Fricker, Jr.
p. ; cm.
Includes bibliographical references and index.
ISBN 978-0-521-19134-0 (hardback)
I. Title.
[DNLM: 1. Biosurveillance – methods.   2. Bioterrorism – prevention & control.
3. Communicable Disease Control – methods.   4. Disease Outbreaks – prevention & control.
5. Models, Statistical. WA 950]
363.325′3–dc23   2012035196

ISBN   978-0-521-19134-0   Hardback

*Dedicated to all who are
working to protect the world
from disease and terrorism.*

Contents

Part V   Appendices

Preface

This book is about basic statistical methods useful for biosurveillance. The focus on basic methods has a twofold motivation. First, there is a need for a text that starts from the fundamentals, both of public health surveillance and statistics, and weaves them together into a foundation for biosurveillance. Only from a solid foundation can an enduring edifice be built.

Second, while there is a large and growing literature about biosurveillance that includes the application of some very complicated and sophisticated statistical methods, it has been my experience that more complicated methods and models do not always result in better performance. And even when they do, there is often an inherent trade-off made in terms of transparency and interpretability.

Indeed, a real challenge in today's data-rich environment is deciding when enough complication is enough. More is not always better, whether we're talking about eating dessert or building a model or developing a detection algorithm. There is a rich history that speaks to this point:

> Occam's razor: "All other things being equal, a simpler explanation is better than a more complex one."

> Blaise Pascal (1623–1662): "Je n'ai fait cette lettre – ci plus longue que parce que je n'ai pas eu le loisir de la faire plus courte." (I have made this letter longer than usual, only because I have not had time to make it shorter.)

> Albert Einstein (1879–1955): "Make everything as simple as possible, but not simpler," and "Any intelligent fool can make things bigger, more complex. . . . It takes a touch of genius . . . to move in the opposite direction."

Note the theme in these quotes is not one of just simplicity but also that it takes effort and insight to *appropriately* simplify. Hence, I do not claim that the methods in this book are necessarily the best or most correct ones for biosurveillance. Most of the research necessary to reach such a determination is yet to be done. However, the philosophy on which this book is predicated is that biosurveillance should start with basic methods such as those described herein and, only after *empirically demonstrating the added value of more complicated methods*, extend from there.

This text presumes a familiarity with basic probability and statistics at the level of an advanced undergraduate or beginning graduate-level course. For readers requiring a probability refresher, Appendix A provides a brief review of many of the basic concepts used throughout the text. However, the text also uses some statistical methods that are often not taught in introductory courses, such as ROC (receiver operating characteristic) curves, imputation, and time series modeling. In presenting these and other methods, the goal has been to make the exposition as accessible and as relevant to the widest audience possible. However, this inevitably means that some of the concepts and methods will be insufficiently explained for some readers, while others may have preferred a more advanced treatment. In an attempt to accommodate all levels of interest, the end of each chapter contains an "additional reading" section with pointers to other resources, some providing more background and introductory material and others providing a more advanced treatment of the material.

That said, this book is largely focused on univariate temporal data. More complicated data, whether multivariate or spatio-temporal, will by definition require more complicated statistical methods. In this book, I touch on these types of data, but they require a treatment more in depth than a text of this length will allow.

As a statistician with a background in industrial quality control, I approach the problem of biosurveillance early event detection from the perspective of statistical process control (SPC). This is, of course, only one way to approach the problem, and different disciplines have different viewpoints.

SPC methods were first developed to monitor industrial processes, which are generally more controlled and for which the data are often easier to distributionally characterize than biosurveillance data. Nonetheless, I am of the opinion that, appropriately applied to biosurveillance data, these methods have much to offer in terms of (1) their performance and (2) a rich, quantitatively rigorous literature that both develops the methods and describes their performance characteristics. Thus, returning to a previous point, my motivation for starting from an SPC perspective is that it provides biosurveillance with a solid methodological foundation on which to build.

It is also important to note that I tend to look at biosurveillance as a tool for guarding against bioterrorism. Of course, a system designed to detect a bioterrorism attack is also useful for detecting natural disease outbreaks, but it's not necessarily true that a biosurveillance system designed for natural disease detection will be optimal for bioterrorism applications. Just as the person who tries to please everyone ends up pleasing no one, so it is with biosurveillance. Thus, while these systems do have dual-use possibilities, I am of the opinion that first and foremost they should be designed for thwarting bioterrorism.

Additional material related to this book, including errata, can be found at http://facultly.nps.edu/rdfricke/biosurveillance_book/. Please feel free to e-mail me at rdfricker@nps.edu with any comments, thoughts, or material that might be relevant and useful in the next revision.

In conclusion, I hope this book contributes to the effective design and implementation of biosurveillance systems. Given the increasingly dangerous threats that face humankind, some of natural origin and some not, and all magnified by our increasingly interconnected world, biosurveillance systems are truly a first line of defense.

Monterey, California
September 2012

R. D. Fricker, Jr.
Associate Professor

Acknowledgments

This book has benefited from discussions and interactions with, and the assistance of, many people. The following is surely an incomplete list.

In the academic community: Bill Woodall, Dan Jeske, Howard Burkom, David Buckeridge, Doug Montgomery, Ken Kleinman, Galit Shmueli, Lance Waller, Karen Kafadar, Mike Stoto, Kwok Tsui, Yajun Mei, Al Ozonoff, and Abel Rodriguez.

In the public health community: Henry Rolka, Taha Kass-Hout, Lori Hutwagner, Jerry Tokars, Myron Katzoff, Wendy Wattigney, and Kathy O'Connor of the Centers for Disease Control and Prevention and Krista Hanni, Suzie Barnes, Kristy Michie, and Bryan Rees of the Monterey County Health Department (MCHD).

I would particularly like to thank Krista Hanni and the MCHD for sharing data. One of the major impediments to improving biosurveillance is the lack of access to real data. Krista and the MCHD were uncommonly forward leaning; rather than finding reasons why something could not be done, they constantly looked for ways to make things work. The rest of the public health community would do well to follow their lead.

A large portion of the research for this book was conducted while I was on sabbatical at the University of California, Riverside (UCR). My thanks to Dan Jeske, chair of the UCR Department of Statistics, for hosting my sabbatical. Thanks also to the Naval Postgraduate School (NPS) for sponsoring the sabbatical.

While on sabbatical, I taught a course using an early version of this book. I am very appreciative of the UCR students who took the class: Tatevik Ambartsoumian, Fei He, Quan Tuong Truong Le, Rebecca Phuonganh Le, Xin Zhang, Joyce Yingzhuo, Anne Hansen, and Judy Li. Their involvement and comments helped significantly improve the text.

At NPS, I also used a draft for a reading course, and the material was again improved with the feedback of those who participated in that course: Krista Hanni, Suzie Barnes, Manny Ganuza, Katie Hagen, and Randi Korman. And much of the material in Chapters 9 and 10 is the result of joint research with NPS students, including Katie Hagen, Ben Hegler, Matt Knitt, Andy Dunfee, and Cecilia Hu.

I am indebted to many people who, over the years, have supported and nurtured my research and academic career, including Randy Spoeri, who first introduced me to statistics and sparked my interest in the field; Joe Chang, advisor and researcher extraordinaire, without whose patience and support I would not have survived the dissertation process; and Nancy Spruill, a great friend and mentor, whose leadership, management, and organizational abilities I admire and to which I can only aspire.

Many thanks also to Lauren Cowles, my editor at Cambridge University Press. Lauren's encouragement and calm patience are major reasons this book actually made it to completion.

For many reasons I will always be beholden to and grateful for my spouse, Christine Arruda. In terms of this book, she good-naturedly endured, and often encouraged, my research and writing efforts. The time invested in this book often came at the expense of time we would otherwise have spent together.

Finally, I would be terribly remiss if I did not acknowledge the broader community of researchers and practitioners from whom I've benefited over the years and on whose work this book is based. Of course, any errors or omissions – and all opinions – are my own.

Part I

Introduction to Biosurveillance

1

Overview

While the public health philosophy of the 20th Century – emphasizing prevention – is ideal for addressing natural disease outbreaks, it is not sufficient to confront 21st Century threats where adversaries may use biological weapons agents as part of a long-term campaign of aggression and terror. Health care providers and public health officers are among our first lines of defense. Therefore, we are building on the progress of the past three years to further improve the preparedness of our public health and medical systems to address current and future BW [biological warfare] threats and to respond with greater speed and flexibility to multiple or repetitive attacks.

Homeland Security Presidential Directive 21

Bioterrorism is not a new threat in the twenty-first century – thousands of years ago, the plague and other contagious diseases were used in warfare – but today the potential for catastrophic outcomes is greater than it has ever been. To address this threat, the medical and public health communities are putting various measures in place, including systems designed to proactively monitor populations for possible disease outbreaks. The goal is to improve the likelihood that a disease outbreak, whether artificial or natural, is detected as early as possible so that the medical and public health communities can respond as quickly as possible.

The ideal biosurveillance system analyzes population health-related data in near-real time to identify trends not visible to individual physicians and clinicians. As they sift through data, many of these systems use one or more statistical algorithms to look for anomalies and trigger investigation, quantification, localization, and outbreak management. This book is focused on the design, evaluation, and implementation of the statistical algorithms, as well as other statistical tools and methods for effective biosurveillance.

Before discussing the statistical methods, however, this chapter first puts them in the perspective of the systems and the data upon which they are based. It begins by first defining the term "biosurveillance" and various associated terms followed by a brief look at some biosurveillance systems currently in use and concluding with a discussion about what is known about biosurveillance utility and effectiveness.

Chapter Objectives

Upon completion of this chapter, the reader should be able to:

- Define the terms *biosurveillance, epidemiologic surveillance*, and *syndromic surveillance.*
- Explain the objectives of biosurveillance: early event detection and situational awareness.
- Describe biosurveillance systems in terms of system functions and components.
- Discuss biosurveillance system utility and effectiveness, including the ongoing research challenges.
- Compare and contrast biosurveillance to traditional public health surveillance and to statistical process control.

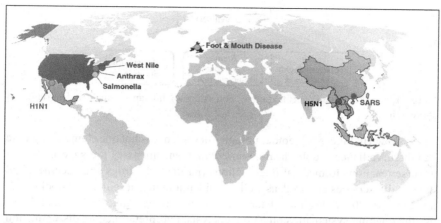

Figure 1.1. A map of select worldwide disease outbreaks in recent decades (GAO, 2010).

1.1 What Is Biosurveillance?

In the *National Biosurveillance Strategy for Human Health*, the US Centers for Disease Control and Prevention (CDC) says, "Biosurveillance in the context of human health is a term for the science and practice of managing health-related data and information for early warning of threats and hazards, early detection of events, and rapid characterization of the event so that effective actions can be taken to mitigate adverse health effects" (CDC, 2010a, p. 11). As discussed in the introduction, early detection has become an important focus as globalization and the threat of bioterrorism make the spread of highly virulent diseases an increasing threat to human health. For example, Figure 1.1 is a map of select worldwide disease outbreaks in recent decades (GAO, 2010).

Homeland Security Presidential Directive 21 (HSPD-21) defines *biosurveillance* as "the process of active data-gathering with appropriate analysis and interpretation of biosphere data that might relate to disease activity and threats to human or animal health – whether infectious, toxic, metabolic, or otherwise, and regardless of intentional or natural origin – in order to achieve early warning of health threats, early detection of health events, and overall situational awareness of disease activity" (US Government, 2007).

As shown in Figure 1.2, *biosphere data* can be divided into information about human, animal, and agricultural populations, and biosurveillance thus consists of health surveillance on each of these populations.

One particular type of biosurveillance is *epidemiologic surveillance*, which HSPD-21 defines as "the process of actively gathering and analyzing data related to human health and disease in a population in order to obtain early warning of human health events, rapid characterization of human disease events, and overall situational awareness of disease activity in the human population." Thus, epidemiologic surveillance addresses that subset of biosurveillance as it applies to human populations.

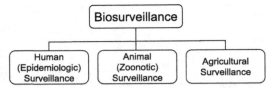

Figure 1.2. A biosurveillance taxonomy consisting of human, animal, and agricultural surveillance.

As shown in Figure 1.3, epidemiologic surveillance is but one element of public health surveillance. Public health surveillance encompasses the surveillance of adverse reactions to medical interventions (particularly drugs and vaccines) and how health services are used, as well as epidemiologic surveillance. Brookmeyer and Stroup (2004, p. 1) quote Thacker (2000) in defining public health surveillance as "the ongoing systematic collection, analysis, interpretation, and dissemination of health data for the purpose of preventing and controlling disease, injury, and other health problems."

Syndromic surveillance is a specific type of epidemiologic surveillance that Sosin (2003) defines as "the ongoing, systematic collection, analysis, interpretation, and application of real-time (or near-real-time) indicators of diseases and outbreaks that allow for their detection before public health authorities would otherwise note them." Thus, syndromic surveillance is epidemiologic and public health surveillance restricted to using leading indicators of disease. In particular, syndromic surveillance is based on the notion of a *syndrome*, which is a set of nonspecific prediagnosis medical and other information that may indicate the release of a bioterrorism agent or natural disease outbreak. See, for example, Syndrome Definitions for Diseases Associated with Critical Bioterrorism-associated Agents (CDC, 2003).

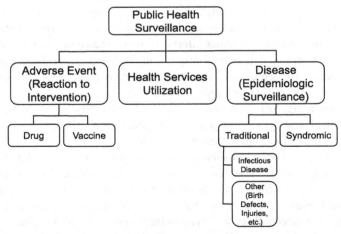

Figure 1.3. A taxonomy of public health showing that epidemiologic surveillance is but one part of a broader set of surveillance activities. (Adapted from Rolka & O'Connor, 2010.)

Table 1.1. A comparison of the categories of data used in biosurveillance, epidemiologic surveillance, and syndromic surveillance

Category of data	Biosurveillance	Epidemiologic surveillance	Syndromic surveillance
Prediagnosis			
• ER chief complaint	X	X	X
• OTC medicine sales	X	X	X
• EMS call rates	X	X	X
• Absenteeism records	X	X	X
• Lab results	X	X	X
• Other	X	X	X
Medical diagnoses	X	X	
Lab results	X	X	
Water and air monitoring	X		
Zoonotic	X		
Agricultural	X		

Syndromic surveillance differs from traditional epidemiologic surveillance in a number of important ways. For example, whereas syndromic surveillance often uses nonspecific health and health-related data (e.g., daily number of individuals reporting with sore throats to an emergency room), traditional notifiable disease reporting is based on suspected or confirmed cases (e.g., daily number of individuals diagnosed with the flu).[1] In addition, although in traditional public health surveillance, routine surveillance is conducted on specific, well-defined diseases, and non-routine surveillance is generally not initiated without a known or suspected outbreak, syndromic surveillance systems actively search for evidence of possible outbreaks[2] well before there is any suspicion of an outbreak.

As shown in Table 1.1, syndromic surveillance tends to use the least medically specific data. Often it is based on data derived from "chief complaints" of people presenting at hospital emergency rooms (ERs). Chief complaints are broad categories that capture the main reason or reasons an individual goes to the ER. Syndromic surveillance may also be based on over-the-counter (OTC) medicine sales, emergency medical services (EMS) calls, absenteeism records, and other health-related data. Epidemiologic surveillance, in comparison, uses all of these data types as well as other data from actual diagnoses and diagnostic laboratory

---

[1] For example, during the flu season, the *United States Influenza Sentinel Physicians Surveillance Network*, which consists of individual doctors throughout the United States, reports weekly to the CDC the total number of patients seen and the number of patients with influenza-like illness by age group.

[2] Although discussions throughout the text focus on the detection of disease outbreaks, the more general concept is detection of an adverse event, in which a disease outbreak is but one type of adverse event that may be of interest to the public health community. The term "outbreak" is used simply to make the discussion concrete and should not be taken as a limit on the application of biosurveillance.

results. Biosurveillance adds to these sources of data with information from water and air monitoring stations as well as zoonotic and agricultural data.

For the purposes of this text, biosurveillance is discussed within the context of epidemiologic surveillance and often even within the more specific context of syndromic surveillance. However, because the statistical methods discussed in this book clearly apply to a broad class of public health surveillance problems, the general term "biosurveillance" is used throughout.

1.1.1 Biosurveillance Objectives

Syndromic surveillance has also been defined as ". . . surveillance using health-related data that precede diagnosis and signal a sufficient probability of a case or an outbreak to warrant further public health response" (Fricker & Rolka, 2006; CDC, 2006a). This definition focuses on a number of ideas important to biosurveillance.

- First, biosurveillance is health surveillance, not military, regulatory, or intelligence surveillance. It may use a wide variety of types of data, from case diagnoses to health-related data such as chief complaint counts.
- Second, the data and associated surveillance are generally intended to precede diagnosis or case confirmation in order to give early warning of a possible outbreak. Clearly, after a definitive diagnosis of a bio-agent has been made, the need for detection becomes moot, although tracking the location and spread of a potential outbreak are still important whether an outbreak has been confirmed or not.
- Third, the process must provide a signal of "sufficient probability" to trigger "further public health response." Often the goal is not to provide a definitive determination that an outbreak is occurring but rather to signal that an outbreak *may* be occurring. Such a signal indicates that further investigation is warranted in the form of a more detailed investigation by public health officials.

Biosurveillance systems have two main objectives: to support public health *situational awareness* (SA) and to enhance outbreak *early event detection* (EED). The CDC (2008) defines them as follows:

- **Situational awareness** is the ability to utilize detailed, real-time health data to confirm or refute and to provide an effective response to the existence of an outbreak. It also is used to monitor an outbreak's magnitude, geography, rate of change, and life cycle.
- **Early event detection** is the ability to detect, at the earliest possible time, events that may signal a public health emergency. EED is composed of case and suspect case reporting along with statistical analysis of health-related data. Both real-time streaming of data from clinical care facilities as well as batched data with a short time delay are used to support EED efforts.

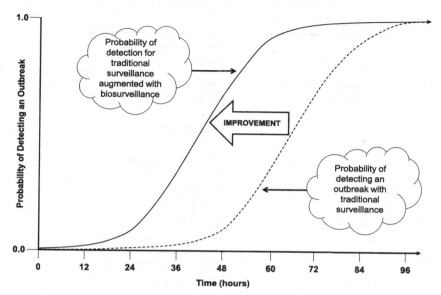

Figure 1.4. An illustration of how biosurveillance is intended to improve the probability of detecting a disease outbreak, whether artificial or natural.

As illustrated in Figure 1.4, biosurveillance systems are supposed to improve the chances the medical and public health communities catch a disease outbreak early. The more biosurveillance improves the probability of detecting an outbreak, the more a biosurveillance system is likely to enhance SA and EED. The goal is "...deployment of surveillance systems that can rapidly detect and monitor the course of an outbreak and thus minimize associated morbidity and mortality" (Bravata *et al.*, 2004).

The vertical axis in Figure 1.4 is in terms of probability specifically because early event detection is a stochastic[3] phenomenon, in which a variety of circumstances drive if and whether either a clinician or a biosurveillance system first detects a particular outbreak. In a given situation, whether a clinician will be faster than a biosurveillance system or vice versa is a function of both the aspects of the specific situation and chance.

When assessing biosurveillance systems, speed of (true positive) detection is one of three dimensions critical for completely characterizing performance. The other two dimensions are the rate of false positives and the probability of successfully detecting an outbreak. In the biosurveillance literature, these dimensions are often generically referred to as timeliness, specificity, and sensitivity.

All three dimensions are necessary, and they trade off. For example, for a given EED methodology, improving the speed of detecting an outbreak generally

---

[3] The term "stochastic" means the outcome involves an element of chance.

Table 1.2. Bioterrorism diseases, agents, and pathogens
and associated symptoms. (Adapted from Grey & Spaeth,
2006, Table 5-2, p. 77)

Symptoms	Disease, agent, or pathogen
Respiratory distress and fever	Anthrax Plague Ricin Staph enterotoxin B
Rash and fever	Smallpox Viral hemorrhagic fevers
Flu-like	Tularemia Brucellosis Q Fever
Neurologic	Botulism Venezuela equine encephalitis Eastern equine encephalitis Western equine encephalitis
Blistering	T-2 mycotoxin Arsenicals Mustards Phosgene oxime

comes at the cost of increasing the rate of false positives. Similarly, increasing the probability of detection usually comes at the expense of the speed of detection. These trade-offs are similar to the Type I and Type II error trade-offs inherent in classical hypothesis testing, although the sequential decision-making aspect of biosurveillance adds an additional level of complexity.

Chapter 6 discusses the appropriate metrics for assessing biosurveillance systems as well as how to evaluate biosurveillance system performance.

The motivation for biosurveillance and syndromic surveillance systems in particular is that some bio-agents have symptoms in their prodromal stages similar to naturally occurring diseases. For example, in the first week or two after exposure to smallpox, individuals tend to have symptoms similar to those of the flu such as fever, malaise, aches, nausea, and vomiting (Zubay, 2005). Table 1.2 lists various bio-agent pathogens by the syndromes corresponding to the most likely symptoms of the pathogens. The idea of syndromic surveillance, then, is that detecting an anomalous increase in one or more syndromes might correspond to a bioterrorism incident. Similarly, geo-spatial displays of one or more syndromes can provide additional situational awareness on the spread of a pathogen.

1.2 Biosurveillance Systems

As HSPD-21 states, "A central element of biosurveillance must be an epidemiologic surveillance system to monitor human disease activity across populations.

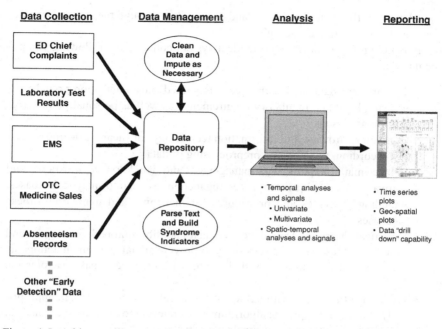

Figure 1.5. A biosurveillance system has four main functions: data collection, data management, analysis, and reporting. Raw data enter the system at the left and flow through the system to become actionable information at the right.

That system must be sufficiently enabled to identify specific disease incidence and prevalence in heterogeneous populations and environments and must possess sufficient flexibility to tailor analyses to new syndromes and emerging diseases."

The use of biosurveillance, particularly in the form of syndromic surveillance, is widespread. In 2003, it was estimated that approximately 100 state and local health jurisdictions were conducting some form of syndromic surveillance (Sosin, 2003). In 2004, Bravata *et al.* (2004) conducted a systematic review of the publicly available literature and various websites from which they identified 115 surveillance systems and of which they found 29 that were designed specifically for detecting bioterrorism. In 2007 and 2008, Buehler *et al.* (2008) sent surveys to public health officials in 59 state, territorial, and large local jurisdictions. Fifty-two officials responded (an 88 percent response rate) representing jurisdictions containing 94 percent of US population. They found that 83 percent reported conducting syndromic surveillance for a median of three years, and two-thirds said they are "highly" or "somewhat" likely to expand the use of syndromic surveillance in next two years.

1.2.1 Components

As depicted in Figure 1.5, a biosurveillance system has four main functions: data collection, data management, analysis, and reporting. As illustrated in the figure, raw data enter the system at the left and as they flow through the system becomes actionable information at the right.

Expanding on Rolka (2006), the ideal system contains the following components:

- The original data, to which access is gained only after appropriately addressing legal and regulatory requirements, as well as personal privacy and proprietary issues
- Computer hardware and information technology for (near) real-time assembly, recording, transfer, and preprocessing of data
- Subject-matter experts, data management and data knowledge experts, and software and techniques for processing incoming data into analytic databases, including processes and procedures for managing and maintaining these databases
- Statistical algorithms to analyze the data for possible outbreaks over space and time that are of sufficient sensitivity to provide signals within an actionable time frame while simultaneously limiting false-positive signals to a tolerable level
- Public health experts with sufficient statistical expertise who can appropriately choose and apply the algorithms most relevant to their jurisdictions and appropriately interpret the signals when they occur
- Data display and query software, as well as the necessary underlying data, that facilitate rapid and easy investigation and adjudication of signals by public health experts, including the ability to "trace back" from a signal to a likely source
- Other data displays, combined with decision support and communication tools, to support situational awareness during an outbreak to facilitate effective and efficient public health response

Mandl *et al.* (2004), in *Implementing Syndromic Surveillance: A Practical Guide Informed by the Early Experience*, provide a detailed discussion of what is required and guidance about how to implement biosurveillance systems.

1.2.2 Examples

Below are brief descriptions of three biosurveillance systems chosen to illustrate large-scale systems. The first two are true systems in the sense that they are comprised of both dedicated computer hardware and software. The third is more properly described as a set of software programs that can be downloaded and implemented by a public health organization.

- **BioSense**. Developed and operated by the CDC, BioSense is intended to be a United States–wide biosurveillance system. Begun in 2003, BioSense initially used Department of Defense and Department of Veterans Affairs outpatient data along with medical laboratory test results from a nationwide commercial laboratory. In 2006, BioSense began incorporating data

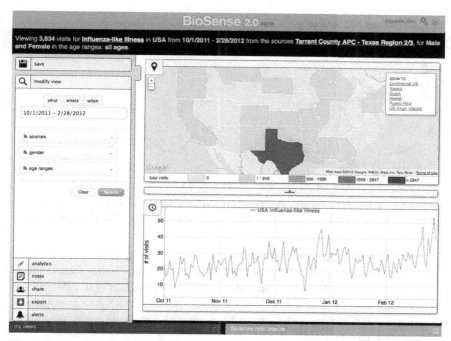

Figure 1.6. BioSense 2.0 data display.

from civilian hospitals as well. The primary objective of BioSense is to "expedite event recognition and response coordination among federal, state, and local public health and healthcare organizations" (Tokars, 2006; CDC, 2006c). In 2010, BioSense was completely redesigned; an example of the new interface is shown in Figure 1.6. Designated BioSense 2.0, the redesign was based on input and guidance from local, state, and federal stakeholders (CDC, 2012a).

- **ESSENCE**. An acronym for Electronic Surveillance System for the Early Notification of Community-based Epidemics, ESSENCE was developed by the Department of Defense (DD) in 1999. ESSENCE IV now monitors for infectious disease outbreaks at more than 300 military treatment facilities worldwide on a daily basis using data from patient visits to the facilities and pharmacy data. For the Washington, DC, area, ESSENCE II monitors military and civilian outpatient visit data as well as OTC pharmacy sales and school absenteeism (DoD, 2006; Lombardo *et al.*, 2004; Office of the Secretary of Defense [OSD], 2005). Components of ESSENCE have been adapted and used by some public health departments.
- **EARS**. An acronym for Early Aberration Reporting System, EARS was developed by the CDC. EARS was originally designed for monitoring for bioterrorism during large-scale events that often have little or no baseline data (i.e., as a short-term "drop-in" surveillance method) (CDC, 2007). For example, the EARS system was used in the aftermath of Hurricane Katrina

United States Flu Activity

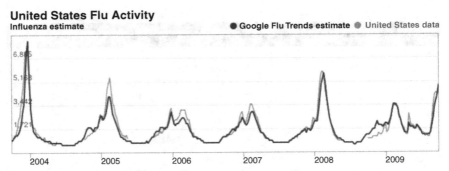

Figure 1.7. A graph of Google Flu Trends results, for Google query-based flu estimates versus sentinel physician influenza-like illness (ILI) data from the CDC (Google, 2012).

to monitor communicable diseases in Louisiana (Toprani *et al.*, 2006), for syndromic surveillance at the 2001 Super Bowl and World Series, and at the Democratic National Convention in 2000 (Hutwagner *et al.*, 2003a). Although developed as a drop-in surveillance system, EARS data management procedures and algorithms have been adapted for use in many syndromic surveillance systems.

State and local biosurveillance systems may use EARS, BioSense, or in some cases ESSENCE, while some localities have instituted their own systems. Other biosurveillance and health surveillance systems include the Real-time Outbreak and Disease Surveillance system (RODS, 2010), the National Notifiable Diseases Surveillance System (CDC, 2010c), and the National Electronic Telecommunications System for Surveillance (CDC, 2010b). Descriptions of some of these state and local systems (as well as other information) can be found in volume 53 of the CDC's *Morbidity and Mortality Weekly Report* and the Annotated Bibliography for Syndromic Surveillance (CDC, 2006b).

Among the more recent and unique surveillance effort is Google Flu Trends, which is designed to track "health-seeking" behavior in the form of search engine queries for flu-related information. As with syndromic surveillance systems using OTC medicine sales, the idea is that sick people first attempt to self-treat before seeking medical attention, and often the first step is a search engine query for information. Figure 1.7 compares Google Flu Trends's estimated flu incidence based on search queries for flu-related terms to the CDC's sentinel physician data. The figure shows a clear correspondence between the two time series. Ginsberg *et al.* (2009, p. 1012) say, "Because the relative frequency of certain queries is highly correlated with the percentage of physician visits in which a patient presents with influenza-like symptoms, we can accurately estimate the current level of weekly influenza activity in each region of the United States, with a reporting lag of about one day."

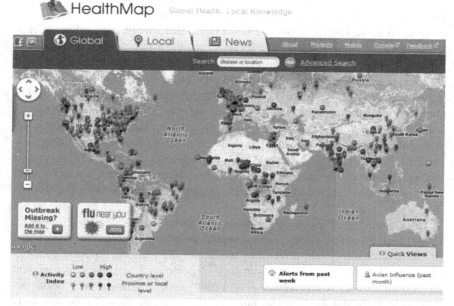

Figure 1.8. Screen shot of HealthMap from April 12, 2012. (HealthMap, 2012)

Another unique surveillance effort is HealthMap, a "multistream real-time surveillance platform that continually aggregates reports on new and ongoing infectious disease outbreaks" (Brownstein *et al.*, 2008). HealthMap extracts information from web-accessible information sources such as discussion forums, mailing lists, government websites, and news outlets. It then filters, categorizes, and integrates the information and, as shown in Figure 1.8, plots the information on a map. The goal of HealthMap is to provide real-time information about emerging infectious diseases and is intended for use by both public health officials and the traveling public (HealthMap, 2012). As Brownstein *et al.* (2008, p. 1019) say, "Ultimately, the use of news media and other nontraditional sources of surveillance data can facilitate early outbreak detection, increase public awareness of disease outbreaks prior to their formal recognition, and provide an integrated and contextualized view of global health information."

1.3 Biosurveillance Utility and Effectiveness

Despite the widespread and potentially expanding use of biosurveillance, questions remain about its utility and effectiveness. Reports and papers that discuss various issues, challenges, and important research needs associated with effective implementation and operation of biosurveillance systems include the Government Accountability Office (GAO) (2011, 2010, 2009), CDC (2010a), Fricker (2010), Shmueli & Burkom (2010), Uscher-Pines *et al.* (2009), Green (2008),

Buehler *et al.* (2008), Fricker & Rolka (2006), Rolka (2006), Stoto *et al.* (2004), Bravata *et al.* (2004), Reingold (2003), and Sosin (2003).

In 2010 in the United States, the GAO found that "While national biodefense strategies have been developed to address biological threats such as pandemic influenza, there is neither a comprehensive national strategy nor a focal point with the authority and resources to guide the effort to develop a national bio-surveillance capability." In 2011, the GAO further identified challenges at the US state and local governments, saying: "State and city officials identified common challenges to developing and maintaining their biosurveillance capabilities: (1) state policies that restrict hiring, travel, and training in response to budget constraints; (2) ensuring adequate workforce, training, and systems; and (3) the lack of strategic planning and leadership to support long-term investment in cross-cutting core capabilities, integrated biosurveillance, and effective partnerships" (GAO, 2011).

In case studies of health departments in eight US states, Uscher-Pines *et al.* (2009) found that fewer than half had written response protocols for responding to biosurveillance system alerts, and the health departments reported conducting in-depth investigations on fewer than 15 percent of biosurveillance system alerts. Furthermore, Uscher-Pines *et al.* (2009) said, "Although many health departments noted that the original purpose of syndromic surveillance was early warning/detection, no health department reported using systems for this purpose. Examples of typical statements included the following: 'I was a big supporter of syndromic surveillance for early warning early on, but now I am more realistic about the system's limitations.'"

In the professional literature, Reingold (2003) suggested that a compelling case for the implementation of biosurveillance systems has yet to be made. Cooper (2006) said, "To date no bio-terrorist attack has been detected in the United Kingdom, or elsewhere in the world using syndromic surveillance systems." Stoto *et al.* (2004) questioned whether biosurveillance systems can achieve an effective early detection capability. And Green (2008) said, "Syndromic surveillance systems, based on statistical algorithms, will be of little value in early detection of bioterrorist outbreaks. Early on in the outbreak, there will be cases serious enough to alert physicians and be given definitive diagnoses."

The research challenges span many disciplines and problems:

- Legal and regulatory challenges in order to gain access to data
- Technological challenges related to designing and implementing computer hardware and software for collecting and assembling data
- Ethical and procedural issues inherent in managing and safeguarding data
- Analytical challenges of assessing the likelihood of outbreaks and of displaying data to enhance situational awareness
- Managerial challenges of effectively assembling and operating the entire system

These research challenges are not necessarily of equal importance nor are they listed in any type of priority order. Furthermore, little is known about how they should be prioritized in terms of their contributions to improving the utility or effectiveness of biosurveillance. However, it is clear that improvements are necessary in all of these disciplines to achieve biosurveillance systems that are maximally useful and effective.

Much of the continuing controversy surrounding biosurveillance stems from its initial focus on early event detection, a use that requires a number of still unproven assumptions, including:

- Leading indicators of outbreaks exist in prediagnosis health-related data of adequate strength such that they are statistically detectable with satisfactory power.
- The leading indicators occur sufficiently far in advance of clinical diagnoses so that, when found, they provide the public health community with enough advance notice to take action.
- Statistical detection algorithms exist that produce signals reliable enough to warrant continued dedication of public health resources to investigate the signals.

Of course, a myopic focus only on EED in biosurveillance systems misses important benefits such systems can provide, particularly the potential to significantly advance and modernize the practice of public health surveillance. For example, whether or not biosurveillance systems prove effective at the early detection of bioterrorism, they are likely to have a significant and continuing role in the detection and tracking of seasonal and pandemic flu, as well as other naturally occurring disease outbreaks. This latter function is echoed in an Institute of Medicine report *Microbial Threats to Health* by Smolinski *et al.* (2003): "[S]yndromic surveillance is likely to be increasingly helpful in the detection and monitoring of epidemics, as well as the evaluation of health care utilization for infectious diseases." In a similar vein, Uscher-Pines *et al.* (2009) quote a public health official: "Health departments should not be at the mercy of alerts; they need to develop their own uses for syndromic surveillance."

In terms of bioterrorism, Stoto (2006) states that biosurveillance systems build links between public health and health care providers – links that could prove to be critical for consequence management if a bioterrorism attack occurs. Furthermore, Sosin (2003) points out that biosurveillance systems can act as a safety net if the existing avenues of detection fail to detect an attack, so countermeasures can be taken swiftly and then can provide additional lead time to public health authorities so they can take more effective public health actions. For example, a Dutch biologist conducting automated *Salmonella* surveillance related that the surveillance system detected an outbreak whose occurrence was somehow missed by sentinel physicians (Burkom, 2006). And unusual indicators in a biosurveillance system (not necessarily a signal from an EED algorithm) may give public health

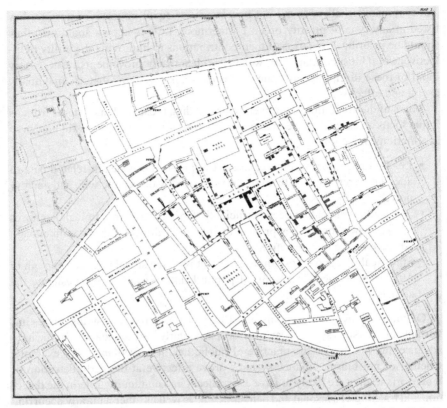

Figure 1.9. Dr. John Snow's map of the 1854 London cholera epidemic was used to link the cholera outbreak to water coming from the Broad Street pump. Pump locations are indicated by the dots (in the streets), and the bars represent the number of deaths at each address. In the center of the map, roughly in the geographic center of the deaths, is the Broad Street pump.

organizations time to begin organizing and marshaling resources in advance of a confirmed case or provide critical information about how and where to apply resources.

1.3.1 Biosurveillance Compared with Traditional Public Health Surveillance

Epidemiology traces its roots back to Dr. John Snow, who used statistical mapping techniques to help determine that cholera was transmitted by a contaminated water supply in the London epidemic of 1854. One way he demonstrated this was to simultaneously plot on a map the number of cholera deaths by city address and the locations of each of the city's water pumps. As shown in Figure 1.9, the result was a clear visual association between areas of higher death rates from cholera and certain water pumps.

Since that time, the field has developed many and varied tools for understanding factors affecting the health and illness of populations. Epidemiologists and public health professionals are often called upon to determine the cause or causes of a particular disease outbreak, much as Dr. Snow first did almost two centuries ago. A defining feature of such an investigation is that the outbreak has already been identified. This is often referred to as *event-based* surveillance. In event-based surveillance the investigation is a *retrospective* effort focused on trying to determine the cause of a known outbreak.

In contrast, biosurveillance, particularly in the form of syndromic surveillance, is often a *prospective* exercise in monitoring populations for possible disease outbreaks. The goal is to routinely evaluate data for evidence of an outbreak prior to the existence of a confirmed case (in fact, even prior to any suspicion of an outbreak). This type of routine prospective monitoring, in which the disease rates or the health care-seeking behaviors of a population are monitored on an ongoing basis for evidence of change, is also part of traditional epidemiologic surveillance. However, in traditional epidemiologic surveillance, the disease or behavior is usually well defined and the surveillance is targeted to measure the particular disease or behavior.

In comparison, with syndromic surveillance the type of outbreak to be detected is generally not well defined. Furthermore, the monitoring is often based on electronic data that may not be specific to any particular type of outbreak and that may be in a form and of a volume not previously encountered. As a result, the public health tools and techniques developed over the past two centuries generally do not apply to the nontraditional epidemiologic surveillance problems. Public health practitioners have thus turned to the field of industrial quality control, sometimes applying and adapting those tools directly to biosurveillance.

1.3.2 Biosurveillance Early Event Detection Compared with Statistical Process Control

Industrial quality control traces its roots to 1931 when Walter A. Shewhart wrote *Economic Control of Quality of Manufactured Product* and when he developed the concept of the control chart, a graphical statistical tool most commonly used to control manufacturing processes. The success of Shewhart's method in the industrial world lies in its simplicity. Essentially, one establishes control limits and as long as a statistic derived from the data, sequentially observed over time, falls within the control limits the manufacturing process is assumed to be "in control." If one or more fall outside the control limits, then the process is examined to determine whether it is "out of control" and requires adjustment. Shewhart's work gave rise to the field of *statistical process control* (SPC) and a large and still growing literature of research about statistical methods for monitoring industrial and other processes.

In industrial quality control, and thus SPC, it is often reasonable to assume that:

- Because one controls the manufacturing process, the in-control distribution is (or can reasonably be assumed to be) stationary.
- Observations can be drawn from the process so they are independent (or nearly so).
- Monitoring the process mean and standard deviation is usually sufficient.
- The asymptotic distributions of the statistics being monitored are known and thus can be used to design appropriate control charts.
- Shifts, when they occur, remain until they are detected and corrective action is taken.
- Temporal (as opposed to spatial) detection is the critical problem.

However, the general biosurveillance problem violates many, if not all, of these assumptions. For example:

- There is little to no control over disease incidence, and thus the distribution of disease incidence is usually nonstationary.
- Observations (often daily counts) are autocorrelated, and the need for quick detection works against the idea of taking measurements far enough apart to achieve (near) independence.
- In biosurveillance, there is little information on what types of statistics are useful for monitoring – one is often looking for anything that seems unusual.
- Because individual observations are being monitored, the idea of asymptotic sampling distributions does not apply, and the data often contain significant systematic effects that must be accounted for.
- Outbreaks are transient, with disease incidence returning to its original state after an outbreak has run its course.
- Identifying both spatial and temporal deviations is often critical.

This gap between existing SPC methods and the biosurveillance problem provides an area ripe for new research and, indeed, quite a bit has been going on for the past decade or so.

1.4 Discussion and Summary

This chapter began with definitions of biosurveillance, epidemiologic surveillance, and syndromic surveillance from HSPD21. This was followed by a discussion of the objectives of biosurveillance, particularly its use for situational awareness and EED, a description of the components of an ideal biosurveillance system, and then a brief description of three specific systems: BioSense, ESSENCE, and EARS. The chapter concluded with a discussion of the utility and effectiveness of biosurveillance.

Most of the material in this chapter is definitional, although not everyone agrees with the specific definitions, which have evolved over time and will undoubtedly continue to evolve. The specific biosurveillance systems discussed are illustrative of some recent larger systems but do not represent all possible types of biosurveillance systems either currently in use or contemplated for future use. In fact, the concept of a biosurveillance "system" is questioned by some, perhaps because of the heterogeneity of the various installations, because the various systems and system boundaries vary considerably in scope, or because some installations are not dedicated systems per se. But these are narrow distinctions that do not detract from the fact that BioSense, ESSENCE, EARS, and related systems exist and are in use despite what they may be called.

Perhaps the most contentious issue, at least at the current time, is whether biosurveillance systems can usefully conduct EED. Yet although some literature cited in Section 1.3 questions the viability and usefulness of biosurveillance, it is important to keep in mind that the field is still young and dynamically developing. Thus, for example, the argument that poor EED performance in existing systems means the public health community should "throw in the towel" and stop using biosurveillance for EED is not convincing. Rather, what is required is the judicious use of EED in current systems while more technical, operational, and policy research is conducted to improve biosurveillance integration and performance. After all, research has been ongoing in the field of SPC since the 1930s – a more than 60-year head start over biosurveillance.

This chapter provides a general overview of biosurveillance, mainly to put the statistical methods in the rest of the book in an appropriate context. The next chapter examines some types of biosurveillance data. For those who would like to delve more deeply into the topics presented in this chapter, the Additional Reading section below provides some suggested references.

Additional Reading

- For more detail on biosurveillance and biosurveillance systems, the *Handbook of Biosurveillance* (Wagner *et al.*, 2006), particularly Parts I and II, describes biosurveillance in detail, including biosurveillance of animals, laboratories, water, food, and pharmaceuticals, as well as the functional requirements for biosurveillance systems. Useful references that further describe biosurveillance and expound upon current issues and challenges include:
  - *BIOSURVEILLANCE: Nonfederal Capabilities Should Be Considered in Creating a National Biosurveillance Strategy* (GAO, 2011)
  - *BIOSURVEILLANCE: Efforts to Develop a National Biosurveillance Capability Need a National Strategy and a Designated Leader* (GAO, 2010)
  - *BIOSURVEILLANCE: Developing a Collaboration Strategy Is Essential to Fostering Interagency Data and Resource Sharing* (GAO, 2009)
- For access to current resources related to public health surveillance and biosurveillance, consider the CDC's Emergency Preparedness and Response

website (http://www.bt.cdc.gov/episurv/), the CDC's BioSense website (http://www.cdc.gov/biosense/), and various professional organizations' conferences and websites, including:

- ○ International Society for Disease Surveillance (ISDS): http://www.syndromic.org
- ○ National Association of County and City Public Health Officials (NACCHO): http://www.naccho.org
- ○ American Public Health Association (APHA): http://www.apha.org
- For more information about bioterrorism pathogens, *Agents of Bioterrorism: Pathogens and Their Weaponization* (Zubay, 2005) contains detailed information about pathogens considered to be major biothreats, including their biology and steps that can be taken to defend against them. *The Bioterrorism Sourcebook* (Grey and Spaeth, 2006) is a clinical and public health guide to preparing for and responding to chemical, biological, radiologic, and nuclear (CBRA) events.
- Readers interested in more information about traditional disease surveillance should consult *Monitoring the Health of Populations* (Brookmeyer and Stroup, 2004). Those interested in epidemiology more broadly may want to refer to *Epidemiology Kept Simple: An Introduction to Classic and Modern Epidemiology* (Gerstman, 2003).

2

Biosurveillance Data

An ounce of prevention is worth a pound of cure.
Benjamin Franklin (1706–1790)

Biosurveillance is based on data but data that may come in many different forms and from many different sources. Most often, biosurveillance uses medical and health-related data. The data may be clinically well-defined and linked to specific types of outbreaks, such as groupings of *ICD-9* diagnosis codes, or they may be less well-defined, such as syndrome counts based on emergency room chief complaint data or only vaguely defined and perhaps weakly linked to specific types of outbreaks, such as over-the-counter (OTC) sales of cough and cold medication or absenteeism rates.

Biosurveillance data may also be based on active air or water sampling. For example, the BioWatch program uses detectors that collect airborne particles onto filters that are subsequently sent to laboratories for analysis. As with syndromic surveillance systems, a goal is early warning of a pathogen release. Biosurveillance may also include agricultural and zoonotic data.

This chapter begins by describing the types of data used in biosurveillance, delving into the specific details of syndromic surveillance data using two sets of actual data. The syndromic surveillance example data illustrate some of the common features of biosurveillance data and are used in subsequent chapters throughout the book. Following this, the chapter focuses on how to prepare data for biosurveillance. Data preparation is particularly important for biosurveillance data – as it is for most messy real-world data – because data typos, errors, and other issues must first be addressed before an analysis is undertaken.

Chapter Objectives

Upon completion of this chapter, the reader should be able to:

- Describe the types and characteristics of biosurveillance data.
- Understand what biosurveillance data look like based on actual clinic-level and hospital-level data, including various systematic effects such as seasonal trends and day-of-the-week effects.
- Be able to calculate correlation and autocorrelation for biosurveillance data, including plotting correlograms showing autocorrelation for various lags.
- Discuss the various steps in data preparation, including data cleaning, coding, and imputation, including:
  - For data cleaning, describe what it is and the various types of checks for catching data errors and inconsistencies.
  - For data coding, understand how to code and recode data, including the use of free text matching and natural language processing for coding chief complaints.
  - For imputation, describe the types of imputation and understand how to implement mean value imputation, retrospective and prospective longitudinal imputation, regression imputation, and hot deck imputation.

Mathematical Notation

$\mathbb{E}(Y\|x)$	Expected value of a random variable Y for a given the value of variable x
i, j	Indices
I_x	Indicator variable ($I = 1$ if x is true, otherwise $I = 0$)
$N(0, s_y^2)$	Normal distribution with mean 0 and variance s_y^2
s_y	Sample standard deviation of variable y
s_y^2	Sample variance of variable y
y_i	ith observation of variable y
$\bar{y}$	Sample mean of variable y
y_i'	Imputed value for missing observation y_i
Z	Random variable (used in stochastic mean imputation)
β_i	ith regression coefficient
$\hat{\beta}_i$	ith estimated regression coefficient
$\hat{\epsilon}_i$	Residual for observation i
$\hat{\mu}_i$	Estimated mean for observation i

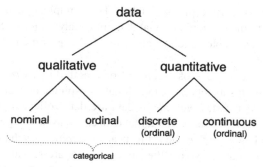

Figure 2.1. A hierarchy showing how the terms describing the data types are related.

2.1 Types of Data

Not all data are alike. As shown in Figure 2.1, the most basic distinction divides data into two categories, quantitative and qualitative. *Quantitative* data can be measured on a numerical scale, but *qualitative* data cannot be so measured. For example, consider demographic data that might be associated with a biosurveillance patient's record: height, weight, and age are all quantitative, but gender and treatment facility are qualitative.

Quantitative data can be either *continuous* or *discrete*. Data are discrete if there are gaps between the values the data can assume. For example, the number of individuals classified with a particular syndrome can be 0, 1, 2, 3, etc. It cannot be 2.7. If there are no gaps between possible data values, then the data are continuous. Another way to think about continuous data is that with an infinitely accurate measuring device, one could express the data to any number of decimal places and it would still make sense. So, for example, height is continuous: someone can be 6 feet tall, 5.97 feet tall, or 5.9722683 feet tall.

Qualitative data can be either *ordinal* or *nominal*. Nominal data occur when the data fall into categories but there is no natural ordering to the categories. For example, gender is a nominal type of data: each individual is classified as "male" or "female," but it does not make any sense to say that "male" is greater than "female." Ordinal data, on the other hand, have a clear ordering. For example, a patient's rating for quality of care is ordinal: an "excellent" rating is better than "good," which is, in turn, better than "poor." Of course, quantitative data are trivially ordinal. For example, the number of people who present at a treatment facility classified with a particular syndrome on a given day is ordinal.

Note that the term *categorical* can refer to data that are either discrete or qualitative. Also, continuous data can be transformed into categorical data by defining categories that correspond to ranges of continuous values. For example, for height, male individuals may be categorized as "short" if they are less than 5 feet tall, "average" if they are between five and six feet, and "tall" if they are six feet or greater in height. Conversely, it is sometimes useful for the purposes of modeling or analysis to represent qualitative data with numeric labels, but care must be taken not to overinterpret such labels. For example, *indicator variables* are sometimes used to incorporate nominal data into analyses in which, for example, one could create a variable called "male gender" that is equal to "1" for men and "0" for women.

Data can also be either cross-sectional or longitudinal. *Cross-sectional* data are data collected on subjects (e.g., individuals, hospitals, or regions) at the same point in time. In contrast, *longitudinal* data are data collected over time. Often referred to as *time series* data, longitudinal data can consist of repeated collections of cross-sectional data (so that the subjects are different at each point in time), or they may be *panel* data in which the same subjects are repeatedly measured or observed over time.

The reason these distinctions are important is that the appropriate statistical analyses, and even the proper way to display data, often depend on the type of data. In terms of biosurveillance, then, the effective display of data for situational awareness, or the selection of the appropriate algorithm for early event detection, (EED) should take into account the type of data being monitored, displayed, or modeled.

2.2 Types of Biosurveillance Data

Biosurveillance data can be of any of the types just described. The data used in this text are predominantly based on counts and are thus discrete data. Examples of such data are the daily number of people presenting at a clinic who are diagnosed and assigned a particular *ICD-9* code and the daily count of people presenting at an ER subsequently classified into a particular syndrome. However, continuous data can also be encountered, such as when doing air or water monitoring, or perhaps if the location of cases are geo-coded in terms of latitude and longitude.

Biosurveillance data are collected from a wide variety of sources. For epidemiologic surveillance, sources of data include hospitals and physicians, laboratories, coroners and medical examiners, pharmacies, emergency medical services (EMS) 911 and other telephone hotlines, and even absenteeism records. For example, Figure 2.2 shows a map of sales of thermometers by county using data from approximately 10,000 retail stores from four national retail chains (Wagner *et al.*, 2003, Fig. 2). Figure 2.3 shows a comparison of "Transport for London" employee absenteeism rates to syndromic surveillance indicators of influenza-like illness (ILI) (Paterson *et al.*, 2011). Zoonotic and agricultural surveillance data sources include federal and state departments of agriculture and veterinary and animal health organizations such as the Fish and Wildlife Service, the US Geological Society, and the American Zoo and Aquarium Association (Wagner *et al.*, 2006, p. 111).

Biosurveillance data may be collected in an automated or near-automated fashion for some surveillance systems and more manually for others, and they may be part of either a one-time or recurring surveillance of various populations. The breadth and depth of specific biosurveillance data are too great to explore in any

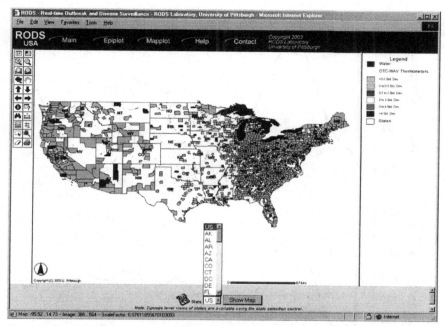

Figure 2.2. An example of using OTC medical sales for surveillance: A map of sales of thermometers by county using data from approximately 10,000 retail stores from four national retail chains. (Wagner *et al.*, 2003, Fig. 2).

detail here. For a more complete list, see Table 1.2 in Brookmeyer and Stroup (2004, pp. 12–32), which provides an extensive list of public health surveillance data sources (but note that even for a list of 20 pages long, Brookmeyer and Stroup label it as "selected data sources"). Also, Chapter 2 of Brookmeyer and Stroup (2007) describes in more detail the types of biosurveillance data and their sources, and Parts II and IV of Wagner *et al.* (2006) more broadly describe the organizations that conduct biosurveillance and the data they collect.

2.2.1 Additional Characteristics of Biosurveillance Data

As just described, biosurveillance data may be quantitative or qualitative and may be cross-sectional or longitudinal. The type and choice of data are driven by both the purpose of the surveillance and what data are available and relevant. In addition to these distinctions about types of data, biosurveillance data frequently have some or all of the following characteristics:

- The distribution of background disease incidence data is usually nonstationary, meaning that the distribution changes over time. For example, the distribution of daily ILI syndrome counts likely changes from season to season during the year.

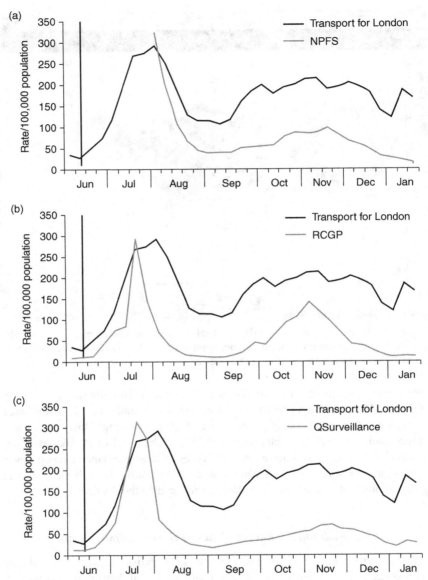

Figure 2.3. A comparison of "Transport for London" employee absenteeism rates with syndromic surveillance indicators of ILI (Paterson *et al.*, 2011). From top to bottom, the surveillance indicators are National Pandemic Flu Service (NPFS), Royal College of General Practitioners (RCGP), and QSurveillance. Vertical black line shows when the World Health Organization declared a pandemic (June 11, 2009).

○ Furthermore, some of the changes in the background incidence have known causes or at least regular cycles, which means that these types of changes are estimable, predictable, or at least somewhat understood. Other background incidence changes are random, not well understood, or unpredictable, but they may also not be of direct interest in terms of being related to particular disease outbreak or outbreaks that are of interest.

○ Compounding this, what is or is not of interest, meaning what is deemed background disease incidence versus what constitutes an interesting or important deviation from the background incidence (as opposed to simply being part of it) may change with time or circumstances.

• Outbreaks are transient, with disease incidence increasing during an outbreak but then returning to an original state after the outbreak has run its course.

○ During an outbreak, the distribution of disease incidence is a mixture of the normal background incidence distribution and the outbreak distribution.

○ So the distribution of outbreak disease incidence is also nonstationary.

○ For most bio-agents, little is known about what their outbreak distributions are likely to look like.

• Both the background disease incidence and outbreak data may be correlated over time and space.

As upcoming chapters will discuss, it is important to account for these biosurveillance data characteristics in both situational awareness and EED. For example, during routine surveillance for natural diseases, an increase in the ILI syndrome during the winter months may be useful for detecting the onset of the flu season. In this situation, an uptick in the daily counts of those classified with ILI syndrome, over and above the natural variation that occurs in such daily counts, is an indicator of a flu outbreak. Thus, the estimation of the background incidence should be based on historical daily ILI syndrome counts observed during nonflu periods, and a potential flu outbreak is signaled when the daily ILI syndrome count is significantly above this background incidence. On the other hand, if the goal is detecting a bioterrorism attack, then during the flu season, the background incidence is the daily ILI syndrome counts, *including* those attributable to a flu outbreak, and a potential bioterrorism attack is signaled when the ILI syndrome count increases significantly above what would be expected during a normal flu season.

2.2.2 Syndromic Surveillance Data

In their 2007–2008 survey of public health officials in 59 state, territorial, and large local jurisdictions (first described in Chapter 1), Buehler *et al.* (2008) found that ER data are most commonly used for syndromic surveillance (84 percent) followed by:

• Outpatient clinic visits (49 percent)
• OTC medication sales (44 percent)

Table 2.1. Typical syndromes used in
syndromic surveillance systems

Botulism-like	Lymphadenitis
Fever	Neurological
Gastrointestinal (GI)	Rash
Hemorrhagic illness	Respiratory
ILI	Unspecified infection

- Calls to poison control centers (37 percent)
- School absenteeism (37 percent)[1]

Syndromic surveillance data are often based on syndromes derived from chief complaint data. Some common syndromes are listed in Table 2.1. A chief complaint is a brief summary of the reason or reasons that an individual presents at a medical facility. Table 2.2 gives some examples of actual chief complaints as taken from a syndromic surveillance system. Written by medical personnel, chief complaints are couched in jargon, acronyms, and abbreviations for use by other medical professionals. To distill the chief complaints down into syndrome indicators, the text is searched and parsed for key words, often of necessity including all the ways a particular key word can be misspelled, abridged, and otherwise abbreviated.

For example, to generate respiratory syndrome counts, the chief complaint text would be searched for terms such as "respiratory" (including common misspellings such as "resparatory," common typos such as "repsiratory," and common abbreviations such as "resp") and related terms such as "apnea," "bronchitis," and "pneumonia," as well as their common misspellings, typos, and abbreviations. This information might then be combined with other information gleaned from the chief complaint text, such as whether the visit was related to pregnancy or a chronic condition, so that the final respiratory syndrome count is based on people who present with a respiratory chief complaint that is unrelated to pregnancy or a chronic respiratory condition.

Depending on the locality, the chief complaint data, such as that shown in Table 2.2, might be preprocessed, and only the daily counts transmitted into the biosurveillance system. Or, the raw data could be sent to the biosurveillance system for processing. In the latter case, the system might also receive additional information at the individual level such as gender, age, race or ethnicity, date of service, diagnoses, and address information.

Example: County-Level Clinic Data

The first set of data consists of patient-level raw chief complaint text and limited demographic information for six public health clinics from one US county for a one-year period from August 1st through July 31st (during which the pandemic

---

[1] Survey respondents could indicate more than one type of data, so the percentages sum to more than 100 percent.

Table 2.2. Typical chief complaint data used in biosurveillance systems

NEWPAT EST CARE/NO MEDS/ NO
   CONDITION
OBCPE/RES PER PT SHE WANTS
   SOONER APPT
DISCHG/MUDGE REV/JP
RASH/LC
CHDP /RV PER MOM RES
+CHLAM JP
NEW PT ER FU PT HAD SAB/LM
WALK IN HEAD ACHE
1WK F/U OK TO ADD
2WK OB CK PER DR L
FOR RTN WCC/LC 2006 PATIENT
FEVER, SORETHROAT, DIARRHEA/LC
NEW/EVAL/SEISURES
wants bcm has pact
F/U RASH IN 1 WEEK
NPE FU HOSPITALIZATION DETOX
FUP ER VISIT
wants bcm/RES PER PT
W/I BCM / ABDL BUMP
NP GYN EVAL
NEW PAT WCC/NO MEDS/NO CONDITON
BOOK PER MD HTN ///R/S FROM
   07/09-NA LFT MESS ON V
NP TONSIL PROBLEMS
FU//JR/ LEFT MESS IN V/M WITH
   TIME CHANGE//MS
C/O STOOL PROB X 1WK//MS
3mth fu sleep apnea
IZ SIBS
WANTS REFILL/ANY PROV AVAIL
DTAP//PER MOM
PAP (MISSED LAST ONE)
WALK IN FEVER W/RESIDENT
NWBRN
FEELING WEAK,DIZZY-OD
RTN 2WK NB EVAL-VS
FU VST 1 WK GDM IN AT 2:30
NPE WCC CCAH
1 WK F/U JAUNDICE
PARTIAL CHDP IN IN 4 WEEKS
   HEPA #A
FEVER/COUGH/LC
F/U IN 3 MONTHS
   CALLED 2 RE-SCH MISS
FP COUNSELING
FOLLOW UP LUNGS,HT-OD
POSSIBLE STD

NPE/////////7 YRS WCC ADVICED
   TO SIGN ROR ror
rtn fu missed 07/17.vs
fever/diarrhea
3:30 PM3-4 DAY WEIGHT CHECK /
   BILI 3:30
TB TEST TWO STEP PRIVATE PAY
NPE FOR WOUND CK //KR
OB CPE/FEW MINUTES LATE/
   PLEASE CHK IF OK
WI R-HAND PAIN
F/U CHANGE BMC
F/U PT MISSED PRV APPT SCC
NEW WCC SIBS PURGED CHART
   (NO MED/ NO CONDITION)
WCC QBI
WI ANXIETY ATTACK
wcc for pre school
F/U NAIL 3-4WK
FEVER/COLDS/SORETHROAT/LC
F/U 2WK/NOT PACT
WALK IN PULLED CHART
stomache ache-vs
#3 GARDASIL--HT
TRIAGE POSS UTI NEW PT/RB
IZ TB TEST
FOLLOW UP WT,HT CHECK-OD
WALK IN /DIARRHEA VOMITTING
   X1 DAY
F/U BACK AND DM
HBG
walk in COUGH
START LTBI CL
INJECTION SCC
PRESUMTIVE ELIG //KR
FOR NEW PT WCC/LC NEEDS
   GATEWAY
FOLOW UP 4 DAYS
WCC IN 2 WEEKER IRIS
NEWBOR
BK PER MD 2 WK FU
NEW BABY ED--HT
SIDE PAIN/ LUMP EVAL
FOLLOW UP DYSMENORRHEA
6WK IUD CK
TRIAGE/MASTITIS
FU C/O NEEDS HEP B AND
   ANXIETY
RV CK EAR

Gastrointestinal Syndrome

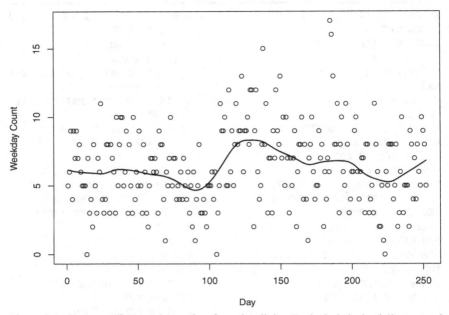

Figure 2.4. One year of GI syndrome data from the clinics. Each circle is the daily count of the number of people presenting who were classified into the GI syndrome. Clinics are not open on most weekends or holidays, so there are 252 daily observations in the data.

2009 H1N1 flu was present). The clinics are not open on weekends and major holidays, resulting in 252 days with syndrome counts for this particular year of data. Figures 2.4 and 2.5 plot the daily counts for gastrointestinal and ILI syndromes. In the plots, the circles are the daily counts, and the line is the estimated daily average count[2] to show time trends.

For the GI syndrome, Figure 2.4 shows that the daily counts range from 0 on three days to a maximum of 17 that occurred on day 185 (April 28). For the year, the average is 6.4 people presenting with GI symptoms per day. The line shows that the daily counts were essentially constant from August through December (days 1–100 or so) followed by an increase in counts from mid-January to mid-March (roughly days 110–150 or so) and a spike in late April (roughly days 185–190), after which the rate essentially returned to the average. This is a pattern consistent with a winter flu season.

---

[2] The estimated daily average is calculated using "lowess," a computationally intensive method for fitting a smooth line to scatterplot data. Lowess stands for locally weighted scatterplot smoother. To calculate it, for each data point in the plot, a low-degree polynomial is fitted to a local neighborhood of the data point using weighted least squares. The value at a point is obtained by evaluating the fitted polynomial. In lowess, the parameter f controls the amount of smoothness of the fitted line; Figures 2.4 and 2.5 use $f = 0.1$, which means 10 percent of the data influence the smoother at each value (Cleveland, 1997).

Influenza–like Illness Syndrome

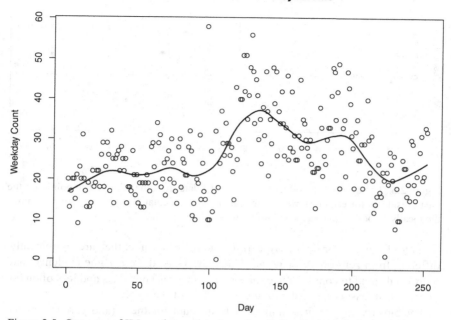

Figure 2.5. One year of ILI syndrome data from the clinics. Each circle is the daily count of the number of people presenting who were classified into the ILI syndrome. Clinics are not open on most weekends or holidays, so there are 252 daily observations in the data.

The ILI syndrome exhibits a similar pattern in Figure 2.5. For this syndrome, the daily counts range from 0 on one day to a maximum that occurred on day 98 (December 22) of 58. Over the entire period, the average is 28.8 people presenting with ILI symptoms per day. The line shows a more pronounced increase in the winter months as well as a spike again in late April. Furthermore, in both figures, the lines clearly demonstrate that because the daily averages are not constant over time, the underlying distributions of the data are not stationary.

In addition to an annual trend or cycle, there may also be other systematic effects in biosurveillance data. For example, although not visible in Figures 2.4 and 2.5, the clinics have a systematic day-of-the-week effect. To see this, Figure 2.6 shows the average daily *residuals* after the trend is removed from the data. That is, if y_i is the daily count for a syndrome, $i = 1, \ldots, 252$, and $\hat{\mu}_i$ is the estimated average daily count (calculated from the line), then the residual for day i is $\hat{\epsilon}_i = y_i - \hat{\mu}_i$. The dots in Figure 2.6 are the average residuals calculated for each day of the week.

So, in Figure 2.6, dots not on the horizontal zero line represent days that are systematically higher or lower than the overall average. Of course, these differences may just be noise, but not all of the differences are attributable to noise. In particular, the residuals for GI syndrome are statistically significantly

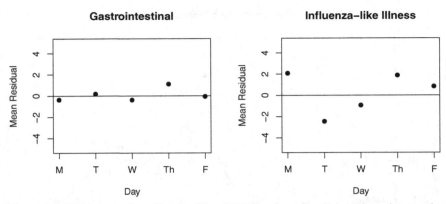

Figure 2.6. The average day effect for GI and ILI data from the clinics. The points are the mean residuals for each day, where the residual $\hat{\epsilon}_i$ is calculated as that day's count minus the locally smoothed average (the lowess lines in Figs. 2.4 and 2.5).

different from zero on Thursday, and for the ILI syndrome, they are significantly different from zero on Tuesday and Thursday. Thus, there is some evidence that individuals tend to come to the clinics more often on Thursdays and less often on Tuesdays, at least compared with the other days of the week.

For biosurveillance, it is important to account for these (and perhaps other) systematic differences in terms of both situational awareness and EED. That is, it is important to be aware of and perhaps adjust for the fact that, on average, on Tuesdays, ILI counts are about 2 less than would otherwise be expected, and on Thursdays, GI and ILI counts are elevated by 1 or 2, respectively, over what would otherwise be expected.

Example: City-Level Hospital Data

The second set of data consists of daily syndrome counts for seven hospitals from a large metropolitan area. Figure 2.7 shows the average daily trends[3] for the GI syndrome for each of the hospitals for slightly more than 2-1/2 years. The actual daily counts are not shown for clarity of the plots.

Figure 2.7 illustrates that even within the same metropolitan area for the same syndrome, the trends and incidence rates can be very different, ranging from an average of 3.2 per day to 22.4 per day. In addition, although there are some common cyclical trends in the smoothed time series, they clearly do not move in "lock step" with one another. Figure 2.8 is a plot of daily counts for respiratory syndrome for the seven hospitals. Note both the similarities and differences between the plots for GI and respiratory chief complaint counts.

Figure 2.9 shows the day effects for the hospital data (calculated in the same way as for the clinic data). Here they tend to be largest on Mondays and then decrease through the week, with the most negative differences on the weekends.

---

[3] As with the clinic data, the lines were calculated using lowess with $f = 0.1$.

Gastrointestinal Syndrome

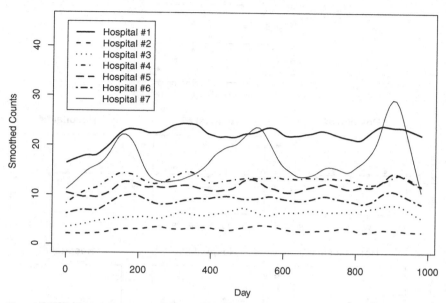

Figure 2.7. Smoothed counts of GI syndrome for seven hospitals in a large metropolitan region over $2\frac{1}{2}$ years.

Respiratory Syndrome

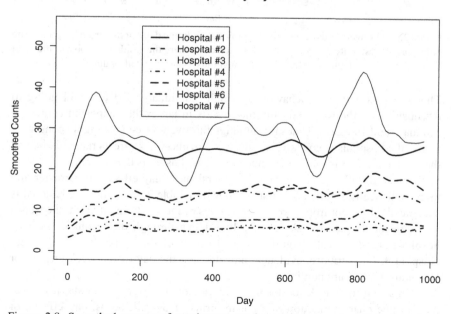

Figure 2.8. Smoothed counts of respiratory syndrome for seven hospitals in a large metropolitan region over $2\frac{1}{2}$ years.

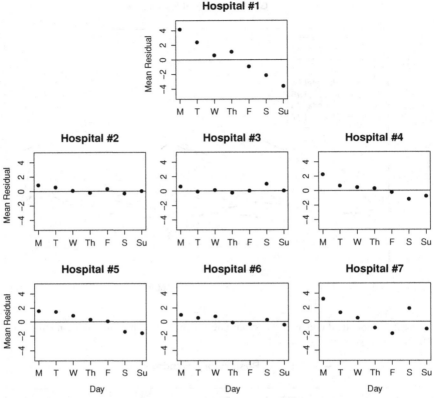

Figure 2.9. The average day effect for respiratory syndrome data for the seven hospitals. The points are the estimated mean residual for each day, where the residual for observation i at hospital j, $\hat{\epsilon}_{ij}$, is calculated as that day's count minus its average daily value: $\hat{\epsilon}_{ij} = y_{ij} - \hat{\mu}_{ij}$.

This suggests a typical behavior in which individuals tend to avoid going to the hospital on the weekends and that results in larger than expected counts on Mondays and Tuesdays. That said, although this overall trend is roughly consistent across the hospitals, some have stronger day-of-the-week effects than others, and the weekend effect is more pronounced in some hospitals than others.

Compared with the clinic data, in general these day effects are stronger and more statistically significant. First, as shown in Table 2.3, the average residual is statistically different from zero for more days of the week. In addition, the trends in the residuals (i.e., the slopes of a line drawn through the residuals for each hospital) are statistically significant (and negative) for all the hospitals except Hospital 3. Furthermore, evidence indicates that the day-of-the-week effects for Hospitals 4 and 7 are nonlinear.

Comparing the city-level hospital and the county-level clinic data, it is clear that no one characterization of data, in terms of overall trends, day effects, or other systematic effects, can be applied to or assumed for all biosurveillance

Table 2.3. Assessing the significance of the day effects for the hospitals: * denotes the average residual is marginally statistically different from zero, ** indicates moderate statistical significance, and *** indicates the difference is highly significant

Hospital	Mon	Tue	Wed	Thu	Fri	Sat	Sun
#1	***	***		**	*	***	***
#2	***	**					
#3	***						***
#4	***	*				**	***
#5	***	***	**			***	***
#6	***	*	***			**	
#7	***	**			***	**	***

data. Furthermore, these are only two specific examples of data, and they do not reflect all the types of biosurveillance data in use nor all the possible systematic effects present in other types of data. For example, OTE pharmaceutical sales data contains systematic effects caused by variations in consumer buying behavior, store operating policies, sales promotions, and so on. Thus, although these data have demonstrated some specific systematic effects, some of the challenges of biosurveillance are identifying, estimating, and perhaps adjusting for such effects so that situational awareness and early event identification are most efficiently and effectively conducted.

2.3 Data Preparation

Biosurveillance data, similar to most real-world data, are rarely in such pristine condition that one can proceed directly to analysis. Rather, it is critical that the data are first appropriately prepared for analysis. This preparation may entail *cleaning* up various errors in the data (e.g., typographical data entry errors), *coding* new variables from the raw data (e.g., creating syndrome indicators from chief complaint text-based data), and perhaps *imputing* missing data. As shown in Figure 2.10, these steps generally occur in a serial fashion, where the data must first be cleaned before they can be coded, and imputation usually follows both cleaning and coding. Although relevant to any data analysis effort, this section describes these data preparation steps as they apply to biosurveillance.

2.3.1 Cleaning

Cleaning (also sometimes referred to as *cleansing*) is the process of examining data to detect errors and inconsistencies, either to possibly correct the errors or perhaps to delete the record containing the error or errors. The errors and inconsistencies can be due to input or transactional problems and often can be corrected by contacting the data source for updated information. Iteratively working to correct such errors often has the dual benefit of fixing the erroneous data and improving

DATA PREPARATION STEPS

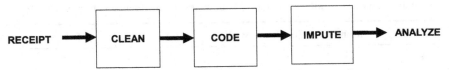

Figure 2.10. Prior to conducting an analysis, biosurveillance data often need to be cleaned, coded, and imputed.

the data acquisition process so that similar errors are reduced in the future. If obtaining corrected data from the original source is not possible, as described in Section 2.3.3, imputation may be an alternative for missing or incorrect data. If those methods fail, then deleting the erroneous record is always possible, although deletion should be used only as a last resort because records with partial data are often preferable to no data at all.

Cleaning should be conducted on the raw data as it comes into the biosurveillance system. The goal is to sanity check the data to catch and correct errors prior to conducting analyses. After all, an analysis is only as good as the data upon which the analysis is based. The adage "garbage in, garbage out" applies just as much to biosurveillance as to any other type of statistical analysis, and perhaps more so, because in biosurveillance, the goal is to detect an outbreak signal in the presence of noisy background information. To the extent that the background noise can be reduced via cleaning, the signal detection will be that much more effective.

Identifying data that may need cleaning is most fundamentally accomplished using different kinds of checks, including:

- *Missing data checks*: Are some fields empty for individual records, or has a site failed to submit its data?
- *Range checks*: Does the data fall within an expected range? For example, if the data are received at the individual level and the data include an age variable, then it would be reasonable to check that the values in the age field lie between 0 and 100 years.
- *Outlier checks*: Are one or more observations very different in some dimension from the other data? For example, do some of the observations have zip codes from far outside of the local area?
- *Logic and consistency checks*: Are the data within records internally consistent? For example, data might be checked to see if all those with a pregnancy indicator are female.

In addition to the above checks, graphical plots may be useful for identifying unusual data. For continuous data, useful plots include histograms and scatterplots. For discrete data, bar charts and contingency tables can be helpful. These and other plots are described in Chapter 4.

Note that data cleaning may be a manual, partially automated, or completely automated process. In all cases, periodic reviews should be conducted to ensure that as the data change over time, the cleaning process and rules are best for capturing and handling errors. Particularly if the process is semiautomated or completely automated, in which the cleaning logic is coded into software as rules, then that logic should periodically be evaluated by comparing the cleaned data with the raw data to ensure that the rules are still operating as desired. Ideally, these reviews should be part of a continuous improvement effort focused both on eliminating as many of the errors on the "front end" where the data are generated and, for those that slip through, that they are being most appropriately and effectively handled at the "back end" upon receipt of the data by the biosurveillance system.

2.3.2 Coding

Coding is the process of turning text-based answers into numerically coded variables. In biosurveillance, this might include creating syndrome indicator variables from chief complaint text. It might also include creating indicator or other numeric variables for categorical demographics such as gender, race or ethnicity, and so on.

For example, consider data with a *gender* variable coded as either "male" or "female." Ignoring the issues of missing data and other possible errors, the following pseudo-code[4] could be used to create a 0/1 *gender_ind* variable:

```
if gender = "male" then gender_ind = 0
   else gender_ind = 1
```

The *gender_ind* variable now equals 0 for males and 1 for females. However, note that *gender_ind* is set to 1 whenever *gender* is not equal to "male," which could introduce errors if, say, "m" and "f" are sometimes used to denote gender. Similarly, whenever the *gender* variable is left blank, *gender_ind* is set to 1, or if the *gender* variable contains a typo (say "mael"), then *gender_ind* is set to 1. More sophisticated code to address these issues is:

```
if gender = {"male" or "m" or "mael"}
   then gender_ind = 0
   else if gender = {"female" or "f" or "femail"}
      then gender_ind = 1
   else gender_ind = 99
```

This type of coding also facilitates data cleaning because observations with *gender_ind* = 99 can now be reviewed to determine why they were not coded as either male or female. Thus, good coding can improve the process of data cleaning.

---

[4] Pseudo-code expresses the logic of computer code using a generic syntax rather than the syntax of a specific computer language.

As another example, the following pseudo-code creates the *GI_ind* indicator variable for the GI syndrome by searching for keyword substrings within chief complaint text:

```
loop from i = 1 to number of data records
set GI_ind(i) = 0
    loop from j = 1 to number of GI keywords
        {
        if GI_keyword(j) is a substring in chief_complaint(i)
            then GI_ind(i) = 1
        }
}
```

The above is perhaps the simplest way to identify whether a set of terms is contained in a free-form text block and is relatively easy to implement if the software being used has a text search function to find specific substrings within a given text string. It requires a list of GI terms to be searched for, a list that should also include abbreviations, acronyms, and common misspellings of the terms. Creating such a list that is complete, and then subsequently maintaining the list, is not a trivial task, however.

This is the approach used in the Early Aberration Reporting System (EARS) system, where "symptom" indicators are first created by searching chief complaint free text for various "words." For example, in one installation, if any of the words COLD, OE, DISCH, or OM (or 91 other words) matches a character sequence in an individual's chief complaint text, then the cold symptom is set to one for that individual: *cold_symptom_ind* = 1. Once all the symptoms are coded, syndromes are coded based on various combinations of the symptoms. For example, the flu syndrome is set to one (*flu_syndrome_ind* = 1) if any of the following symptoms are positive: flu, cold, cough, fever, chills, muscle pain, or headache.

Note that depending on the particular substring to be searched for, without more sophisticated text parsing, simple text-matching algorithms are subject to spurious false positives. For example, "D" is sometimes used in chief complaints as shorthand for diarrhea, and diarrhea is a symptom associated with the GI syndrome. But simply setting *gastro_syndrome_ind* to 1 whenever a "D" occurs anywhere in the chief complaint text will result in the syndrome indicator is being incorrectly set to 1 more often than not (e.g., in Table 2.2, "NO MEDS," "POSSIBLE STD," and "DISCH" are unrelated to the GI syndrome).

Similarly, the existence of the word "FLU" in chief complaint free text is used in the EARS system as an indicator for various symptom indicators. However, those symptom indicators would be incorrectly set for chief complaint text that reads "FLU SHOT" because those going for a flu shot are likely to be healthy, not sick. This type of simple text matching has been referred to as the "bag-of-words" approach; "natural language processing" allows for more nuanced and complex text processing.

A more sophisticated text coding algorithm would set *gastro_ind*=1 when, for example, "D" occurs as a separate "word" in the chief complaint text (as in "D AND VOMITING" or "D&V") but not as part of a longer word (as in "DISCHARGE" or "DEAD"). In addition, the text-coding algorithm must be flexible enough to flag when the requisite root word is found in the text string (e.g., "VOMIT" within the text "VOMITING"). Also note that, as a practical matter, if the software used for the text coding is case sensitive, both the search terms and chief complaint text should be either converted to all uppercase or lowercase to facilitate matching.

Coding, or perhaps more properly *recoding*, also includes the process of creating new or alternative numerical variables from other numerical variables. Usually this is done to facilitate the analysis. For example, perhaps when the data were received, the gender variable is coded 1 for male and 2 for female, but the analysis requires a 0/1 coded gender variable. Then, upon receipt of the data, the biosurveillance system software might execute an instruction similar to the following pseudo-code:

```
if gender = 1 then new_gender = 0
    else if gender = 2 then new_gender = 1
    else new_gender = 99
```

In the *new_gender* variable, males are now coded 0 and females 1, and all other values, including missing values, are coded as 99. This latter choice of coding missing values the same as any other numeric entry not equal to 1 or 2 may or may not be appropriate. If during data preparation, numeric entries not equal to 1 or 2 will be cleaned while missing values will be imputed (as described in the next subsection), the following pseudo-code would be preferred:

```
if gender = 1 then new_gender = 0
    else if gender = 2 then new_gender = 1
    else if gender = "" then new_gender = 99
    else new_gender = 98
```

In general, explicit coding such as the above is to be preferred, particularly for missing values and nonmatches, so that the various types and causes of the errors can be determined. This facilitates data and software code corrections and improvements.

2.3.3 Imputing

Imputation is the process of correcting missing data by estimation. For biosurveillance, imputation may be used to substitute an appropriate value for the missing data within an individual-level observation using within-sample inference, or it can be used to impute missing aggregate count data. An example of the former is a biosurveillance system that receives data on individuals, and the records for some individuals are incomplete. An example of the latter is a biosurveillance system that receives aggregate counts, say of number of individuals presenting with a particular syndrome per day, but the counts are not received from a facility for one or more time periods.

The advantage of imputation is that it maximizes the use of all the available data. One disadvantage, however, is that some think of imputed data as "made-up" data. In fact, it is made-up data, but if done correctly, the data are not arbitrarily or capriciously made up. Rather, the imputation is conducted in a careful, principled way so that:

- The benefits of using the information in partial records more than makes up for the efforts involved in and the effects of using the imputed data.
- The information from the actual data is not compromised and can be used directly in any analysis.
- The imputed data can always be distinguished from the actual data.

Although naive analysts sometimes ignore all records that are not complete (referred to as *casewise deletion* in the statistical imputation literature), this can result in a significant waste of data. After all, why ignore a whole record just because one field is missing? For example, consider a model-based estimate of the number of individuals expected to present with a particular syndrome in the next time period. Such an estimate is useful for judging whether the actual number that present in that period is unusually large. The model could require the use of many covariates drawn from the data and, without imputation, all records with data missing for one or more covariates cannot be used. If the amount of missing data is non-negligible, this could result in the "deletion" of a significant number of records in the model, perhaps resulting in biased estimates of the number of individuals expected to present.

The following subsections describe four methods of imputation, proceeding from easiest to most difficult: mean value imputation, regression imputation, hot deck imputation, and multiple imputation.[5]

Mean Value Imputation

The basic idea of *mean value imputation* is to replace the missing observations of a variable with the average calculated from the nonmissing observations of that same variable. The main advantages of mean value imputation are that it is easy to do and that it does not affect the average. Its disadvantages include that it is only useful for numeric data, that it distorts the distribution of the data (resulting in a spike at the average value), that it can result in underestimation of standard errors, and that using the same average value for all the missing observations may not be appropriate.

---

[5] Note that this material requires some familiarity with basic numerical summary statistics (sample mean, standard deviation, and variance) and linear regression. Readers requiring a refresher may wish to first read Section 4.1.1 of Chapter 4 (particularly the parts related to Equations 4.2 and 4.6) and Section 5.3.1 of Chapter 5. Also, for a brief review of some of the fundamental concepts from probability and statistics, see Appendix A.

To illustrate the idea of mean value imputation, consider a biosurveillance system that receives data at the individual level, one variable of which is age. Denote the age of the ith observation on a particular day as y_i. Imagine on one day that the last two observations out of n are missing age and that during data cleaning that actual age values could not be determined. Then, using mean value imputation, the missing ages could be imputed as

$$y'_{n-1} = y'_n = \bar{y},$$

where in this example

$$\bar{y} = \frac{1}{n-2} \sum_{i=1}^{n-2} y_i.$$

For the nonmissing observations (in this case, $i = 1, \ldots, n-2$), set $y'_i = y_i$. As appropriate, the calculation of the mean could be extended to include data from adjacent time periods.

Example 2.1. Table 2.4 contains eight observations for 10 time periods. The observations for periods 9 and 10 are missing. Using mean value imputation, impute y_9 and y_{10} from the rest of the data.

Solution: The imputed values are $y'_9 = y'_{10} = \frac{1}{8} \sum_{i=1}^{8} y_i = 37.4$. Note that the sample mean is unaffected by the imputation, $\bar{y} = \bar{y}'$, but the standard deviation incorrectly calculated from the imputed age data (using $n = 10$) results in a sample standard deviation that is too small ($s_{y'} < s_y$), and thus any statistical inference conducted using that standard error would be inappropriately precise. Also note the imputation flag indicating which of the ages were imputed is included in Table 2.4.

Stochastic mean value imputation can be used to mitigate the distortion of the distribution of the data. It does so by adding "noise" to the imputed value for the ith observation,

$$y'_i = \bar{y} + Z_i,$$

where Z_i is randomly drawn from some appropriate probability distribution. For example, it might be appropriate to assume Z_i is randomly distributed according to a normal distribution with mean zero and variance the same as the variance of the observed data: $N(0, s_y^2)$. Appropriately applied, stochastic mean value imputation helps correct the standard deviation (and thus the standard error) underestimation problem.

Table 2.4. Illustrating mean value imputation on a hypothetical data set. The dots for observations 9 and 10 denote that data are missing. Note that mean value imputation does not affect the average because, as shown in the table, $\bar{y} = \bar{y}' = 37.4$. However, this type of imputation does affect the estimated standard deviation by making it smaller than it would be if it were calculated without inclusion of the imputed values

Observation (i)	Zip code	Gender	Observed age (y_i)	Imputed age (y_i')	Imputation flag
1	90001	M	63	63	0
2	90001	F	57	57	0
3	90002	F	22	22	0
4	90001	M	78	78	0
5	90002	M	31	31	0
6	90002	M	16	16	0
7	90002	F	6	6	0
8	90002	M	26	26	0
9	90001	M	.	37.4	1
10	90002	F	.	37.4	1
			$\bar{y} = 37.4$	$\bar{y}' = 37.4$	
			$s_y = 25.5$	$s_{y'} = 22.5$	

Example 2.2. Returning to the Example 2.1 data, use stochastic mean value imputation to impute y_9 and y_{10} from the rest of the data.

Solution: Calculate $y_i' = \bar{y} + Z, i = 9, 10$, where Z is a random variable and for this data $Z \sim N(0, s_y^2) = N(0, 25.5^2)$. Table 2.5 shows the observed random draws for Z and the resulting imputed values for y_9 and y_{10}. Note that the resulting estimated standard deviation of imputed age is now closer to the estimated standard deviation for the $n = 8$ actual observations in Table 2.4.

If there are systematic differences among various subgroups in the population (e.g., by gender), then conducting mean value imputation or stochastic mean value imputation within each subgroup can sometimes provide more appropriate imputed values. For example, if it is necessary to impute the height or weight for some patients missing that information in their records, it would make more sense to do so by gender because men tend to be both taller and heavier than women. Similarly, it might be better to impute after grouping by, say, zip code if the distribution of the variable of interest varies by zip code.

Example 2.3. Again returning to the Example 2.1 data, given that the age distribution between the two zip codes is different, with 90001 residents generally older than 90002 residents, impute the missing data using mean imputation by zip code subgroup.

Table 2.5. Illustrating stochastic mean value imputation for the data from Table 2.4

Observation (i)	Zip code	Gender	Observed age (y)	$\bar{y}_i$	Z	Imputed age (y'_i)	Imputation flag
1	90001	M	63			63	0
2	90001	F	57			57	0
3	90002	F	22			22	0
4	90001	M	78			78	0
5	90002	M	31			31	0
6	90002	M	16			16	0
7	90002	F	6			6	0
8	90002	M	26			26	0
9	90001	M	.	37.4	7.2	44.6	1
10	90002	F	.	37.4	−27.1	10.3	1

$$\bar{y} = 37.4 \qquad \bar{y}' = 35.4$$
$$s_y = 25.5 \qquad s_{y'} = 24.2$$

Solution: Table 2.6 shows imputed age now calculated using the sample mean by subgroup, in this case zip code. Note that because the number of observations from the zip codes is not equal, the mean of imputed age no longer equals the sample mean of the observed ages.

Imputation by subgroup can also be extended to multiple subgroup categories, although so doing can quickly become excessively complex. For example, returning to the question of imputing height and weight, not only does it differ by gender, but also by age, race or ethnicity, and perhaps geographic location. Imagine that is appropriate to use 20 age categories and 5 race or ethnicity categories and that

Table 2.6. Illustrating mean value imputation by subgroup on the hypothetical data set from Table 2.4

Observation (i)	Zip code	Gender	Observed age (y)	Imputed age (y')	Imputation flag
1	90001	M	63	63	0
2	90001	F	57	57	0
4	90001	M	78	78	0
9	90001	M	.	66.0	1
3	90002	F	22	22	0
5	90002	M	31	31	0
6	90002	M	16	16	0
7	90002	F	6	6	0
8	90002	M	26	26	0
10	90002	F	.	20.2	1

$$\bar{y}_{90001} = 66.0 \qquad \bar{y}' = 38.5$$
$$\bar{y}_{90002} = 20.2 \qquad s_{y'} = 25.0$$

there are 10 geographic location categories. Then, along with the two gender categories, one would have to calculate $20 \times 5 \times 10 \times 2 = 2,000$ averages. In these cases, it is usually easier to use regression imputation (see the next subsection).

Up to this point, mean value imputation has been applied to cross-sectional data – that is, data from one time period within which missing values have been imputed from data in that same time period. This is the typical imputation problem. It arises in the context of biosurveillance with data at the individual level. However, some systems receive and operate on aggregate data such as counts per time period. In this situation, imputation may be required for missing counts in which, for example, a facility may fail to submit its counts for a day. This is imputation for longitudinal data, and the appropriate imputation strategy depends on whether the imputation is being done prospectively or retrospectively.

In *retrospective imputation* for longitudinal data, a historical time series data set is available and, within that data set, some values are missing. In this situation, strategies for imputing the missing values can use data that occurred both before and after the missing value. In contrast, *prospective imputation* (more commonly referred to as *forecasting* or *prediction*) only uses historical data to impute the next unobserved observation in a series. Forecasting methods are discussed in detail in Chapter 5.

One simple retrospective method is longitudinal mean value imputation. Given a sequence of data, $y_1, y_2, \ldots, y_{n-1}, y_n$, where the subscript represents the order the data was received in the biosurveillance system, let y_j be missing. Then, for some positive integer k, impute y_j as

$$y'_j = \frac{1}{2k} \left(\sum_{i=j-k}^{j-1} y_i + \sum_{i=j+1}^{j+k} y_i \right).$$

When used for imputation of biosurveillance data, the choice of k should be based on the seasonal and other systematic variability in the data and should generally be fixed at some multiple of the smallest systematic cycle in the data. For example, if the data exhibit a weekly cycle resulting from systematic day-of-the-week effects, perhaps with monthly and annual cycles as well, k should be set as a multiple of 7 (assuming the data comes in seven days a week). In addition, the more variable the data, the smaller k should be set so that the resulting imputed values are not oversmoothed and, if the data sequence has multiple missing values, k should be set to be at least as small as the smallest distance between missing values.

Example 2.4. Consider the following daily counts of individuals presenting at local community clinics on weekdays and subsequently classified into the ILI syndrome.

Time (t):	1	2	3	4	5	6	7	8	9	10	11
y_t:	8	9	4	3	8	–	13	9	7	4	12

Using longitudinal mean value imputation, impute y_6 for $k = 2$ and $k = 5$.

Solution: For $k = 2$,

$$y'_6 = \frac{1}{4}\left(\sum_{i=4}^{5} y_i + \sum_{i=7}^{8} y_i\right)$$

$$= \frac{3 + 8 + 13 + 9}{4}$$

$$= 8.25.$$

And, for $k = 5$,

$$y'_6 = \frac{1}{10}\left(\sum_{i=1}^{5} y_i + \sum_{i=7}^{11} y_i\right)$$

$$= \frac{8 + 9 + 4 + 3 + 8 + 13 + 9 + 7 + 4 + 12}{10}$$

$$= 7.7.$$

Regression Imputation

Regression imputation is useful for estimating mean values and is easier to implement than mean value imputation when the value to be imputed depends on multiple other variables. The idea is to use the information from observations with complete data to estimate a regression model and then use the model to estimate the mean value for observations with missing dependent variables. Consider the case of data with two continuous variables, one of which has some missing values (the y) for which the other variable (the x) can usefully be used for prediction. Then, for observations that have both x and y, fit the model

$$\mathbb{E}(Y|x) = \beta_0 + \beta_1 x$$

and then use that model to predict the missing ys using

$$y'_i = \hat{\beta}_0 + \hat{\beta}_1 x_i.$$

Regression imputation is particularly useful when there are multiple independent variables, where mean value imputation can become overly complicated to implement, and it can be applied to categorical data using indicator variables. For example,

$$y'_i = \hat{\beta}_0 + \hat{\beta}_1 x_i + \hat{\beta}_2 I_{\text{Mon}} + \hat{\beta}_3 I_{\text{Tue}} + \hat{\beta}_4 I_{\text{Wed}} + \hat{\beta}_5 I_{\text{Thu}} + \hat{\beta}_6 I_{\text{Fri}} + \hat{\beta}_7 I_{\text{Sat}}$$

incorporates indicator variables to accommodate day-of-the-week effects.

However, regression-based imputation tends to have limited utility for individual-level data in biosurveillance applications because the variable being predicted must be numeric. In addition, when using multiple regression, data must be available on all independent variables in the model. This is sometimes either too hard or results in too few observations available with all data to build an effective model. To work around this problem, sometimes a series of regression-based imputations is conducted in which the imputed values from one model are then used as independent variables in the next regression imputation model.

Regression (and time series methods) can also be useful for prospective longitudinal imputation, particularly when the data come from a process that has a significant trend. In this situation, estimates based on mean value imputation will either systematically over- or underestimate the quantity of interest. These methods will be discussed in more detail in Chapter 5.

Hot Deck Imputation

Hot deck imputation (also known as the *last value(s) carry forward* approach in the imputation literature) is often used for large-scale imputation processes, in which the name *hot deck* dates back to the use of computer punch cards. A stack of punch cards (the "deck") was "hot" because it was currently being processed. Thus, hot deck imputation uses information drawn from the data currently in use. Cold-deck imputation, by contrast, selects information from a deck of cards (i.e., other data) not currently in use.

Hot deck imputation fills in missing values on incomplete observations using values from similar but complete records. Generally, the easiest way to accomplish this is to first sort the data by the variables that are most related to the outcome of interest and then, starting at the top, replace any missing data with value or values of the immediately preceding observation. If numeric data in the first observation are missing, they are replaced with appropriate mean values. If non-numeric data are missing, they are replaced with the data from appropriately selected random observations.

Hot deck imputation has a number of advantages. First, it can be used for non-numeric data, which means that in biosurveillance applications it can be used to impute missing chief complaint text and other non-numeric demographic or text-based data. Second, it is fast because it only requires data sorting and not model fitting. Third, unlike mean value and regression imputation, it incorporates the inherent variability in the data so that standard error estimation is less affected.

Example 2.5. Consider a biosurveillance system that receives gender, age, race, and chief complaint data on individuals presenting at a hospital ER. As shown in Table 2.7, sometimes the race and chief complaint data are missing. Impute the missing values using hot deck imputation, in which the missing values are related to gender and age.

Solution: Because chief complaint is most related to gender and age, the data are first sorted by gender and then age within gender. Then, missing race and chief complaint data are imputed by starting at the top of the sorted list and replacing any missing data with value or values of the immediately preceding observation.

Table 2.7. Illustrating hot deck imputation on a hypothetical data set where race and chief complaint data are sometimes missing

Gender	Age	Race	Imputed race	Race imputation flag	Chief complaint	Imputed chief complaint	Chief comp. imputation flag
F	68	Black	Black	0	RTN/FLP	RTN/FLP	0
F	62	White	White	0	f/u	f/u	0
F	60	White	White	0	RTN/FLP	RTN/FLP	0
F	59	Asian	Asian	0	MED REFILL	MED REFILL	0
F	53	Black	Black	0	RTN/FLP	RTN/FLP	0
F	54	White	White	0	F/U	F/U	0
F	45	White	White	0	WWE	WWE	0
F	45	White	White	0	dizziness	dizziness	0
F	36	Asian	Asian	0	FU/NEEDS IZ'S	FU/NEEDS IZ'S	0
F	31	White	White	0	RTN RV	RTN RV	0
F	30		White	1	OBCPE/RB	OBCPE/RB	0
F	30	White	White	0	RTN/FLP/BC	RTN/FLP/BC	0
F	30	White	White	0	FOR PAP AND DEPO	FOR PAP AND DEPO	0
F	19	White	White	0	PN/RV	PN/RV	0
F	15	White	White	0	LROB //KR	LROB //KR	0
F	15	White	White	0	WCC	WCC	0
F	14	White	White	0	FLU SHOT	FLU SHOT	0
F	14	White	White	0	SEIZURES	SEIZURES	0
F	11	White	White	0	FLU SHOT HPV #2	FLU SHOT HPV #2	0
F	10	White	White	0	rash around neck	rash around neck	0
F	7	White	White	0	allergy test	allergy test	0
F	6	White	White	0	F/U	F/U	0
F	4	White	White	0	RTN/WCC	RTN/WCC	0
F	1		White	1		RTN/WCC	1
F	1	White	White	0	FLU SHOT	FLU SHOT	0
F	1	White	White	0	FEVER	FEVER	0
M	74	Asian	Asian	0	RTN/FLP	RTN/FLP	0
M	67	White	White	0		RTN/FLP	1
M	65	Asian	Asian	0	rtn/flp	rtn/flp	0
M	59	White	White	0	RTN/FLP	RTN/FLP	0
M	57	White	White	0	RTN/FLP	RTN/FLP	0
M	57	White	White	0	FU	FU	0
M	49	White	White	0	F/U	F/U	0
M	38	White	White	0	F/U	F/U	0
M	27	White	White	0	NEW/STD CHK	NEW/STD CHK	0
M	10	White	White	0	STOMACH ACHE	STOMACH ACHE	0
M	10	White	White	0	FLU SHOT	FLU SHOT	0
M	9	White	White	0	rtn/wcc	rtn/wcc	0
M	9	White	White	0	CONGESTION	CONGESTION	0
M	5	White	White	0	RTN/WCC	RTN/WCC	0
M	4	White	White	0	triage	triage	0
M	2		White	1	COUGH 15 DAYS	COUGH 15 DAYS	0
M	1	White	White	0	TRIAGE	TRIAGE	0
M	0	White	White	0	RTN/WCC	RTN/WCC	0

There are many variants on hot deck imputation. The main idea is to fill in missing data from observations with data that are similar to those that are missing the data. In the previous example, this was accomplished by sorting the data by variables that are correlated with those missing data. This is a somewhat crude way to identify similar observations, but it has the advantage of being fairly easy to implement. A more sophisticated method is nearest neighbor hot deck. With this method, the observations are first separated into a "donor" class (observations not missing data) and a "recipient" class (observations missing data). These two classes may be defined by subgroups, say, geographically by zip code. Then, for each observation in the recipient class, a "nearest neighbor" is found in the donor class, in which the nearest neighbor is computed using some sort of distance measure on characteristics that are correlated with the variable missing data.

Multiple Imputation

Multiple imputation is an even more sophisticated (and complicated) imputation methodology. It creates multiple imputed data sets (hence the name), and variation across the multiple data sets allows for estimation of overall variation, including both sampling and imputation variance. Multiple imputation requires the specification of an "imputation model" and the use of specialized software and methods that are beyond the scope of this text.

2.4 Discussion and Summary

This chapter described the various types of data used in biosurveillance, data that are often based on counts, and it used two syndromic surveillance data sets to illustrate. The chapter then described the steps in preparing data for use in a biosurveillance system. As with any data analysis effort, the "garbage in, garbage out" principle applies to biosurveillance. Indeed, good data preparation is critical for good EED because the more sources of extraneous noise that are minimized or removed from the data, the more sensitive the system will be at detecting outbreaks.

Hence, the discussion on cleaning focused on detecting and removing errors and inconsistencies from incoming biosurveillance data. Part of cleaning – and any good data analysis – is simply to carefully look at the data, both individually and using various summary measures and plots. In biosurveillance, this will pay double dividends. First, carefully looking at the data will both familiarize the user with the data itself, particularly its idiosyncrasies and potential errors. Second, regularly identifying and correcting the sources of errors in the data collection, assembly, and transmission processes will improve the overall operation and sensitivity of the biosurveillance system.

Depending on the intended use of the biosurveillance system, it may be important to extend data cleaning to identifying and removing data associated with outbreaks as well. Specifically, if the purpose of the biosurveillance system is to detect natural disease outbreaks, then such a system will likely be more sensitive to detecting such outbreaks if it is only calibrated using non-outbreak data. In industrial quality control and statistical process control, this is akin to what is called "Phase I" control charting, in which control charts are used to identify data associated with out-of-control conditions in order to remove those data from subsequent analyses.

Coding is used for transforming data into forms useful for biosurveillance monitoring and analysis. In so doing, it is important to ensure that the coding schemes are appropriately implemented so that both unexpected data are identified (for cleaning) and missing data are flagged (for potential imputation). One critical aspect of the coding process is to periodically compare the coded values with the original data to ensure the codes match the data as intended. This is particularly important when coding chief complaints to syndrome categories, in which it is critical to routinely examine sets of chief complaints within a particular syndrome category to ensure the syndrome definition logic continues to identify the requisite conditions.

Conventional imputation methods are designed to address information missing at the individual record level in cross-sectional data. To the extent that this problem occurs in biosurveillance systems, existing methods apply directly. However, imputation in the context of aggregated biosurveillance data, such as daily syndrome counts, and its effect on biosurveillance system EED and SA performance is unique. In particular, determining how to impute missing daily counts, for example, such that EED is not degraded, is an open research question. Similarly, it is not clear how much imputation is useful and operationally relevant in the practice of biosurveillance, the answer to which requires additional research and likely depends on the data quality within a particular system.

Additional Reading

To read more about biosurveillance data, consider the following:

- Chapter 1 of *Monitoring the Health of Populations* (Brookmeyer & Stroup, 2004) provides a 20-page extensive list of "selected" public health surveillance data sources in the United States, listing the surveillance system, the populations targeted for surveillance, the frequency of monitoring, and relevant references.
- Chapter 2 of *Disease Surveillance: A Public Health Informatics Approach* (Lombardo & Buckeridge, 2007) describes in more detail the types of biosurveillance data and their sources, including data from hospitals and physicians, pharmacies, EMS, 911 and telephone hotlines, absenteeism, as well as environmental and animal data.
- Part II of *Handbook of Biosurveillance* (Wagner *et al.*, 2006) more broadly describes the organizations that conduct biosurveillance and the data they collect, including the government; human health care providers; animal health organizations; laboratories, coroners and medical examiners, and water, food, and pharmaceutical providers.

In terms of data cleaning, recoding, and imputation, there are few general references and none directly related to public health surveillance. For example, after describing the sources of data, texts such as Brookmeyer and Stroup (2004), Lombardo & Buckeridge (2007), Wagner *et al.* (2006), Lawson & Kleinman (2005), and M'ikanatha *et al.* (2007) jump right to detection and other statistical algorithms, essentially ignoring the issue of data preparation. That said, to read more about data cleaning and imputation, consider the following:

- *Cody's Data Cleaning Techniques Using SAS* (Cody, 2008) discusses how to check and clean both text and numeric data, including identifying missing data and duplicate observations. The text is intended for SAS statistical software users, but software syntax aside, the book provides many useful tips and ideas for cleaning up messy data.
- *Missing Data: A Gentle Introduction* (McKnight *et al.*, 2007) delves more deeply into most of the imputation methods discussed in this chapter, as well as others. For a more statistically advanced treatment of hot deck methods, see Andridge and Little (2010), who discuss the pros and cons of hot deck imputation in the context of survey research.

Part II

Situational Awareness

3

Situational Awareness for Biosurveillance

He who loves practice without theory is like the sailor who boards ship without a
rudder and compass and never knows where he may be cast.

Leonardo da Vinci (1452–1519)

Situational awareness (SA) is one of the two main functions of a biosurveillance system. As Homeland Security Presidential Directive 21 (HSPD-21) states, biosurveillance is "the process of active data-gathering with appropriate analysis and interpretation of biosphere data that might relate to disease activity and threats to human or animal health – whether infectious, toxic, metabolic, or otherwise, and regardless of intentional or natural origin – in order to achieve early warning of health threats, early detection of health events, and *overall situational awareness of disease activity*" [emphasis added] (US Government, 2007).

Intuitively, most interpret the term "situational awareness" to mean that one is cognizant of one's surroundings. But awareness in this sense is actually only one part of situational awareness. A solid understanding of, and rigorous definition of, situational awareness in a biosurveillance context is critical for being able to assess whether a biosurveillance system, in fact, provides situational awareness, how such systems should be modified to improve biosurveillance situational awareness, and whether one system or method provides better situational awareness and thus should be preferred.

This chapter begins by defining situational awareness and then describing a general theoretical model of situational awareness that has been used in many nonbiosurveillance decision-making contexts. The chapter discusses how the general model applies to biosurveillance and then connects data and statistical methods to where and how they are required to support situational awareness.

Chapter Objectives

Upon completion of this chapter, the reader should be able to:

- Define situational awareness, including the three levels of situational awareness: perception, comprehension, and projection.
- Describe why maintaining situational awareness in a dynamically changing environment is important.
- Explain the difference between situational awareness and situation assessment.
- Give examples of how good situational awareness enhances good decision making and how decision making can be degraded with poor situational awareness.
- Apply Endsley's theoretical situational awareness model to biosurveillance.
- In a biosurveillance context, discuss what types of data and statistical methods are required to support the three levels of situational awareness.
- Describe how the situated cognition model extends the theoretical situational awareness model and what the implications are for biosurveillance system design.

3.1 What Is Situational Awareness?

Situational awareness (SA) is often a critical prerequisite for successful decision making, particularly in complex, dynamically changing situations. Endsley (1995, p. 36) defines situational awareness as "the perception of elements in the environment within a volume of time and space, the comprehension of their meaning, and the projection of their status in the near future." Thus, SA is not only about being aware of the current state of events but also about being able to put those events in the context of what is expected so one can understand what they mean, and it involves being able to understand what is likely to occur in the near future given current events. Endsley (1995) goes on to say that "it is important to distinguish the term situation awareness, as a state of knowledge, from the processes used to achieve that state. These processes, which may vary widely among individuals and contexts, will be referred to as situation assessment or the process of achieving, acquiring, or maintaining SA." SA is thus a state of knowledge, and situational assessment is the process or processes necessary to achieve SA.

It is important to recognize that achieving SA requires more than having lots of data or information available. In fact, although a lack of information can impede SA, excessive, irrelevant, or disorganized information can also result in the lack or loss of SA. Think about the problem in terms of driving a car in an unfamiliar location and trying to get to a particular destination. If the location is out in a very rural area without street signs, then it is pretty easy to get lost because of a lack of information about the roads. On the other hand, if the location is New York City and you are driving through Times Square, it is also easy to get lost because of all the visual distractions, the busy traffic, and general information overload.

Data are not necessarily information and, as Endsley (2001) notes, more data do not necessarily provide more information. Similarly, more information does not necessarily translate into more or better SA. Human beings are limited by nature and experience in terms of how much information we can process; certain forms of information are easier to process and understand, and internalizing, integrating, and understanding the meaning of information can be made easier or harder depending on how the information is presented. Thus, the challenge of improving SA is one of identifying what information is needed, and when it is needed, within the context of a particular decision-making problem or scenario.

Situational awareness has been carefully and deeply studied in a number of contexts. For example, in aviation, the focus is on pilots maintaining appropriate SA of the aircraft, including its location in space, whether it is on the correct flight path, its material condition and status, and so on. Designing nuclear plant operations consoles is another example, in which significant effort has been invested in designing interfaces that help facilitate SA.

3.2 A Theoretical Situational Awareness Model

A well-known theoretical model for SA was defined by Endsley (2001, 1995). It posits three distinct levels of SA: (1) perception of the elements in the environment,

(2) comprehension of the current situation, and (3) projection of the future status of the situation. These levels are defined as follows.

- Level 1 SA, *perception of the elements in the environment*: Discerning the relevant elements in the environment, including their attributes, status, and dynamics, is the most basic level of SA. It is awareness of the elements (which may be objects, events, people, systems, environmental factors) and their current states (e.g., locations, conditions, modes, actions). Thus, level 1 SA involves not only recognition of the relevant elements but also ongoing monitoring of the elements because they may change over time.
- Level 2 SA, *comprehension of the current situation*: The next level of SA involves a synthesis of the elements to comprehend the situation. That is, level 2 SA requires integrating the information perceived in level 1 in order to understand significance of the those elements on the desired goals or outcomes. Through the processes of pattern recognition, interpretation, and evaluation, level 2 SA results in a holistic understanding of the environment that allows for the comprehension of the significance of elements and events.
- Level 3 SA, *projection of future status of the situation*: The third and highest level of SA involves the ability to project the future status of the elements in the environment. Given perception and comprehension of the situation (levels 1 and 2 SA), as well as knowledge about how the elements interact dynamically, level 3 SA is achieved by using this information to project likely future states of the environment that are important or useful for decision making.

What it means to achieve each of these levels is highly context dependent for a given situation or scenario. That is, the information necessary for a pilot to achieve SA is completely different from what is required for a nuclear plant operator, and certainly the information necessary for a public health official to maintain SA during a pandemic is similarly quite different from the other two occupations.

As shown in Figure 3.1, in a dynamically changing environment, these three levels of SA are embedded in a loop where the situation is ever changing, both in response to external influences and to changes that result from prior decisions that subsequently affect the current state of the situation. That is, changes in the environment can affect SA, sometimes improving it and other times perhaps degrading it. Similarly, the decisions made with some level of SA can make the situation either better or worse, ultimately feeding back upon the decision maker and perhaps affecting his or her SA for the better or worse.

Returning to the driving example, anyone driving in a large, unfamiliar city has been in the situation in which as they are driving they start to lose track of their location – i.e., their situational awareness starts to degrade. To attempt to recover, they make decisions about where to turn, and those choices either result in getting back on track and thus an improved SA or perhaps getting lost and further degradation of SA. A key idea is that SA is a mental construct of the actual situation. To the extent that the mental construct matches the actual situation,

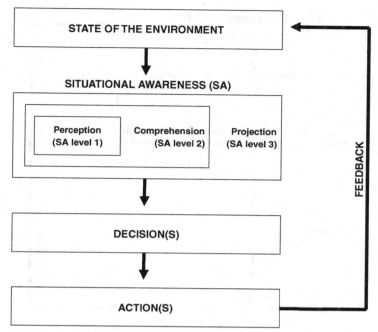

Figure 3.1. Situational awareness in Endsley's model has three levels: perception, comprehension, and projection. In a dynamic situation, SA is embedded in a loop in which
the environment affects SA and decisions made under a particular level of SA affect the
environment (and hence future SA). (Adapted from Endsley, 1995)

good decisions can be made. The more the mental construct departs from the
actual situation, the more likely that inappropriate or incorrect decisions will be
made.

Of course, these days, one strategy many drivers use to improve situational
awareness is a GPS receiver that provides visual maps showing current location
and verbal directions about the route to follow. In terms of the three levels of
SA, GPS units can improve perception by showing the car's location on a map, it
can improve comprehension by displaying the location with respect to the desired
route, and it can improve projection by giving advance notice of future actions the
driver will need to take to say on the route.

In the driving example, note that SA involves both a temporal and a spatial
component ("Am I on time?" and "Am I on track?"). Time in SA is important
because, in a dynamic situation such as flying a plane or managing the public health
response to a pandemic, things are constantly changing. Thus, it becomes critical to
be able to appropriately update one's mental construct of the situation in response
to changing conditions. In terms of biosurveillance, the spatial component is often
of importance as well. It is not enough to know when an outbreak is occurring; one
must also know where, and one must keep track of the outbreak region or regions
as the pandemic evolves over time.

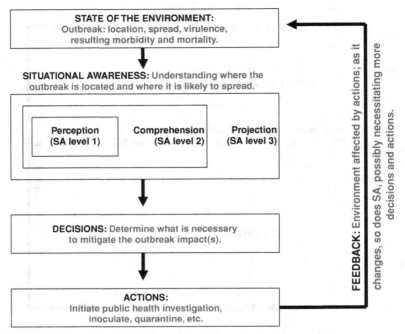

Figure 3.2. Endsley's model of SA applied to biosurveillance.

3.3 Biosurveillance Situational Awareness

Figure 3.2 illustrates how Endsley's theoretical model applies to biosurveillance. The environment is the human, zoonotic, or agricultural population of interest, including their heath status, disease vectors, and the status of intervention assets. During an outbreak, it includes the location, spread, virulence, and resulting morbidity and mortality of a disease or an agent. The SA is what a decision maker (in terms of either a public health individual or an organization) believes he or she knows about the environment. Decisions and their subsequent actions, including initiating epidemiological investigations and public health interventions, then affect the environment and complete the loop.

In terms of the three levels of SA, a recent Government Accountability Office (GAO) report states,

Officials at CDC with key biosurveillance responsibilities subscribe to a definition that includes three components:

1. awareness that a situation has occurred (e.g., detection of a biological condition that differs from the norm),
2. comprehension of its meaning (e.g., characterization of the nature and scope of a biological event), and
3. projection of its likely course in the near future (e.g., how its nature and scope will evolve and the decision implications of that evolution, particularly whether it may have catastrophic consequences).

The projection aspect of situational awareness, sometimes overlooked in other definitions, is crucial in the biological context, because of the high degree of uncertainty and instability as the event unfolds over a period of time, which is not necessarily encountered in more discrete disaster events. (GAO, 2010, p. 13)

Thus, at least in broad terms, the application of the Endsley model to biosurveillance problems seems clear. Perception is detection of an event. Comprehension is understanding the event, both in terms of type and scope, as well as the availability of resources to intervene. And projection is being able to extrapolate what will happen in the near future in terms of how the situation is likely to evolve. Note that, according to this definition, early event detection (EED) is actually part of SA.

Bolstad *et al.* (2011, Fig. 4.2) also discuss the three levels of SA in terms of the broader biosurveillance problem, characterizing them in terms of answering questions:

- SA Level 1, perception: "Which information do I need?"
- SA Level 2, comprehension: "What does this mean to me?"
- SA Level 3, projection: "What do I think will happen?"

Following this approach, Figure 3.3 puts the three levels of SA in the context of the necessary data and statistical methods. SA level 1 is the acquisition of the necessary and appropriate data, which may include current and historical data on syndrome or case counts as well as other types of data from laboratories, 911 calls, over-the-counter (OTC) drug sales, and current population demographic and public health information.

Building on level 1, SA level 2 is the application of descriptive and summary statistics and plots to the raw data to facilitate an understanding of the data. At this level, the goal is to turn the raw data into information that helps a decision maker understand what the current state of affairs is, both in terms of historical norms and whether, how much, and where the existing situation deviates from those norms. Thus, SA level 2 involves the use of maps and plots to display the expected and observed status of the population, including expected disease or syndrome counts or rates for time of year and location and the deviation of the observed data from what would be expected.

Finally, SA level 3 requires the use of statistical models and forecasts to provide a spatio-temporal projection of disease spread and severity along with forecasts of morbidity and mortality given particular assumptions and interventions. In addition to forecasting the disease, other types of forecasts may be required, such as the projected level or amount of resources available to respond to the event(s).

3.4 Extending the Situational Awareness Model: Situated Cognition

Endsley's model is focused on the decision maker and, as presented in Figures 3.1 and 3.2, implicitly assumes that the decision maker has the necessary, correct, and

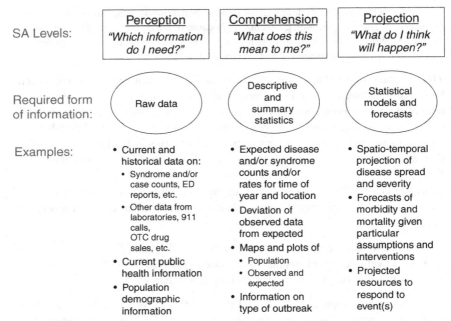

SA Levels:	Perception *"Which information do I need?"*	Comprehension *"What does this mean to me?"*	Projection *"What do I think will happen?"*
Required form of information:	Raw data	Descriptive and summary statistics	Statistical models and forecasts
Examples:	• Current and historical data on: • Syndrome and/or case counts, ED reports, etc. • Other data from laboratories, 911 calls, OTC drug sales, etc. • Current public health information • Population demographic information	• Expected disease and/or syndrome counts and/or rates for time of year and location • Deviation of observed data from expected • Maps and plots of • Population • Observed and expected • Information on type of outbreak	• Spatio-temporal projection of disease spread and severity • Forecasts of morbidity and mortality given particular assumptions and interventions • Projected resources to respond to event(s)

Figure 3.3. The three levels of SA each depend on specific types of data and statistical methods for their information requirements. Level 1, perception, depends on the collection of the correct raw data. Level 2, comprehension, depends on appropriately summarizing the raw data via descriptive and summary statistics. And, level 3, projection, depends on having good statistical models and forecasting methods to project what is likely to happen in the near future. (Adapted from Kass-Hout & Zhang, 2011, Fig. 4.2)

appropriate data available from which to make decisions. It also does not seem to address the issue that different decision makers may reach different decisions based on their particular situation. Shattuck and Miller's situated cognition model incorporates these real-world SA considerations.

In terms of data, for example, the decision maker can only have a subset of all possible data in the environment, and thus it is important to recognize that a decision maker's mental model of the situation will be both limited by unavailable data and shaped by the available data. This includes how the data are parsed and presented and how then are interpreted by the decision maker. This is an important consideration when designing and operating a biosurveillance system because design and operation directly affect the information available to the decision maker.

As Shattuck and Miller (2006) discuss, one issue is how technology and system design either enhances or degrades information. As shown in Figure 3.4, at the far left (1) are all the data that are available in the environment. Of all these data, not all of it is "detected" in (2), which could mean that it is literally not detected, as in an individual who is sick but only self-medicates and so is not visible to the public health system, or perhaps the biosurveillance system's coverage of the

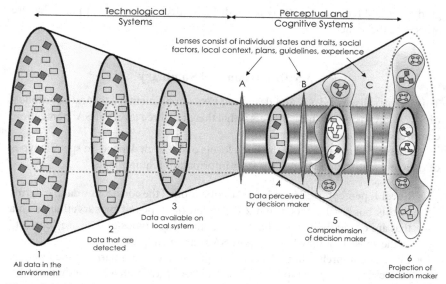

Figure 3.4. Situational awareness depends not only on how a human being interprets data but also on what data are actually available to be interpreted. The dynamic model of situated cognition illustrates that the way data are handled in and filtered through technological systems affects SA. (Source: Shattuck & Miller, 2006, Fig. 1)

population is incomplete either because some providers are not providing data or perhaps that some types of data are not in a convenient electronic form and thus not able to be captured in a biosurveillance database. Whatever the reason, not all of the data that exist in the environment will be available or in a form that it useful for the biosurveillance system.

Now, of all the data that are detected, only a subset will be available or visible on the local biosurveillance system in (3). For example, choices in how the data are filtered in the system; how the data are processed, including the choice of EED algorithms; and how the data are displayed (e.g., the types of maps and plots available) may reduce the data that can be locally displayed. In addition, depending on the system structure, it may limit access to the raw data, perhaps for privacy reasons, or the ability to sort or conduct *ad hoc* analyses. Thus again, perhaps for a variety of reasons, the data available to the decision maker are reduced from all that exists in the environment.

It should thus be clear that in the real world, system design has the potential to dramatically affect biosurveillance effectiveness. However, decisions are affected by more than system design. In Figure 3.4, Shattuck and Miller (2006) use a lens metaphor to illustrate the decision maker's perception, comprehension, and projection (the three SA levels) are shaped by his or her personal experience as well as the local context and response plans and guidelines. Shattuck and Miller refer to these as the "perceptual and cognitive systems." Simply stated, different people with different types of experience or operating in an environment with different guidelines and requirements may reach different decisions even with data that are otherwise the same.

3.5 Discussion and Summary

This chapter discussed SA and described two complementary theoretical models of SA. A key insight of these models is that there are three levels of SA: perception, comprehension, and projection.

As described in Figure 3.3, the three levels of SA each depend on specific types of data and statistical methods for their information requirements:

- Level 1, perception, depends on the collection of the correct raw data. In terms of this book, Chapters 1 and 2 described the types of biosurveillance data that are currently being collected. Whether these types of data are "correct" in the sense that they best support SA is an open question.
- Level 2, comprehension, depends on appropriately summarizing the raw data via descriptive and summary statistics. Descriptive statistical methods useful for situational comprehension will be discussed in Chapter 4.
- Level 3, projection, depends on having good statistical models and forecasting methods to project what is likely to happen in the near future, which will be developed in Chapter 5.

The GAO defines biosurveillance SA as "information that signals an event might be occurring, information about what those signals mean, and information about how events will likely unfold in the near future" (GAO, 2010, p. 6). Although these three steps follow Endsley's model, clearly biosurveillance is more than just an event-focused activity. Event (i.e., outbreak) detection and tracking is one of the main goals of biosurveillance, but one cannot judge whether an event might be occurring unless one also has SA of the biosphere *prior to the event*. As Rolka *et al.* (2008, p. 2) say,

> Public health situation awareness is needed by public health leaders in three different types of settings that can occur simultaneously or in sequence: 1) pre-event/threat situations where a wide range of public health events and threats are assessed, 2) emergency response situation awareness in which detailed assessments of a specific event or threat and the public health responses to that threat are monitored, and 3) recovery operations during which the on-going mitigation and preventive efforts to a specific event or threat are monitored.

Compared with EED, some argue that SA is the more important function because it is something a biosurveillance system needs to continuously support. That is, as just described, it is important to maintain SA of the biosphere whether an outbreak is present or not, but EED is only necessary given an outbreak. However, as described in this chapter, EED is actually a part of level 1 SA, and thus the two cannot be separated.

Some have also argued that EED is more effectively performed by individual medical professionals during the treatment of patients rather than by a statistical algorithm, but SA is inherently better performed by aggregating information across doctors and hospitals, hence within some sort of biosurveillance system. Given that this is a book about statistical methods in support of biosurveillance, statistical methods for EED are developed in Chapters 6–8. However, even before discussing the statistical methods for EED, it should be clear that one approach does not rule out the other, so some appropriate combination of the two approaches is to be preferred over just one or the other.

Although not the focus of this book, one thing this chapter should have brought to mind is that biosurveillance system design is critical to acquiring and maintaining SA, particularly in the midst of a major outbreak. Unfortunately, to date it appears that system designs have been driven more by technology and the convenient availability of certain types of data than by deliberate design in support of biosurveillance SA. As Toner (2009) says,

> While these surveillance efforts undoubtedly provide information flows that did not exist before, it is not clear to what extent they have enabled a more robust understanding of a rapidly unfolding event. How do, or how can, these diverse systems, programs, and centers work together to provide an integrated picture? Can decision makers use these systems effectively to direct action in a crisis? Do these systems provide the necessary information in real time? It seems overall that there has been much more emphasis placed on systems to detect outbreaks rather than on systems to manage outbreaks. It appears that there is a lot of technology, but relatively little science. Systems exist without a clear concept of operation. (p. 3)

However, the beginnings of change are appearing; SA in the context of system design is starting to be discussed in the literature. See, for example, Bolstad *et al.* (2011) and Toner (2009). However, compared with fields such as aviation, the discussion has barely begun. Furthermore, discussion is not sufficient. Those public health organizations operating biosurveillance systems need to sponsor studies of whether and how the systems support SA and facilitate system improvements to enhance their SA functionality.

Additional Reading

Although SA is one of the two main foci for biosurveillance systems, surprisingly little has been written about SA in a biosurveillance context. For those who would like to delve more deeply into the material presented in this chapter, consider:

- For more information about Endsley's theoretical model, see the original paper, *Toward a Theory of Situation Awareness in Dynamic Systems* (Endsley, 1995) as well as *Situation Awareness: Analysis and Measurement* (Endsley & Garland, 2000). For a more in-depth discussion of the situated cognition model, see Shattuck and Miller's original paper, *Extending Naturalistic*

Decision Making to Complex Organizations: A Dynamic Model of Situated Cognition (Shattuck & Miller, 2006).

- Returning to the issue of designing biosurveillance systems to support SA, Chapter 4 of *Biosurveillance: Methods and Case Studies* (Bolstad *et al.*, 2011) describes a notional process for conducting SA requirements analyses. The process uses goal-directed task analysis to identify a system's major goals and then to delineate the dynamic information requirements to support each of the goals.

Bolstad *et al.* (2011) also summarize a series of SA-oriented design principles that should be applied to the design of biosurveillance systems. See also *Designing for Situation Awareness: An Approach for Human-Centered Design* (Endsley *et al.*, 2003) and *Designing for Situation Awareness in Complex Systems* (Endsley, 2001) for more detail.

4

Descriptive Statistics for Comprehending the Situation

... while the individual man is an insoluble puzzle, in the aggregate he becomes a mathematical certainty. You can, for example, never foretell what any one man will do, but you can say with precision what an average number will be up to. Individuals vary, but percentages remain constant. So says the statistician.

Sherlock Holmes in *The Sign of Four* (Sir Arthur Conan Doyle, 1890)

The purpose of summary statistics is to take a mass of raw data and condense it in some useful manner. With biosurveillance, the goal is to facilitate an understanding of some aspect of the biosphere. In terms of situational awareness (SA), biosurveillance systems must summarize the data in ways that facilitate an understanding of historical trends, the current state, and how the current state compares with historical trends. That is, as the chapter title says, they must effectively display the situation for the decision maker.

Whereas medical practitioners operate at the individual datum level, meaning they see the biosphere one patient at a time, the point of biosurveillance is aggregation of data in order to see events that may not be evident at the individual level. In terms of early event detection (EED), both views are necessary for effective biosurveillance because some types of events are best detected on a case-by-case basis by individual medical practitioners, and other types of events are best detected in the aggregate.

This chapter focuses on statistical tools and methods useful for the perception and comprehension steps of SA. In statistical terms, they would be described as descriptive statistics and exploratory data analysis. Descriptive statistics are first presented in terms of various types of numerical summary statistics followed by types of plots for graphically displaying the data. Exploratory data analysis (EDA) is an interactive approach to exploring and analyzing data, often using the summary statistics just described. The purpose is to explore the data with the purpose of generating insights and hypotheses.

Chapter Objectives

Upon completion of this chapter, the reader should be able to:

- Define and calculate numerical descriptive statistics for cross-sectional data, including the following:
    - Measures of central tendency: mean, trimmed mean, median, and mode
    - Measures of variation: variance, standard deviation, standard error, covariance, and correlation
    - Other summary statistics: percentile, quantile, quartile, interquartile range, range, and mode
- Define and calculate numerical descriptive statistics for longitudinal data, including repeated cross-sectional statistics, statistics based on moving windows of data and the moving average, and autocorrelation.
- Identify and interpret graphical descriptive statistics for cross-sectional data, including bar charts, histograms, lattice plots, box plots, and scatterplots and scatterplot matrices.
- Identify and interpret graphical descriptive statistics for longitudinal data, including time series plots, repeated cross-sectional plots, and lattice plots conditioned on time.
- Identify and interpret graphical descriptive statistics for spatial and spatio-temporal data, including maps applied to cross-sectional data and repeated with longitudinal data.
- Define EDA, discuss how a biosurveillance system should support EDA, and why effective interface design and data display is important for effective SA.

Mathematical Notation

$\mathrm{cov}(x, y)$	Sample covariance for variables x and y
i, j	Indices for either time or the observations
k	Lag
n	Sample size
N	Population size
r	Sample correlation
r_k	Sample autocorrelation for lag k
R	Range
s	Sample standard deviation
s^2	Sample variance
$\mathrm{s.e.}(\bar{y})$	Standard error of the sample mean
$\widehat{\mathrm{s.e.}(\bar{y})}$	Estimated standard error of the sample mean
$\widehat{\mathrm{s.e.}(\tilde{y})}$	Estimated standard error of the median
$\widehat{\mathrm{s.e.}(s)}$	Estimated standard error of the sample standard deviation
y	An observation
t	Time index
$y_{(i)}$	ith ordered observation
$\bar{y}$	Sample mean
$\bar{y}_t$	Moving average at time t
$\bar{y}_{tr(p)}$	$100p$ percent trimmed mean
$\tilde{y}$	Median
$\tilde{y}_t$	Moving median at time t
μ	Population mean
σ	Population standard deviation
σ^2	Population variance

4.1 Numerical Descriptive Statistics

Numerical descriptive statistics, as should be clear from the name, describe or summarize a set of data in terms of numbers – statistics calculated from the data. Typically, the goal is to efficiently summarize a set of data, which is often in terms of where the data are located and how variable they are using statistics such as the average and standard deviation. However, depending on what one is interested in learning about the data, these two statistics may or may not be the most appropriate or effective.

In particular, because biosurveillance data are typically longitudinal and trends over time are often of interest, simple cross-sectional statistics may be insufficient. Hence, this section is divided into two parts, starting with numerical descriptive statistics that are typically used on cross-sectional data. It then proceeds on to how those statistics can be applied to longitudinal data, as well as numerical descriptive statistics defined explicitly for longitudinal data.

4.1.1 Descriptive Statistics for Cross-sectional Data

As discussed in Chapter 2 (see page 26), cross-sectional data are collected on subjects (e.g., individuals, hospitals, or regions) at the same point of time. Statistics may then be used to summarize these data, with the intention of reducing the mass of data into a few numbers that usefully provide information about the situation at a particular point in time.

4.1.1.1 Measures of Central Tendency

Measures of central tendency or *measures of location* are typically used to quantify where the "center" of the data is located. The word "center" is in quotes because there are a number of common measures of central tendency, each of which quantifies the "center" in a different way. The most common measure is the *mean*, which is the average of a set of observations in either a sample or a population. That is, the mean is the sum of the observations divided by the total number of items in the sample or population.

Mathematically, for data from an entire population of size N, where each observation is denoted y_i and $i = 1, 2, 3 \ldots, N$, the *population mean* μ is

$$\mu = \frac{1}{N} \sum_{i=1}^{N} y_i. \tag{4.1}$$

For data from a sample of size n, the *sample mean* $\bar{y}$ is

$$\bar{y} = \frac{1}{n} \sum_{i=1}^{n} y_i. \tag{4.2}$$

Note that the calculation is really the same. The difference is simply a matter of what is being averaged: the entire population or some subset (i.e., sample) of the population. In terms of the notation, a capital letter N is typically used to indicate the number of observations in a population, and the small letter n denotes the number of observations in a sample down from the population. In a similar way, the population mean is denoted by the Greek letter μ, and the sample mean is denoted by $\bar{y}$. Often μ is unobserved and the sample mean $\bar{y}$ is used to estimate the population mean. Also note that the mean does not have to be one of the observed data points and, in fact, it need not even be close to any particular observed value.

A common alternative to the mean as a measure of central tendency is the median. For a sample of data, the median, denoted $\tilde{y}$, is the observation that divides the sample in half. For an odd number of observations, it is literally the value of the middle observation of the *ordered* data. For an even number of observations, it is the average of the middle two points of the ordered data.

To define the median mathematically, let $y_{(i)}$ denote the ith ordered observation (which is also sometimes referred to as the ith order statistic). Using this notation, then the sample median is

$$\tilde{y} = \begin{cases} y_{(\frac{n+1}{2})}, & \text{if } n \text{ is odd} \\ \left[y_{(\frac{n}{2})} + y_{(\frac{n}{2}+1)} \right] \big/ 2, & \text{if } n \text{ is even.} \end{cases} \qquad (4.3)$$

With n replaced by N, the calculation for the population median is the same as the sample median.

Although both the median and the mean are measures of central tendency, they are distinctly different. In particular, when the data contain one or more *outliers*, meaning data points that are unusually large or small compared with the rest of the data, the median is sometimes preferred to the mean. This is because the median is less affected by the outliers.

To illustrate, consider a sample of the following seven ordered observations: $\{0, 1, 2, 2, 2, 3, 4\}$. These might be, for example, daily influenza-like illness (ILI) counts at a small community hospital for one week. Here the mean equals the median, which equals 2. When data are symmetric about the mean, as with the data in this simple example, the mean is equal to the mean. But what if by accident a typo resulted in the first entry being 70, so that the observed ordered observations became $\{1, 2, 2, 2, 3, 4, 70\}$? Even with the typo, the median remains unchanged at 2, but the mean becomes 12 – clearly a big difference for a change in one data point.

In addition, the use of the mean as a measure of central tendency in the second case with the typo outlier should seem a bit dubious because the resulting sample average of 12 is larger than all but one of the observations. In contrast, the median is the same regardless of whether the last observation is 4, 70, or 1,000,000. Whenever data are very *skewed*, either in the direction of one or more significantly larger or smaller observations, then the median may be preferred as the measure of central tendency.

The point is that the median is *robust* with respect to outliers, meaning that it is generally not affected much by their presence, but the mean can be very sensitive to one or more outliers. Thus, if the data are likely to contain large or small values atypical of most of the data, then the median may be the preferred measure of central tendency. Similarly, if by the term "central tendency" one means a typical value in the middle of the data, then it often makes sense to use the median. If, on the other hand, what is of interest is the average value in the data, then the mean is the appropriate measure.

Example 4.1. Using the clinic data introduced in Chapter 2 (see page 30), describe the typical age of a patient presenting for the month of January.

Solution: In January, 13,223 individuals presented at the clinics. The mean age was $\bar{y} = 23.8$ years, and the median age was $\tilde{y} = 23$ years. Thus, the average patient was almost 24 years old, but roughly half of those presenting were younger than 23 years and half were older than 23 years.

Note that the mean and median for these data are quite close, but the mean is greater than the median. This occurs because there are some ages quite a bit larger than the median, but ages cannot be less than 0, so the data are moderately skewed toward older ages, resulting in the mean being larger than the median. However, the difference between the two is modest; thus, in this case, it matters little which is used to describe the location of the data.

The *trimmed mean* is another measure of central tendency that can be a useful compromise between the mean and the median. For $0 \le p \le 0.5$, the $100p$ percent trimmed mean is calculated by first discarding the $100p$ percent largest and smallest observations in the data and then averaging the remaining observations.

Mathematically, let $y_{(1)} \le y_{(2)} \le \ldots \le y_{(n)}$ be the order statistics of n observations. Then the trimmed mean $\bar{y}_{tr(p)}$ is defined as

$$\bar{y}_{tr(p)} = \frac{1}{n - 2m} \sum_{i=m+1}^{n-m} y_{(i)}, \tag{4.4}$$

where $m = p \times n$. If $p \times m$ is not an integer, simply round it down to the nearest integer.

Note that the $100p$ percent trimmed mean actually deletes $2 \times 100p$ percent of the data. Also note that $\bar{y}_{tr(0)} \equiv \bar{y}$ and $\bar{y}_{tr(0.5)} \equiv \tilde{y}$, but for any other value of $0 < p < 0.5$, there is no guarantee that the trimmed mean will be between the mean and median.

Example 4.2. Calculate the 20 percent trimmed mean for the previous community hospital example data, both with and without the typo, and then for the clinic data of Example 4.1.

Solution: First, for the community hospital example, $n = 7$. With $p = 0.2$, $0.2 \times 7 = 1.4$, so $m = 1$. Thus, the original set of ordered data

$\{0, 1, 2, 2, 2, 3, 4\}$ is trimmed to $\{1, 2, 2, 2, 3\}$. So

$$\bar{y}_{tr(0.2)} = \frac{1+2+2+2+3}{5} = 10/5 = 2.0 \text{ patients/day.}$$

In a similar way, the ordered data with the typo $\{1, 2, 2, 2, 3, 4, 70\}$ is trimmed to $\{2, 2, 2, 3, 4\}$. Thus,

$$\bar{y}_{tr(0.2)} = \frac{2+2+2+3+4}{5} = 13/5 = 2.6 \text{ patients/day,}$$

which, although somewhat larger than $\tilde{y} = 2$, is not nearly as large as $\bar{y} = 12$.

Now, for the clinic data $0.2 \times 13,223 = 2,644.4$, so $m = 2,644$. From the data, then,

$$\bar{y}_{tr(0.2)} = \frac{1}{7,935} \sum_{i=2,645}^{10,579} y_{(i)} = 20.6 \text{ years.}$$

This is an example in which the trimmed mean turns out to be smaller than both the mean (23.8 years) and the median (23 years).

Note that the mean, median, and trimmed mean are all appropriate to use with either continuous or discrete data. For example, imagine some discrete data composed of the number of children in a sample of families. Although it does not make sense to say that any particular family has $2\frac{1}{2}$ children, it is perfectly fine to say that the average number of children per family is 2.5. However, when data are nominal, none of these measures work. For nominal data, the *mode*, which is the data category with the largest number of observations, is the appropriate measure.

Example 4.3. Using the clinic data, summarize the patients who presented in January in terms of race and ethnicity.

Solution: The most complete way to summarize the data is in a table, as in Table 4.1. As it shows, Hispanic is the modal ethnicity, comprising 82.9 percent (10,963 of 13,223) of those presenting for whom ethnicity was recorded. Similarly, the modal race is white, comprising 80.6 percent (10,653 of 13,223) of those presenting, again for those for whom race was recorded. And white Hispanics are the modal race-ethnic category, comprising 72.3 percent (9,560 of 13,223) of those presenting.

Thus far, the discussion has focused on calculating means and medians for cross-sectional data from one population. However, rate-based information is often important in public health surveillance, particularly when the population of interest is changing, either in terms of size or composition, or when comparing between two or more disparate populations. Thus, rather than simply comparing the number

Table 4.1. Counts for the clinic data by race and ethnicity for
January 2009

	Ethnicity			
Race	Hispanic	Non-Hispanic	Unknown	*Total*
Asian	11	402	15	428
Black	212	294	2	508
Other	8	59	1	68
White	9,560	1,044	49	10,653
Unknown	1,172	235	159	1,566
Total	10,963	2,034	226	13,223

of people with a particular disease or syndrome, the appropriate comparison is the rate: the number of people with the disease or syndrome per some appropriate population unit (e.g., per 100,000 people).

There are various types of rates depending on the medically appropriate way to characterize the prevalence of a disease or event. A *crude rate* consists of a numerator, which is the total number of observed or estimated events, and a denominator, which is the total population at risk, multiplied by a useful population unit such as 100,000. This then gives the event rate in terms of the average number of events per 100,000 people in the population. There are also various adjusted rates. For example, because many health conditions are related to age, *age-adjusted rates* are often of interest. See Chapters 2.2 and 2.3 of Waller and Gotway (2004) for a more detailed discussion.

Details of calculating the various types of rates aside, the salient point here is that all of the descriptive statistics discussed thus far (and to follow in the rest of this chapter) are appropriate for use on, and can be useful for summarizing, rate data. The calculations are all the same. The difference is that the rates become the data and the resulting statistics are expressed in the units of the rate. Thus, for example, the mean of some rate data is simply the average rate, and the median of the rate data is the median rate.

4.1.1.2 Measures of Variation

When describing or summarizing a set of data, providing measures of both location and variation is important. That is, although the mean or median provides information about the average or typical observation in the data, it does not give any information about how the rest of the data are dispersed around that location. But often knowledge about whether the rest of the data tend to be near or far from the center of the data is important. Section 4.2 presents graphical means that allow one to visually assess variation in data. This section presents useful numerical summary measures of variation.

The most common measure is the sample standard deviation. It is based on the *sample variance*, s^2, which is defined as

$$s^2 = \frac{1}{n-1} \sum_{i=1}^{n} (y_i - \bar{y})^2 \tag{4.5}$$

The formula for the sample variance in Equation 4.6 is a bit more complicated than for the sample mean in Equation 4.2. Starting within the parenthesis, the formula says to take the difference between each observation in the sample and the sample mean, square the differences, sum them up, and then divide the sum by $n - 1$.

The sample variance is basically the average squared distance of the observations from the mean. The larger the sample variance, the more the observations are spread out around the mean. The smaller the sample variance, the tighter they are around the sample mean.

The calculation for the population variance, σ^2, is slightly different from the sample variance in that the population mean replaces the sample mean in the formula and the sum of the squared differences is divided by N, not $n - 1$:

$$\sigma^2 = \frac{1}{N} \sum_{i=1}^{N} (y_i - \mu)^2 \tag{4.6}$$

For both the sample and population calculations, the standard deviation is simply the square root of the variance. So, for a sample, it is $s = \sqrt{s^2}$, and for the population, it is $\sigma = \sqrt{\sigma^2}$. Typically, the standard deviation is used to characterize variation because it is in the same units as the mean. So, returning to the example of summarizing the number of children per family, if the mean is in units of the number of children per family, then so is the standard deviation.

The *range*, R, is another measure of variation. The range has the advantage that it is easy to calculate because it is just the difference between the largest and smallest observations. Using the order statistic notation, the range for a sample is $R = y_{(n)} - y_{(1)}$, and for a population, it is $R = y_{(N)} - y_{(1)}$.

Example 4.4. Returning to the clinic age data, summarize the variation in ages of those presenting for the month of January.

Solution: In January, the standard deviation of age for those presenting was $s = 20.7$ years. The standard deviation is so large because there was a wide variety of ages, from the minimum of $y_{(1)} = 0$ years (where 0 years denotes a child younger than 1 year) to a maximum of $y_{(13,223)} = 95$ years. Thus, $R = 95 - 0 = 95$ years.

Another important measure of variation is the *standard error*, which is the standard deviation of a sample statistic. It is a measure of how variable the statistic itself is (compared with the standard deviation, for example, which is a measure of the variability of the data). The idea is that different samples from the population result in different data and thus different sample statistics. It is frequently important to know how much a statistic could vary from sample to sample.

Of course, population statistics have zero standard error because the population mean μ and standard deviation σ are fixed quantities.

Typically, the standard error of the sample mean is of most interest. For a sample of size n, if the population standard deviation σ is known, then the standard error of the sample mean is

$$\text{s.e.}(\bar{y}) = \frac{\sigma}{\sqrt{n}}. \tag{4.7}$$

However, it is frequently the case that the population standard deviation is not known. In this case, the standard error is estimated by "plugging in" the sample standard deviation in place of the population standard deviation:

$$\widehat{\text{s.e.}(\bar{y})} = \frac{s}{\sqrt{n}}. \tag{4.8}$$

Assuming that the data are normally distributed and the sample size is reasonably large ($n \geq 30$), then the estimated standard errors of the median and the sample standard deviation are approximately

$$\widehat{\text{s.e.}(\bar{y})} = 1.25 \frac{s}{\sqrt{n}} \tag{4.9}$$

and

$$\widehat{\text{s.e.}(s)} = 0.71 \frac{s}{\sqrt{n}}. \tag{4.10}$$

Equation 4.10 may seem strange in the sense that it is calculating a measure of variation (the standard error) of a measure of variation (the standard deviation). However, note that s is a sample statistic and, similar to all other sample statistics, will vary from sample to sample. Thus, while s is a measure of the variation in the data, the standard error of s is a measure of the variation of the statistic.

Now, if the assumption that the data is normally distributed does not hold, then it is incorrect to use Equations 4.9 and 4.10. Although beyond the scope of this book, an alternative is a computationally intensive methodology called the bootstrap that avoids having to make any distributional assumptions.

4.1.1.3 Other Numerical Summary Statistics

There are other useful summary statistics in addition to measures of location and variation. One is the *percentile*. The pth percentile is the value of an observation in the data such that p percent of the data is less than or equal to that value. For a given observation, the information communicated by its percentile is where that observation ranks with respect to the rest of the data. That is, it specifies how much of the rest of the data is less than or equal to that observation.

A standardized testing example will make the idea more concrete. If a person scores 720 on the SAT, the 720 score is only somewhat informative because it provides no information about where that places the person among the rest of those who took the test. But if it turns out that a score of 720 corresponds to the 96th percentile, then it is now clear what the score means: 96 percent of the other test takers scored 720 or less or, conversely, only 4 percent of the test takers did better.

There are some special percentiles. The 100th percentile is the largest (maximum) observation in the data. The median is the 50th percentile.[1] Finally, the 0th percentile is defined to be the smallest (minimum) observation, and thus the range is equal to the 100th percentile minus the 0th percentile.

Quantiles are often used in the statistical literature instead of percentiles. Quantiles are simply percentiles divided by 100. That is, whereas percentiles are on a scale of 0 to 100 (percent), quantiles are on a scale from 0 to 1. Those quantiles that divide the data into fourths are called *quartiles*, where the first quartile is the same as the 25th percentile or the 0.25 quantile. The second quartile is the median, and the third quartile is the same as the 75th percentile or the 0.75 quantile. The *interquartile range* or IQR is defined as the 75th percentile minus the 25th percentile.

Example 4.5. Returning to the clinic age data, further summarize the distribution of ages of those presenting for the month of January.

Solution: The ages varied from the 0th percentile of 0 years to the 100th percentile of 95 years. The 25th percentile (first quartile) of the data is 4 years, and the 75th percentile (third quartile) is 34 years, so 50 percent of the patients are between those two ages. A first quartile of 4 years also means that fully one-quarter of the clinic patients are babies and very young children. What fraction are older patients, say, 65 years or older? For January, 64 years was the 94.2 percentile, so 5.8 percent of the patients were 65 years or older.

4.1.1.4 Measures of How Two Variables Co-vary

When looking at a data set with more than one variable, it is often natural to ask whether they seem to be related in some way. For two variables x and y, one such measure is the *sample covariance*, denoted by $\text{cov}(x, y)$ and defined as

$$\text{cov}(x, y) = \frac{1}{n-1} \sum_{i=1}^{n} (x_i - \bar{x})(y_i - \bar{y}). \qquad (4.11)$$

Covariance is a measure of how two variables *co-vary* about their means. Note that the data come in pairs, a pair consisting of one x observation and one y

---

[1] Per Equation 4.3, this is precisely true when n is even, and it is approximately true when n is odd. However, for an odd number of observations, as n gets larger, the fraction of observations less than or equal to the median approaches 50 percent.

observation. In Equation 4.11, each pair is indexed from 1 to n. So, x_1 goes with y_1, x_2 goes with y_2, on up to x_n with y_n. The equation, then, calculates the average of the product of the differences between each x in the pair from the mean of the xs and each y in the pair from the mean of the ys.

Covariance is a measure of both the strength and direction of the *linear* relationship between x and y. If the covariance is a large number (either positive or negative), then the strength of linear association is large; if the covariance is near zero, then the strength of linear association is weak or nonexistent. Similarly, if the sign of the covariance is positive, then the association is positive (meaning that the xs tend to vary in the same direction as the ys); if the sign is negative, then the association is negative (meaning that the xs tend to vary in the opposite direction as the ys).

The difficulty is determining when to call a covariance "large" because the covariance depends on how the observation is measured. That is, changing the measurement units changes the value of the computed covariance. This is troublesome because changing the measurement units (inches instead of feet; grams instead of kilograms) does not change the association between the x and y. And if the association is the same, the numerical measure describing that association should be the same.

The *sample correlation* solves this problem. Sample correlation is the sample covariance divided by the standard deviation of the x values and the standard deviation of the y values. Denoted by r, the sample correlation is thus

$$r = \frac{\text{cov}(x, y)}{s_x \times s_y} = \frac{\sum_1^n (x_i - \bar{x})(y_i - \bar{y})}{\sqrt{\sum_1^n (x_i - \bar{x})^2}\sqrt{\sum_1^n (y_i - \bar{y})^2}}. \tag{4.12}$$

Dividing by the standard deviations of x and y makes the correlation independent of the measurement scale, so that the correlation is always between -1 and 1. That makes interpretation much easier. A correlation near 1 is a strong positive linear association, and a correlation near -1 is a strong negative linear association, where a correlation of either $+1$ or -1 is a perfect linear relationship. And, a correlation of 0 means that there is no linear association between x and y.

The words "association" and "linear" are used purposely in this explanation. It is possible for two variables to be related in a non-linear fashion yet have zero correlation. So, observing a correlation of 0 does not mean there is no association between two variables, only that there is no linear relationship. Also, a non-zero correlation does not mean there is a causal relationship between the variables. The correlation between the two variables can occur for reasons not associated with direct causality, so in the absence of other information, the most that can be said if a non-zero correlation is observed is that there is an association between the variables.

Table 4.2. Gastrointestinal syndrome daily count correlation matrix for the seven metropolitan hospitals

Correlation (r)	Hospital #1	Hospital #2	Hospital #3	Hospital #4	Hospital #5	Hospital #6	Hospital #7
Hospital #1	1.00	0.14	0.13	0.21	0.19	0.14	0.16
Hospital #2		1.00	0.00	0.08	0.07	0.08	0.05
Hospital #3			1.00	0.11	0.19	0.11	0.15
Hospital #4				1.00	0.09	0.12	0.13
Hospital #5					1.00	0.10	0.14
Hospital #6						1.00	0.28
Hospital #7							1.00

Example 4.6. Using the hospital data introduced in Chapter 2 (see page 34), assess the correlation between each pair of hospitals for daily counts of those presenting with gastrointestinal (GI) and respiratory syndromes.

Solution: As shown in Table 4.2, the GI syndrome data are weakly positively correlated across the hospitals.

Note that because $cov(x, y) = cov(y, x)$, there is no need to fill in the lower left part of the table because it would be duplicative of the upper right. Also, the diagonal contains all ones because each hospital's syndrome is perfectly correlated with itself. This should also be clear from Equation 4.12, where if all the ys are changed to xs, then the numerator and the denominator are the same and thus the ratio is 1.

Table 4.3 shows that the correlations are somewhat stronger for the respiratory syndrome compared with GI. However, although both sets of correlations are weak, the syndromes are clearly correlated across the hospitals, and this makes sense because the hospitals are all from the same geographic area.

Table 4.3. Respiratory syndrome daily count correlation matrix for the seven metropolitan hospitals

Correlation (r)	Hospital #1	Hospital #2	Hospital #3	Hospital #4	Hospital #5	Hospital #6	Hospital #7
Hospital #1	1.00	0.11	0.20	0.27	0.24	0.21	0.20
Hospital #2		1.00	0.14	0.12	0.12	0.07	0.08
Hospital #3			1.00	0.16	0.20	0.21	0.23
Hospital #4				1.00	0.18	0.10	0.15
Hospital #5					1.00	0.15	0.13
Hospital #6						1.00	0.19
Hospital #7							1.00

Table 4.4. Monthly summary statistics for GI syndrome using the clinic data

Statistic	Aug	Sep	Oct	Nov	Dec	Jan	Feb	Mar	Apr	May	Jun	Jul
Maximum ($y_{(n)}$)	9.0	11.0	10.0	10.0	8.0	13.0	15.0	13.0	17.0	11.0	11.0	10.0
3rd Quartile	7.0	8.0	7.0	7.0	5.0	9.0	10.5	9.0	8.0	8.3	8.0	8.0
Mean ($\bar{y}$)	5.6	6.7	5.7	5.8	4.2	7.6	8.3	7.5	7.1	7.0	5.2	6.0
Std Deviation (s)	2.4	2.5	2.2	2.1	1.6	3.2	3.4	2.8	4.0	2.5	2.8	2.5
Median ($\tilde{y}$)	5.0	7.0	6.0	6.0	4.0	8.0	8.0	7.5	6.5	6.5	5.0	5.5
1st Quartile	4.0	5.0	3.5	4.0	3.0	5.0	6.5	6.3	4.3	5.8	3.0	4.3
Minimum ($y_{(0)}$)	0.0	3.0	2.0	1.0	1.0	0.0	2.0	2.0	1.0	3.0	0.0	2.0

4.1.2 Descriptive Statistics for Longitudinal Data

The previous location and variability measures can be applied to longitudinal data just as well as cross-sectional data. The only real difference is that when applied to longitudinal data, one is summarizing the data in terms of one or more statistics per time period. This should seem rather natural for biosurveillance because the goal is to monitor data for changes in disease incidence over time. Indeed, this is precisely what Figures 2.4 and 2.5 in Chapter 2 show, although the statistic plotted in those figures is simply the total number of patients presenting each day who were classified into a particular syndrome category.

Example 4.7. Assess the longitudinal trends in GI syndrome by calculating monthly summary statistics for the clinic data.

Solution: Table 4.4 gives the minimum, first quartile, median, standard deviation, mean, third quartile, and maximum monthly values for the GI syndrome data.

The table shows trends similar to those in Figure 2.4. In particular, the monthly mean is quite similar to the lowess line, with a mean of about six GI syndrome cases per day from August through November, then a slight dip in December, followed by elevated daily averages of seven to eight GI syndrome cases per day from January through May, after which the average drops back to an average of around six per day. All of the other statistics follow a similar pattern, showing increases from January to April or May, which is consistent with the winter flu season.

Thus, one approach to longitudinal data is the repeated calculation of summary statistics for separate subsets of data that correspond to different periods of time. As Example 4.7 shows, comparison of the statistics can usefully help discern trends and patterns in the data.

Although doing the calculations in Table 4.4 on a monthly basis is a bit crude, it hints at EED ideas that we will return to in later chapters, namely observing data over time with the objective of trying to determine as early as possible when a disease incidence shows an unusual increase. For example, the jump in the mean and median statistics from December or January is an indication that the flu season started sometime in that period.

Now, in addition to calculating statistics for repeated cross sections of data, there are methods specifically created for longitudinal data. Many of these come in the form of statistical models, and they are described in the next chapter. In terms of numerical descriptive statistics, the next two subsections focus on statistics calculated from moving "windows" of data and quantifying correlation over time.

4.1.2.1 Statistics from Moving Windows of Data

One issue with the Example 4.7 approach for summarizing longitudinal data, at least in terms of trying to detect changes, is that the statistic is only updated monthly. As a result, changes are only visible at the end of the month so that, for example, if a flu outbreak occurred in the first week of a month, it would not be visible for three or more weeks.

One solution to this is to decrease size of the temporal "window" over which the calculations are conducted. That is, instead of calculating the statistics each month, calculate them every two weeks or perhaps weekly or even daily. This will mitigate the reporting delay problem, but it does not eliminate it because there can still be a delay of up to the size of the temporal window, whatever that may be.

In addition, there is an inherent trade-off made between the size of the temporal window and the variability of the resulting statistics. Specifically, as the window size is decreased, so is the sample size, and as Equations 4.7 to 4.10 make clear, as n gets smaller, the standard errors get larger. Thus, the smaller the window, the more variable (i.e., the noisier) the statistics become.

Calculating the statistics using a moving window of the most recent n time periods is one way to address this problem. Now, rather than only calculating a statistic once every n time periods, the statistic is calculated every time period using the n most recent periods. For example, at time t, the *moving average* $\bar{y}_t$ is calculated as

$$\bar{y}_t = \frac{1}{n} \sum_{i=t-n+1}^{t} y_i, \qquad (4.13)$$

where in Equation 4.13 it is assumed there is only one observation per time period. For example, y_i may be the daily ILI syndrome count on day i, so $\bar{y}_t$ is the mean ILI syndrome count for the n days prior to and including day t. At each new time period, the average is recalculated only using the most recent n periods so that, for example, at time $t + 1$, the moving average $\bar{y}_{t+1}$ is calculated using observations $y_{t-n+2}, \ldots, y_{t+1}$.

If there is more than one observation per time period, then there are two options. First, the parameter n in Equation 4.13 can be redefined to be in terms of observations rather than time, and thus the moving average will be based on the most recent n observations. Alternatively, if there are m_i observations in time

Table 4.5. Moving average and standard deviation for GI syndrome using the March clinic data with $n = 10$

	3/2	3/3	3/4	3/5	3/6	3/9	3/10	3/11	3/12	3/13	3/16	3/17	$\cdots$
$\bar{y}$	7.1	7.6	7.8	8.2	7.6	7.6	7.8	8.2	8.5	8.3	9.0	8.8	$\cdots$
s	3.8	3.6	3.5	3.8	3.0	3.0	3.3	2.8	2.8	3.0	2.4	2.5	$\cdots$

	3/18	3/19	3/20	3/23	3/24	3/25	3/26	3/27	3/30	3/31
$\cdots$	8.4	7.9	7.5	7.4	7.0	6.5	6.1	6.4	6.2	6.5
$\cdots$	3.1	2.8	2.9	2.9	2.3	2.8	2.5	2.5	2.3	2.5

period i, calculate

$$\bar{y}_t = \left(\sum_{i=t-n+1}^{t} \sum_{j=1}^{m_i} y_{ij} \right) \Big/ \sum_{i=t-n+1}^{t} m_i, \qquad (4.14)$$

where y_{ij} is the jth observation in the ith time period.

The generalization of this idea to other statistics should be fairly obvious. For example, again assuming there is only one observation per time period, the moving median at time t, $\tilde{y}_t$, is calculated as

$$\tilde{y}_t = \begin{cases} y_{\left(\frac{n+1}{2}\right)}, & \text{if } n \text{ is odd} \\ \left[y_{\left(\frac{n}{2}\right)} + y_{\left(\frac{n}{2}+1\right)} \right] \Big/ 2, & \text{if } n \text{ is even,} \end{cases} \qquad (4.15)$$

which looks exactly like Equation 4.3. The difference is that the order statistics in Equation 4.15 are calculated from $y_{t-n+1}, \ldots, y_t$.

Example 4.8. Show how the moving average and standard deviation compare with the monthly statistics for March from Example 4.7.

Solution: From Table 4.4, the mean and standard deviation for March are $\bar{y} = 7.5$ and $s = 2.8$. Setting $n = 10$, so the immediate last two weeks of data are used in the calculation. Table 4.5 shows the GI syndrome moving average and standard deviation for March 2nd (March 1st was a weekend day) through the 31st.

Note how the moving averages in Table 4.5 show more subtle trends. For example, returning to Table 4.4, the monthly mean GI syndrome rate was down slightly in March from February (from an average of 8.3 per day to 7.5 per day), and the aggregation in that table gives the impression that the GI syndrome rate peaked in February. However, Table 4.5 shows that, in fact, the GI syndrome rate was still increasing though mid-March after which it dropped dramatically.

The choice of n is critical to the behavior of the moving average or any other statistic based on a moving window of data. Specifically, the larger n is, the smoother the statistics will be from time period to time period, which may help make trends in the data more visible by smoothing out the inherent variation in the data. However, the smoothness comes at the cost of adding inertia to the statistic because the larger n is, the more historical data are included in the statistic's calculation. Thus, with the choice n, there is an explicit trade-off to be made between the desired smoothness in the sequence of statistics and the responsiveness of the statistic to changes in the data.

Another consideration when choosing n is whether the data contain regular cycles or other periodicities. For example, Figure 2.9 in Chapter 2 shows that the hospital respiratory syndrome data have a day-of-the-week effect that occurs on a repeating seven-day cycle. In the presence of such cycles, it is important to choose n as a multiple of the cycle periodicity in order to mitigate its effects. Otherwise, the statistic will vary according to the cycle. In the case of the hospital respiratory syndrome data, that means choosing a value for n that is a multiple of 7.

Finally, the choice of a moving window using the past n time periods or observations is based on the presumption of prospective monitoring or analysis. A prospective analysis is one that only looks forward in time and, in such cases, the only data available are those that are prior to the current time period. However, with a retrospective analysis, in which one is looking back in time, the window can be centered around the time period of interest using data from both before and after it. For example, assuming n is odd, the moving average calculation in Equation 4.13 could be modified for a retrospective analysis as follows:

$$\bar{y}_t = \frac{1}{n} \sum_{i=t-\frac{n-1}{2}}^{t+\frac{n-1}{2}} y_i. \tag{4.16}$$

Retrospective analyses can be useful and appropriate, for example, when studying how a disease progressed through a population or when comparing how various biosurveillance early event detection algorithms would have performed on real, but historical, data. Of course, actual early event monitoring can only be conducted prospectively.

4.1.2.2 Autocorrelation

Autocorrelation is the correlation of a longitudinal data set with itself. Autocorrelation quantifies the similarity between longitudinal observations as a function of the time separation (or "lag") between them. For some lag k, $k = 1, 2, \ldots$, the sample autocorrelation function r_k is

$$r_k = \frac{\sum_{i=k+1}^{n} (y_i - \bar{y})(y_{i-k} - \bar{y})}{\sum_{i=1}^{n} (y_i - \bar{y})^2}, \tag{4.17}$$

where $\bar{y}$ is the sample mean taken over the entire sample. Perfect positive or negative autocorrelation at lag k occurs with $r_k = +1$ or $r_k = -1$; $r_k \approx 0$ indicates little to no autocorrelation for lag k.

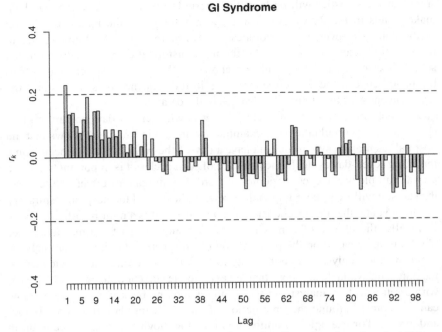

Figure 4.1. Correlogram for the clinic GI syndrome data for various lags, $1 \leq k \leq 100$.

A plot of r_k versus sequential values of k, called a *correlogram*, helps to show whether there are dependencies present in the data such as long-term linear or other trends, short- and/or long-term cycles, etc. Figures 4.1 and 4.2 are the correlograms for the clinic GI and ILI syndrome data for $1 \leq k \leq 100$.

As the plots show, overall the autocorrelation for the GI syndrome is less than that for the ILI syndrome, and both are relatively modest. The roughly linear decrease in r_k is indicative of long-term trends in the data (which are visible in the raw data, as shown in Figures 2.4 and 2.5). There is no evidence of weekly or monthly cycles in the data, which would have manifested as regular spikes at 5- or 20-day increments (because these clinics operate on a 5-day week).

4.2 Graphical Descriptive Statistics

In addition to numerical summaries of data (statistics), which can be very useful for condensing the information from a lot of data down into one or a few numbers, graphical summaries are important for visualizing data. Much like the old saying that "a picture is worth a thousand words," a good graph can be worth a thousand summary statistics.

Furthermore, properly designed graphics can effectively provide insight into large masses of data, and they can help reveal connections and relationships in the data that might otherwise be hard to detect. As John Tukey said, "The greatest

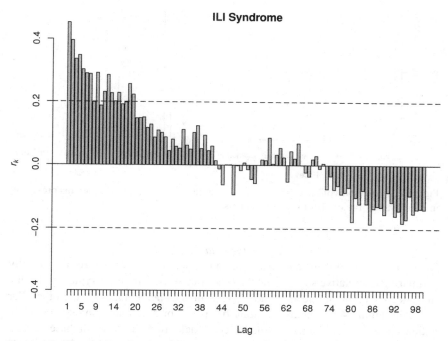

Figure 4.2. Correlogram for the clinic ILI syndrome data for various lags, $1 \leq k \leq 100$.

value of a picture is when it forces us to notice what we never expected to see" (Tukey, 1977).

This section examines graphics useful for summarizing categorical data, such as the bar chart, and graphics useful for continuous data, such as the histogram, the box plot, the scatterplot, and the time series plot. As with the numerical summary statistics, the graphics are presented in terms of their application to cross-sectional and longitudinal data, as well as a third category: spatial data.

Many types of statistical graphics, such as bar charts and scatterplots, are now familiar to the average reader. Not only are they fairly commonly used in the popular media, particularly the financial pages of many major newspapers, but ubiquitous software such as Microsoft Excel makes it easy to generate such plots. On the other hand, more specialized plots, such as box plots, histograms, and bubble charts, may be less familiar.

4.2.1 Graphical Methods for Cross-sectional Data

Section 4.1.1 introduced numerical descriptive statistics for cross-sectional data. The graphical methods presented in this section are useful complements, particularly for further summarizing and displaying cross-sectional data. Appropriately designed, implemented, and presented, these graphical methods give the user intuitive insights into the data that may not be achievable otherwise.

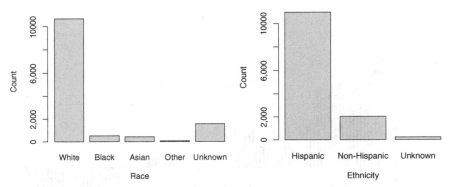

Figure 4.3. Examples of bar charts: Plots of race and ethnicity for clinic patients presenting in January. See Table 4.1 for the exact counts.

Bar Chart

Bar charts are useful for summarizing categorical data, particularly for visually comparing the relative sizes of the various categories. Bar charts typically display the category titles on one axis and either counts or percentages on the other. For example, Figure 4.3 contains separate bar plots for race and ethnicity for clinic patients presenting in January using the count data from Table 4.1. In these figures, the bars are plotted vertically, although they could just as well have been plotted horizontally. In fact, when the category names are long, it is often preferable to plot the bars horizontally so that the names can also be written out horizontally on the y-axis.

As shown in Figures 4.4 and 4.5, bar charts can also display subgroupings, either by breaking the bars up to show the constituent subgroups in a stacked bar chart or

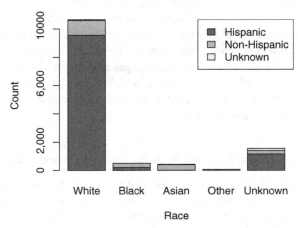

Figure 4.4. A stacked bar chart of ethnicity by race for clinic patients presenting in January for the data from Table 4.1.

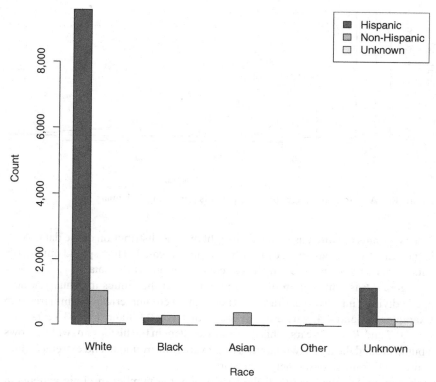

Figure 4.5. A side-by-side bar chart of ethnicity by race for clinic patients presenting in January for the data from Table 4.1.

by showing each main group as a set of bars in a side-by-side bar chart. Stacked bar charts facilitate comparing between the main groupings (race in the figures) while also allowing for comparison of the relative sizes of the subgroupings within each main group (ethnicity in the figures). In contrast, side-by-side bar charts allow direct comparison of the sizes of the subgroupings between the main groupings, but this comes at the cost of not being able to directly compare the sizes of the main groups.

Histogram

A histogram is akin to a bar chart but for continuous data. As just discussed, bar charts are for discrete data, and hence each bar in the chart corresponds to a distinct category in the data. In contrast, histograms are applied to continuous data by dividing the real line up into contiguous ranges (typically called "bins") for which the numbers of observations that fall into each bin are summed up. Then bars are plotted, where the height of each bar corresponds to the observed values that fall in the range of the bar.

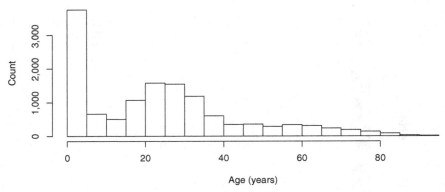

Figure 4.6. A histogram of age for clinic patients presenting in January.

Histograms are often used to gain insight into the distribution of the data. What is its shape? Where are most of the observations located? How spread out are the data? Are there any unusual outliers or concentrations of the data?

Figure 4.6 is a histogram of those presenting at the clinics in January, where age is divided into five-year ranges. These data were numerically summarized in Examples 4.1 and 4.4, where it was found that $\bar{y} = 23.8$ and $\tilde{y} = 23$ years with $s = 20.7$ and $R = 95$ years. This is visually evident in the histogram, which shows a bump around the mean, with quite a bit of variation around it, and extreme values that extend from zero to ninety-five years.

In Figure 4.6, the heights of the bars denote the number of clinic patients in each age range. Visually prominent in the plot is a spike at the 0- to 5-year age range, clearly showing that a large number of clinic patients are young children. Note that the vertical axis can also be expressed in terms of the percentage or fraction of the total observations that fall within the range of each bar.

If examining the distribution of young patients is of most interest, then it can be useful to plot the data with age rescaled. That is, one way to make the distribution of such data easier to "see" is to transform it and plot the transformed values. For example, Figure 4.7 shows the square root transformation of age, which compresses the older ages and spreads out the younger ages. What the histogram of the transformed data shows is that the majority of the young patients are, in fact, younger than one year. So, a large fraction of the clinic effort is devoted to newborn health care.

The point here is that there can be utility in plotting data in units other than the natural units. For example, with data that contain outliers or that are highly skewed, most of the data can end up being compressed into one or only a few bars. In such cases, transformations can reveal interesting aspects of the data. Another alternative is to restrict the horizontal axis plotting range to focus only on the region of interest.

Given the ubiquity of statistical software, the details of how to manually construct histograms will be ignored here. However, be aware that every software

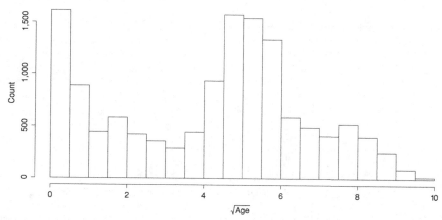

Figure 4.7. A histogram of square root transformed age for clinic patients presenting in January.

package makes certain choices when drawing a histogram based on default values in the software. Two important choices that need to be made when drawing a histogram are (1) how many "bins" should be used and (2) where those bins should be located. A common choice is to begin the first bin at the data's minimum value and end the last bin at the maximum value. In terms of the right number of bins, when n is relatively small, a good choice is often $\sqrt{n}$, and when n is large, a good choice is often $10 \log_{10} n$.

Although the software within the biosurveillance system will likely have defaults, it is important to allow the user to make alternative choices, not only in terms of transformations but also in terms of bin choices because the information communicated with the plot can vary with these choices. For example, Figure 4.8 shows what the same-age data looks like with alternative histograms, where the left plot only has two bins, the middle plot has five bins, and the right plot has ninety-six bins. The plot with only two bins shows almost no details in the data

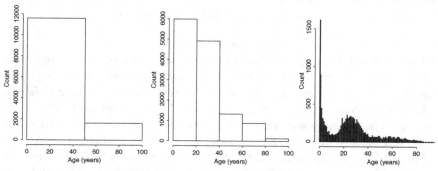

Figure 4.8. Alternative histograms for the same-age data shown in Figure 4.6 using two bins in the left plot, five in the middle plot, and ninety-six in the right plot. The right plot is really just a bar chart because there is a discrete bar for each age year.

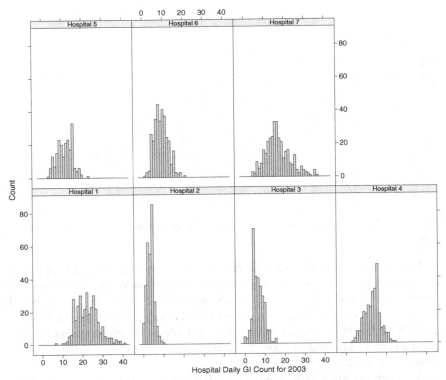

Figure 4.9. Lattice plot of hospital respiratory data for 2003. Here the conditioning variable is the hospital number, which results in a lattice of seven histograms, one for each hospital.

except that the vast majority of clinic patients are younger than 50 years. The histogram with five bins also obscures most of the data and, in fact, is somewhat misleading in the way it shows a fairly constant decrease in counts across the 20-year age bands. The right plot shows the most details and is really just a bar chart because there is a discrete bar for each age year. However, using so many bins is really only effective because the sample size is so large.

Lattice (or Trellis) Plots

Lattice plots (also known as trellis plots) are an array of some type of statistical graph of one variable subset according to the values of one or more categorical variables. The categorical variables are also referred to as conditioning variables. The idea is to create a series of plots of one variable, say histograms for the counts of some syndrome, by separate levels of some categorical variable such as zip code or gender or ethnicity. For example, Figure 4.9 is a lattice of histograms of hospital respiratory data for 2003. Here the conditioning variable is hospital number, which results in a lattice of seven histograms, one for each hospital.

Figure 4.9 shows that the distributions of respiratory syndrome counts differ by hospital. For example, Hospitals #2 and #3 tend to have much smaller daily counts than the other hospitals. On the other hand, Hospitals #1 and #7 have "right tails" that extend much further than the other hospitals, which means those hospitals can have much larger daily respiratory counts than the other hospitals.

In some ways, a lattice plot is nothing more than a set of repeated graphs, one for each category of the conditioning variable or set of categories of the conditioning variables. Three things make lattice plots more useful than simply manually repeating some plot by variable levels. The first is that good software facilitates exploring the data by making it easy to generate lattices. Second, and more importantly, the graphs in the lattice are all plotted with the horizontal and vertical axes on the same scale. This makes the plots easier to compare across the various categories. Third, the lattice can be conditioned on more than one categorical variable, which allows for the discovery of more complicated relationships in the data.

Example 4.9. Create and interpret a lattice plot of clinic patient age histograms conditioned on gender and ethnicity.

Solution: Figure 4.10 is the lattice plot of clinic patient age histograms conditioned on gender and ethnicity. The plots clearly show that there is little to no difference in age distributions by ethnicity but there is by gender.

The difference by gender arises because the clinics provide a significant amount of maternity and well-baby care, and for all ethnic categories, most of the patients between their late teens and mid-30s are female. These are the mothers coming to the clinics for maternity care. Similarly, for both gender categories, there is a pronounced spike at the younger ages. These are the newborns and young children being brought to the clinic for well-baby care.

Note that the spike for male children is much higher than the spike for female children. This does *not* mean that there are more male children than female children because the bars in each of the plots reflect the percentage of those who fall in each bar out of the total of patients in that gender–ethnicity category. Thus, because both the mothers and female babies fall into the same-gender category, the female babies are a much smaller fraction of the total than the males.

Box Plot

Box plots are useful for depicting the distributions of continuous data. They do so by displaying summary statistics of the data, including the median and the quartiles. As a result, box plots require only one dimension (unlike histograms that need two dimensions). Because the box plot is based on summary statistics, some information is lost, but box plots can still be very informative, particularly when comparing the distributions of two or more sets of data.

As shown in Figure 4.11, to construct a box plot, first calculate the median and the quartiles of a set of data. A box is then plotted that connects the first and third quartiles (the 25th and 75th percentiles), and a line is added inside the box

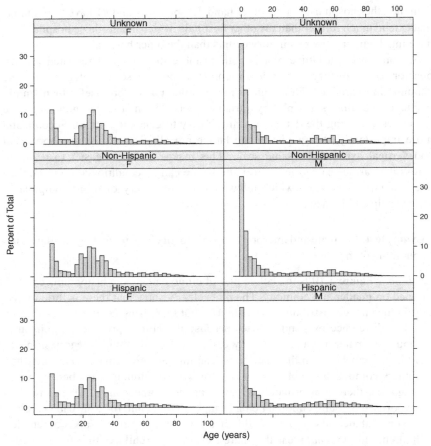

Figure 4.10. A lattice plot of clinic patient age histograms conditioned on gender and ethnicity.

to show the median. At each end of the box, "whiskers" are added by extending lines right and left from the box that are $1\frac{1}{2}$ times the interquartile range. These lines are then truncated back to the last point contained within the line. Each whisker thus terminates at an actual data point, which means the whiskers will likely be of different lengths. Finally, observations that fall outside of the whiskers are indicated by dots and are designated outliers.

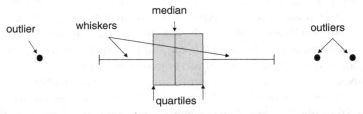

Figure 4.11. An illustration of how a box plot is constructed from summary statistics. Box plots are useful for depicting the distribution of continuous data in one dimension.

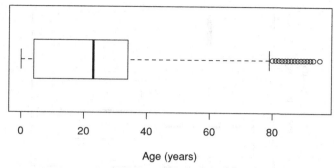

Age (years)

Figure 4.12. A box plot of age for clinic patients presenting in January. Note that box plots cannot show multiple modes in data which means, for example, that the spike from 0 to 5 years evident in the Figure 4.6 histogram is invisible when the data are depicted with a box plot.

So, a box plot displays a lot of information: a measure of central tendency, the median; measures of how variable the data are as indicated by the IQR (shown via the width of the box) and the length of the whiskers; and potentially unusual points, the outliers. Note that how box plots are drawn can vary by software package. For example, when drawing the whiskers, some packages allow the user to choose multiples other than $1\frac{1}{2}$ times the IQR, and some extend the whiskers all the way to the minimum and maximum values in the data. In addition, sometimes the box is based on statistics called "hinges" that are similar to but not precisely the same as quartiles.

Example 4.10. Create and interpret a box plot of the ages of the clinic patients who presented in January.

Solution: Figure 4.12 shows a box plot of the ages of clinic patients who presented in January. As with the histogram in Figure 4.6, the box plot shows that the distribution of ages is skewed, with the median age in the low twenties. The right end of the box, which is the third quartile, looks to be somewhere in the mid-30 year range, indicating that 75 percent of the patients are younger than about 35 years or so. On the other hand, Figure 4.12 also shows a long right whisker that extends out to around 80 years, with lots of outliers, indicating that there is a long and not inconsequential "right tail" of significantly older patients.

A very useful way to compare populations is via side-by-side box plots in which, similar to lattice plots, a separate box plot is created for each population. Side-by-side box plots require a continuous and a categorical measure on each observation (e.g., age and zip code). Also similar to lattice plots, one of the reasons side-by-side box plots are powerful is that all the box plots are graphed on the same scale, which facilitates comparisons among the categories.

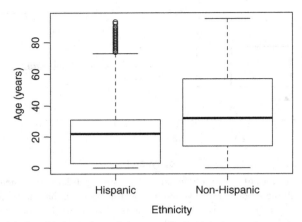

Figure 4.13. Side-by-side box plots of the ages of clinic patients who presented in January by ethnicity. The plot shows that Hispanic patients tended to be younger than non-Hispanic patients.

Example 4.11. Create and interpret side-by-side box plots of age by ethnicity of clinic patients who presented in January.

Solution: Figure 4.13 shows side-by-side box plots of age by ethnicity of clinic patients who presented in January. The plot shows that Hispanic patients tended to be younger than non-Hispanic patients. Note, for example, that the median age of the non-Hispanic patients is roughly equal to the 75th percentile of the Hispanic patients, and the box for Hispanic patients is shifted toward younger ages compared with the non-Hispanic patients. On the other hand, note that the extreme ages are very similar, with the left (lower) whiskers of both groups extending to zero and the right (upper) whisker of the non-Hispanic group extending to about the same age as the greatest outlier for the Hispanic group.

Scatterplot

A scatterplot is a graph of one continuous variable versus another. Scatterplots are useful for summarizing large sets of data, and they are very effective at showing whether there is an association between two variables, where such an association would show up as a pattern in the plot. For example, if a scatterplot shows a distribution of points that fall roughly in an ellipse starting at the lower left corner of the plot and extending to the upper right corner, indicating that larger values of the variable on the horizontal axis are associated with larger values of the variable on the vertical axis, then the two variables will also be positively correlated.

Figure 4.14 is a scatterplot of Hospital #1 versus Hospital #2 respiratory syndrome daily count data. The figure shows there is very little association between the two hospitals in terms of daily respiratory syndrome counts, where large and small counts at Hospital #1 occur with both large and small counts at Hospital

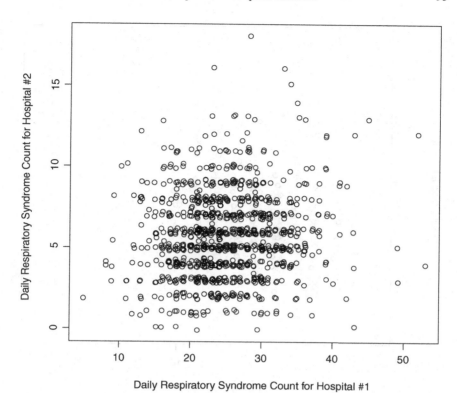

Figure 4.14. Scatterplot of Hospital #1 vs. Hospital #2 respiratory syndrome daily count data. The correlation is $r = 0.11$.

#2. This lack of association most likely exists because the hospitals serve very different populations, and respiratory symptoms are not frequently associated with contagious diseases. The plot is consistent with Table 4.3, which shows that the correlation is only weakly positive ($r = 0.11$). Note that the observations in the plot have been "jittered," meaning a bit of random noise was added to each observation so that days with exactly the same counts for both hospitals did not overplot.

Compare Figure 4.14 with Figure 4.15, which is a scatterplot of clinic GI versus ILI daily count data. Here the correlation is moderately positive ($r = 0.48$), which is visually evident in the plot showing that larger GI values tend to be associated with larger ILI values. This makes clinical sense because flu and GI symptoms often occur simultaneously in patients. Again note that the observations have been "jittered," meaning that a bit of random noise has been added to mitigate over plotting so that all the data are visible.

A correlation of +1 would correspond to all the points in a scatterplot falling perfectly in a straight line, where every "x" value would be precisely equal to its associated "y" value. In contrast, a correlation of -1 would also correspond to all the points falling in a straight line, but the line would go from the upper

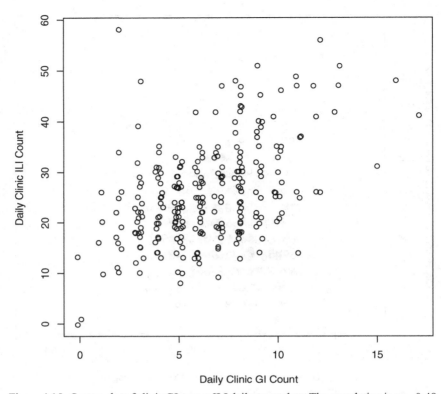

Figure 4.15. Scatterplot of clinic GI versus ILI daily count data. The correlation is $r = 0.48$.

left corner of the plot to the lower right. Note that scatterplots can show other relationships between two variables, perhaps non-linear, that may not be evident in the correlation alone. For example, two variables with a perfect sinusoidal relationship between them would have a correlation of 0.

When there are more than two continuous variables, scatterplot matrices can be used. They display in a lattice-like format scatterplots for all pairs of the data. For example, in the hospital data, there are seven hospitals. Figure 4.14 shows only the scatterplot for Hospital #1 versus #2, but for k variables, there are a total of $k(k-1)/2$ possible pairwise comparisons.

Example 4.12. Create a scatterplot matrix for the hospital respiratory data and interpret it.

Solution: Figure 4.16 is the scatterplot matrix for the hospital respiratory data. There are $7 \times 6/2 = 21$ unique scatterplots, where every plot above the diagonal has an equivalent plot below it, just with the axes reversed. Note how the plot in the first row, second column, is the same as the scatterplot in Figure 4.14.

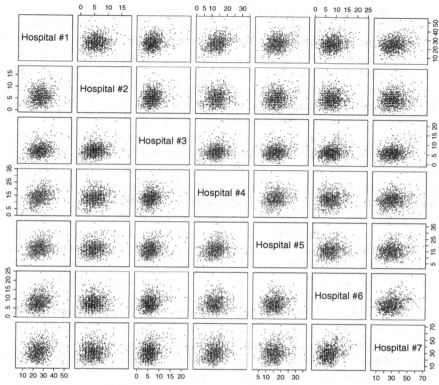

Figure 4.16. A scatterplot matrix of the hospital respiratory data. See Table 4.3 for the associated correlation values for each scatterplot. Note that the plot in the first row, second column, is the same as the scatterplot in Figure 4.14.

Figure 4.16 shows that there are no strong associations between any of the hospitals. This is consistent with the correlations in Table 4.3, where the largest correlation is $r = 0.27$ between Hospitals #1 and #4. As previously described, this lack of strong correlation in daily respiratory counts is clinically plausible. The scatterplot matrix also shows that there are no non-linear relationships that are not evident in the correlation matrix of Table 4.3.

4.2.2 Graphical Methods for Longitudinal Data

Time Series Plots

Time series data consist of observations or other measures taken repeatedly over time, so in that sense, the term "time series" is simply a synonym for longitudinal data. See Chapter 2 (page 26) for additional discussion about types of data. Daily syndrome counts, for example, are time series data, and biosurveillance by its very nature focuses on such data.

Time series plots display longitudinal data plotted with respect to time. By convention, the data are plotted with the magnitude of the observation on the vertical axis and time on the horizontal axis in the appropriate units corresponding to how the data were collected. Time series plots are useful for displaying whether there are trends in the data, such as a regular increase in the number of people presenting at a facility with a particular syndrome (perhaps as a result of regular population growth in the region), or whether there are cycles in the data (perhaps as a result of seasonal or other influences).

Referring to Chapter 2, Figure 2.5 is a time series plot of ILI syndrome data from the clinics, where each point on the plot is the daily count of the number of people presenting who were classified into the ILI syndrome. In this plot, time is represented in terms of days, where the clinics are not open on weekends or holidays, so there are 252 sequential daily observations in the data.

Figure 2.5 displays the time series by plotting the raw data and then overlaying a line that represents the trend in the average daily ILI. This is just one way the data can be displayed, and there are a variety of alternatives depending on what is intended to be emphasized. For example, in Figure 4.17, the upper left plot just shows the data. In the lower left plot, a smoothed line is added to help direct attention to the trends and cycles in the data (much like Fig. 2.5). In contrast, the upper right plot connects all the data with a line, which tends to emphasize the variation in the data from day to day. And the lower right plot adds the smoothing line to try to show both how variable the data are and also the trends and cycles. Which of these is the best or most appropriate display depends on the purpose of the plot and what one is trying to communicate with it.

Another alternative for displaying times series data is shown in Figures 2.7 and 2.8, where only the smoothed lines are plotted and the data are suppressed. In those figures, this was done for the purposes of clarity, where graphing the raw data for all seven hospitals made the plots too busy and virtually unintelligible. However, displaying the time series this way also completely obscures the variation in the data because the data themselves are not even shown.

If adding a smoothing line is desired, that naturally leads to the question of how to calculate it. In Figures 2.4 to 2.5 and 2.7 to 2.8, lowess is used (see the footnote on page 32 for a brief description). Alternatives also include the moving average, the exponentially weighted moving average, and time series models. These are all discussed in more detail in Chapter 5. For now, simply note that adding such smoothers to a plot can help show trends that may be more or less discernible to the unaided eye.

Repeated Cross-sectional Plots

Another way to present time series data is via a series of repeated plots, where each plot represents a different (but sequential) time period. This is simply the graphical equivalent to the approach in Section 4.1.2 for summary statistics. For example, box plots repeated over time can be very informative. Figure 4.18 shows this approach for the clinic ILI data, where each box plot is based on a month of data. Compare Figure 4.18 with Figure 2.5 and the plots in Figure 4.17.

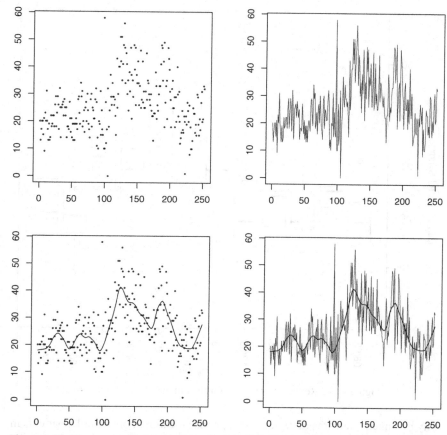

Figure 4.17. Time series plotting variants for the clinic ILI data first presented in Figure 2.5.

Figure 4.18 does show time trends, but the repeated box plots tend to emphasize the variation within each month. An abstraction of the repeated box plots is shown in Figure 4.19, where each of the box plot statistics is joined with a line, the region between the lines corresponding to the first and third quartiles is darkly shaded, and the region between the lines corresponding to the whiskers is lightly shaded. This plot, then, gives some idea of both the overall trends in the data as well as the variation.

Of course, lattice plots can also be used to display repeated cross-sectional plots if the conditioning variable corresponds to time. For example, Figure 4.20 is a lattice plot of the clinic ILI monthly histograms.

4.2.3 Graphical Methods for Spatial and Spatio-temporal Data

Informative displays of spatial data almost by definition require them to be viewed in the context of a map. However, unlike a lot of data that are displayed on geographic information systems (GIS) as precise points on a map, biosurveillance data are frequently areal data. *Areal data* are data that are associated with or can

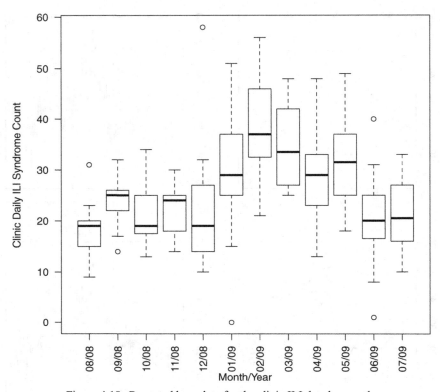

Figure 4.18. Repeated box plots for the clinic ILI data by month.

only be linked to an area or region, not a precise location. For example, patients in the clinic data can only be located to residential zip codes, not to precise residential addresses.

Of course, in some data sets, the precise residential address of the patients is recorded. However, even if they are known, some aggregation across patients and regions is necessary to discern trends and patterns. Furthermore, there is an inherent ambiguity in location because whatever location is precisely recorded for a given patient only corresponds to one location of many that they likely visit over time. That is, employed people spend a significant portion of their time in at least two locations: their residence and their location of employment. Children in school similarly spend much of their time both at home and at school. Thus, whatever location is recorded is at best a proxy for the general location where an individual spends some or more of his or her time.

Maps

Figures 4.21 and 4.22 are examples of maps displaying areal data. Figure 4.21 is a map of the clinic population density by zip code. Clinic locations (which are point data) are denoted by the white diamonds, where it is visually evident

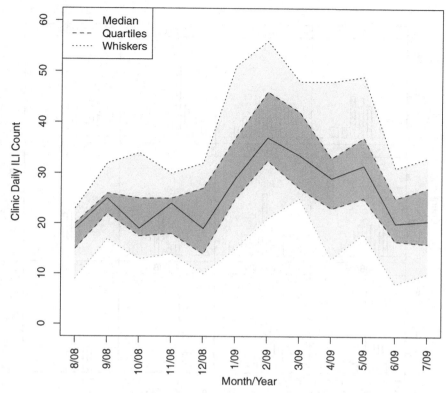

Figure 4.19. An alternate way to display the box plot statistics from the clinic ILI data shown with repeated box plots in Figure 4.18.

that the clinics are located in the more densely populated areas. Figure 4.22 is a map of annual ILI count from the clinics by zip code. Note how, not surprisingly, the distribution of ILI is directly associated with population size and with clinic location shown in Figure 4.21.

These two maps illustrate that care must be taken with how one interprets results (using maps as well as the numerical statistics and other descriptive described in this chapter) from this type of biosurveillance data. At issue is that these data come from what statisticians call *convenience sampling*, which means that there is no control by the public health system of whether or how an individual ends up in the data. For the clinic data, for example, it is likely a complex interaction of socioeconomics and living and working locations that affect whether an individual goes to a clinic. As a result, it is difficult at best, and often impossible, to use results such as that displayed in Figure 4.22 to make inference about ILI incidence in the general population.

Nonetheless, the data can be useful for detecting changes in disease incidence, at least among the populations that use the facilities being monitored. The key is monitoring and displaying data from the same source over time. Figure 4.23

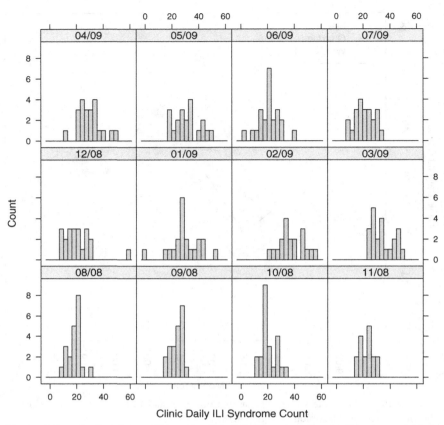

Figure 4.20. A lattice plot applied to the clinic ILI data, where the conditioning variable is the month.

is an example of such a display, where the weekly ILI rates for the clinic are mapped both for a non-outbreak period (8/1/08–12/11/08), a seasonal flu period (12/12/08–2/13/09), and the initial wave of H1N1 in 2009 (4/6/09–5/8/09). The plots show a subtle, yet visible, increase in the weekly ILI for the two outbreak periods compared with the non-outbreak period.

One thing that tends to obscure trends in Figure 4.23 is that different zip codes have different non-outbreak weekly ILI rates because those rates depend on the size and composition of each zip code's population as well as proximity to the clinics. Particularly for low-density regions and regions distant from the clinics, the non-outbreak rate is low, and thus increases from that base rate are difficult to discern on a scale that must span the range of rates across all the regions.

Figure 4.24 solves this problem by plotting the percent change from the base rate, where the base rate was calculated over the non-outbreak period (8/1/08–12/11/08) shown in the top plot of Figure 4.23 and then the percent change is calculated for each week for the flu outbreak from 12/22/08 to 2/16/09 (corresponding to the bottom left plot in Fig. 4.23). Here the increase in ILI is much

County Population Distribution

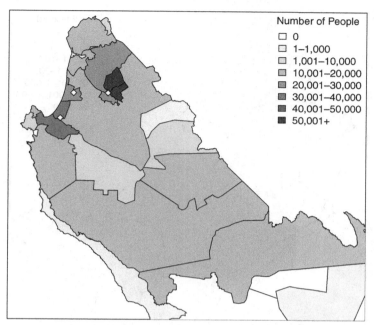

Figure 4.21. Map of clinic population density by zip code. Clinic locations are denoted by the white diamonds, where it is evident that the clinics are located in the more densely populated areas.

more visible, as is the fact that there was an anomalous drop-off in ILI across the region for the week of 1/12/09.

Looking for increases from a base rate, which ostensibly reflects the "normal" state of a population in terms of disease or syndrome incidence, is the fundamental idea of EED. In Figure 4.24, the progression of the flu, as manifested via the proxy measure of ILI syndrome incidence, is quite clear. However, these plots were made *retrospectively* and with the knowledge of the flu period. The challenge in EED and any type of *prospective* monitoring is that one does not know whether the flu period has started or not.

Indeed, the whole point of monitoring is to sequentially observe the data as they unfold over time and determine as early as possible when there is enough evidence to conclude that the flu season (or some other outbreak or attack) has begun. However, such a determination can always turn out to be a false positive, and a major challenge with EED is to appropriately balance how aggressively one makes an outbreak determination with an acceptable rate of false positives. These issues are discussed in more detail in Part III.

Note that Figure 4.24 is essentially just a lattice plot of maps using time (weeks) as the conditioning variable. This often is an effective way to look at spatio-temporal data. However, although these types of plots are useful when

Total ILI Count by Zip Code for 8/08–7/09

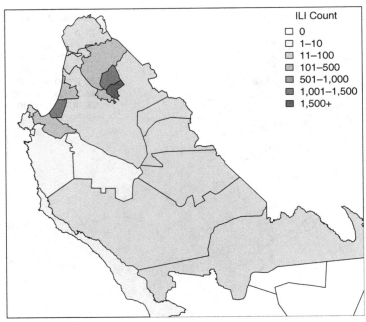

Figure 4.22. Map of annual ILI count from the clinics by zip code. Note that distribution is directly associated with population size and with clinic location shown in Figure 4.21.

viewing the data in a static format, such as on a page in a book, animation is another powerful option when the data can be viewed dynamically. For example, on a computer display, one might have a slider bar under a map that controls what point in time is displayed. By sliding the bar to the right, the user can observe how the incidence rate dynamically changes over time.

Bubble Charts and Other Spatial Displays

Maps, in the strict cartographic sense, are often not necessary to discern important spatial changes in disease incidence. In fact, maps can be limiting in various ways, such as the fact that the map itself uses two dimensions and thus it is challenging to display multidimensional data on a map. Thus, it is difficult to impossible to clearly convey more than one additional dimension on a map. With the addition of animation, it can be increased to two dimensions, where the second is time.

In addition, areal data maps can fool the eye when, as is frequently the case, region size is inversely related to population density. The problem is that the human brain tends to equate size with importance. Thus, changes in color-coded areal maps may be misleading when the least-populated areas are the most noticeable because those areas are the largest.

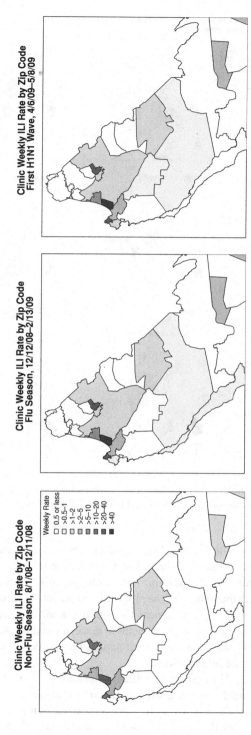

Figure 4.23. Weekly ILI rates for a non-outbreak period, seasonal flu, and the initial wave of H1N1 in 2009. The rate here is simply the total ILI syndrome count for the period of time divided by seven. Note the subtle increase in the weekly ILI for the two outbreak periods compared with the non-outbreak period.

105

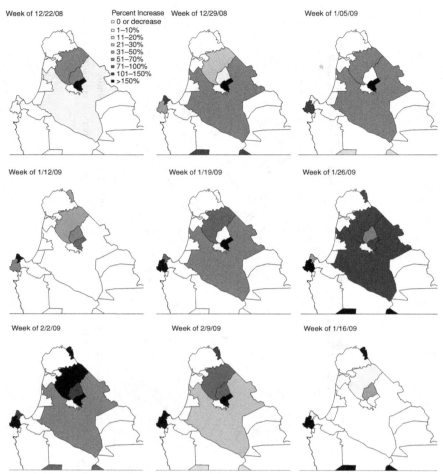

Figure 4.24. Maps for the weeks of 12/22/08 to 2/19/09 showing weekly percent ILI increase from the non-outbreak period of 8/1/08 to 12/11/08 (which corresponds to the top plot in Fig. 4.23).

One solution is a *bubble chart*, which centers bubbles in each area, and the size of the bubble represents the magnitude. For example, Figure 4.25 uses bubbles to display the population size for the clinic data. Compare this plot with Figure 4.21, where the zip codes at the bottom of the plot are large but have comparatively small populations, while some zip codes near the top are small but have much larger populations. This is somewhat more difficult to discern in Figure 4.21 because the size of the zip codes confounds the interpretation, but the bubbles in Figure 4.25 more clearly convey the information.

Other options include *cartograms*, which distort a map by making the area of each region proportional to the measure of interest. The result is a recognizable but distorted shape where the area of each region is resized to match the measure of interest. A cartogram can then convey two-dimensional data, where area represents

Bubble Chart of County Population Distribution

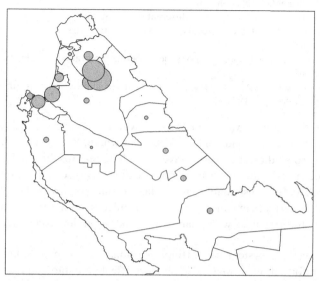

Figure 4.25. Bubble chart of clinic population density by zip code. This is an alternative to Figure 4.21 for displaying the data.

one dimension and color a second. With animation, time can also be added for a total of three dimensions.

4.3 Discussion and Summary

This chapter described numerous numerical and graphical statistical methods for summarizing and displaying data. The goal is to use these methods for enhancing and promoting situational awareness, particularly level 2 situational awareness – comprehension – which depends on appropriately summarizing raw data as they are received by a biosurveillance system.

Although this chapter has presented a suite of useful numerical and graphical statistical methods, how these methods are implemented in a computer interface is also critically important for facilitating SA. That is, although it is beyond the scope of this text, how the biosurveillance system interface is designed in terms of both usability and graphical display can either enhance or inhibit SA.

The general question of effective statistical graphics design has been addressed by Tufte (2001) and others in the statistical literature. For example, Tufte says,

> Excellence in statistical graphics consists of complex ideas communicated with clarity, precision, and efficiency. Graphical displays should
>
> - show the data
> - induce the viewer to think about the substance rather than about methodology, graphic design, the technology of graphic production, or something else
> - avoid distorting what the data have to say

- present many numbers in a small space
- make large data sets coherent
- encourage the eye to compare different pieces of data
- reveal the data at several levels of detail, from the broad overview to the fine structure
- serve a reasonably clear purpose: description, exploration, tabulation, or decoration
- be closely integrated with the statistical and verbal descriptions of the data set (Tufte, 2001, p. 13)

These are critical and relevant guidelines. However, effective interface and graphical design are situation and context dependent where, for biosurveillance, as of this writing, no studies or research have been done that would provide appropriate guidance specific to this particular application. As discussed in Chapter 3 as systems such as BioSense mature, understanding and improving how biosurveillance system interfaces enhance (or degrade) situational awareness – particularly when under stress, such as with a large outbreak – is an important area for future research.

In addition to a system supporting situational awareness through effective display of information, it must also support effective exploratory data analysis (EDA), for example, to help localize possible sources of an outbreak. As with the numerical and graphical methods, effective EDA is as much a function of system and interface design as it is of individual statistical methods.

In the statistics literature, EDA is an approach to data analysis that focuses on summarizing the data so that it is easy to understand, often with visual graphs, without the use of formal statistical models or hypotheses. As described by the National Institute of Standards and Technology (NIST, 2012):

Exploratory Data Analysis (EDA) is an approach/philosophy for data analysis that employs a variety of techniques (mostly graphical) to

- maximize insight into a data set;
- uncover underlying structure;
- extract important variables;
- detect outliers and anomalies;
- test underlying assumptions;
- develop parsimonious models; and
- determine optimal factor settings.

NIST goes on to say,

The particular graphical techniques employed in EDA are often quite simple, consisting of various techniques of:

- Plotting the raw data such as data traces, histograms, bihistograms, probability plots, lag plots, block plots, and Youden plots.
- Plotting simple statistics such as mean plots, standard deviation plots, box plots, and main effects plots of the raw data.
- Positioning such plots so as to maximize our natural pattern-recognition abilities, such as using multiple plots per page.

Promoting and enhancing EDA in biosurveillance requires more than good static summaries of data; it also requires an interface design that allows the user to easily and appropriately explore the data. Important software features include the ability to "drill down" into the data for details to, for example, facilitate easy identification of individual records associated with an EED signal and dynamic and interactive graphics. Good examples of statistical software that emphasize data and graphical interactivity include JMP and the GGobi, Mondrian, and Manet packages in R. Important features include linking plots and "brushing" in which, for example, highlighting one or more data points in one plot also highlights them in the other plots and in the original database and the ability to "tour" through the data, particularly higher dimensional data.

Finally, it is important to recognize that this chapter is focused on descriptive and not inferential statistics. Whereas descriptive statistics are used to quantitatively describe a set of data, inferential statistics are used to learn about some larger unobserved population from an observed sample of data. There are two reasons for the focus on descriptive statistics. The first reason is that the data used in many biosurveillance systems such as BioSense are convenience samples from some larger population. Because they are convenience samples, there is not enough information available to make statistically defensible and quantitatively rigorous inferences from sample to population. The second reason is that often inference from sample to population is not the immediate goal of prospective biosurveillance. Rather, the goal is early detection of SA about an outbreak as it is occurring.

In many traditional health surveillance systems, the goal *is* inference to some larger population using a sample of data. For example, the Behavioral Risk Factor Surveillance System (BRFSS) is designed to track health conditions and risk behaviors and make inferences about these conditions and behaviors to all adults in the United States. This is done via monthly surveys that collect information on health risk behaviors, preventive health practices, and health care access primarily as related to chronic disease and injury. An inferential approach is necessary, reasonable, and appropriate in this situation. It is necessary because it is impossible to survey the entire population; it is reasonable because trends in chronic conditions change slowly; and it is appropriate because the health system is interested in population trends, not just those of a particular sample.

For prospective biosurveillance of a rapidly evolving situation, such as the spread of a virulent contagion, this type of formal sample data collection and analysis is impractical at best. That said, even from a prospective biosurveillance perspective, clearly the more that is known about or that can be inferred to an entire population the better. Information about populations can be obtained either by sampling and then doing statistical inference or by collecting data on the entire population. At least currently, the emphasis seems to be more on acquiring large convenience samples of data that can be transmitted electronically than on ensuring that the data either support formal statistical inference or cover the entire population. Essentially, it is a trade-off of timeliness of data for data coverage, but as electronic sources of data continue to expand, it may well be that eventually electronic data on most of the population is available to biosurveillance. At that point, inference may become irrelevant. Until then, as biosurveillance systems mature, attention should be paid to managing data sources. In so doing, the goal should be clearly articulated, which is either obtaining complete data coverage for entire populations (which, realistically, means obtaining data on as high a fraction of the population as possible) or the careful and appropriate selection of data sources and statistical methods to allow formal inference (including the calculation of margins of error) from sample to population.

Additional Reading

For those who would like to delve more deeply into the material presented in this chapter, consider the following.

- For additional information on, examples of, and further discussion about numerical descriptive statistics, see most standard undergraduate-level statistics textbooks. However, note that such texts vary in the amount of detail devoted to discussing descriptive statistics. Suggested texts include *Statistics* by Voelker *et al.* (2001, chapters 3–9), *Statistics* by Freedman *et al.* (1998, chapters 3–9), *Mathematical Statistics and Data Analysis* by Rice (2006, chapter 10), and *Using R for Introductory Statistics* by Verzani (2005, chapters 2–4).
- For general guidance on design principles for good quantitative graphics, see *The Visual Display of Quantitative Information* by Tufte (2001), *Envisioning Information* by Tufte (1990), *Visualizing Data* by Cleveland (1993), and *The Wall Street Journal Guide to Information Graphics: The Dos and Don'ts of Presenting Data, Facts, and Figures* by Wong (2010). The last book has a decidedly business news orientation, but much of it is also applicable to health surveillance data display. For a discussion of visualizing spatial health data using maps, see Waller and Gotway (2004, chapter 4).
- For more information about exploratory data analysis, the seminal text is *Exploratory Data Analysis* by Tukey (1977).
- To read more about interactive graphics, see *Visual Statistics: Seeing Data with Dynamic Interactive Graphics* by Young *et al.* (2006), *Dynamic Graphics for Statistics* by Cleveland & McGill (1988), and *Interactive and Dynamic Graphics for Data Analysis with R and Gobi* by Cook & Swayne (2007, chapters 1 and 2). Although most of these discuss dynamic graphics in the context of a specific software system, the principles and ideas generalize to any system.
- Finally, although only briefly mentioned in this chapter, the rigorous definition of and appropriate estimation approaches for the risk of contracting a disease and the rate of disease in a population are critical in public health surveillance. Refer to Sections 2.2 and 2.3 of *Applied Spatial Statistics for Public Health Data* by Waller and Gotway (2004) for additional discussion in a traditional health surveillance context.

5

Statistical Models for Projecting the Situation

> Prediction is very difficult, especially about the future.
> Unknown[1]

Statistical models are often used to formally characterize underlying relationships in data. In terms of situational awareness (SA), as the chapter title says, statistical models can be useful for projecting (i.e., forecasting) the current situation into the future. The goal is to provide a decision maker with an understanding of what the near-term trends are likely to be for a particular situation.

A benefit of statistical modeling, appropriately done, is that such models also provide estimates of forecast uncertainty. This is an important part of modeling that is sometimes overlooked or ignored. Simply put, a forecast without some quantification of the uncertainty inherent in the forecast is not particularly useful. Without the uncertainty quantification, a decision maker cannot know how much credence to give the forecast.

This chapter focuses on statistical models useful for the projection step of situational awareness, including time series and regression-based models. As described in Chapter 3, projection is the third and highest level of SA, involving the ability to project the future status of the elements in the environment. Given perception and comprehension of the situation (SA levels 1 and 2), level 3 SA is achieved by using this information in an appropriate model to project likely future states of the environment that are important or useful for decision making.

In addition, the chapter describes how statistical models can also be used for "preprocessing" (also referred to as "preconditioning") biosurveillance data. The terms "preprocessing" and "preconditioning" refer the use of models to account for (as much as possible) the systematic effects present in biosurveillance data. Doing so is important for the appropriate application of many of the early event detection (EED) methods discussed in Chapters 6 to 8.

---

[1] Often attributed to Niels Bohr, although variations of the quote have been traced back to other sources early in the 19th century. Variants of the quote have also been attributed to Yogi Berra, Mark Twain, and Samuel Goldwyn.

Chapter Objectives

Upon completion of this chapter, the reader should be able to:

- Describe how statistical modeling can be used to enhance SA and why forecasting is necessary for achieving SA level 3.
- Explain why it is important to calculate uncertainty bounds for a forecast and calculate the bounds for some simple models.
- Define what it means to preprocess or precondition data and why preprocessing is important for biosurveillance data, particularly with respect to EED. Explain how modeling can be used to preprocess biosurveillance data, particularly in terms of eliminating or mitigating autocorrelation.
- Construct simple smoothing, regression, and time series models of biosurveillance data, including
  - Moving average models, simple exponentially weighted moving average (EWMA) models, and double and triple exponential smoothing models
  - Cross-sectional regression models and autoregressive and adaptive regression models
  - Autoregressive moving average (ARMA) and autoregressive integrated moving average (ARIMA) time series models
- Describe the change point analysis methodology and how it can be used in combination with EED methods to enhance SA.

Mathematical Notation

i, j	Indices for either time or the observations
I	Indicator variable
k	Lag
$MAE(\hat{y})$	Mean absolute error of the forecast $\hat{y}$
$MAPE(\hat{y})$	Mean absolute percent error of the forecast $\hat{y}$
$MSE(\hat{y})$	Mean square error of the forecast $\hat{y}$
n	Sample size
$N(0, \sigma^2)$	Normal distribution with mean 0 and variance σ^2
p	Number of independent variables in a linear regression model or the order of an autoregressive model
q	Order of a moving average model model
r	Sample correlation
r_k	Sample autocorrelation for lag k
S_t	Estimated seasonal component at time t in the Holt-Winters model
t	The current or latest time period
T_t	Estimated trend component at time t in the Holt-Winters model
θ_i	ith coefficient in a moving average model, $i = 1, \ldots, q$
x	An "independent variable" in regression
y	An observation; the "dependent variable" in regression
$\hat{y}_i$	A model's estimate for the ith observation or forecast for time i
β_0	Regression intercept parameter
$\hat{\beta}_0$	Estimated regression intercept
β_i	Regression (partial) slope parameter, $i = 1, \ldots, p$
$\hat{\beta}_i$	Estimated (partial) slope parameter, $i = 1, \ldots, p$
δ	Holt-Winters model seasonal component parameter; order of the integrated part of an ARIMA model
ϵ	Linear regression model error term
$\hat{\epsilon}_i$	Residual for observation i
$\bar{\epsilon}$	Average of the residuals
γ	Holt-Winters model trend component parameter
λ	EWMA parameter; Holt-Winters and Brown's model mean component parameter
ϕ_i	ith coefficient in an autoregressive model, $i = 1, \ldots, p$
σ_ϵ	Standard deviation of the error term ϵ
$\hat{\sigma}_\epsilon$	Estimated standard deviation of the error term ϵ
$\hat{\sigma}_i$	Estimated standard deviation of the ith period forecast

5.1 Modeling Time Series Data

As discussed in Chapter 2, time series or longitudinal data consist of a sequence of observations, often measured in successive time periods spaced at equal time intervals. Examples in biosurveillance include daily syndrome counts and laboratory reports; in sentinel physician systems examples include weekly reports of the number of patients presenting with flu symptoms. Longitudinal data, by definition, have a natural temporal ordering, making time series analysis distinct from other common modeling approaches for cross-sectional data analysis. Time series analysis is also distinct from spatial data analysis in which the observations are typically related by geographical location.

Time series models are generally based on the idea that observations that are close together in time will be more closely related than observations further apart. That is, time series models are based on and try to exploit autocorrelation. In addition, time series models are often prospective, where they use the natural ordering of time to forecast the value in some future period in terms of past values. This is important in prospective monitoring, where the incorporation of information from future observations is clearly impossible.

Models for time series data can have many forms in order to represent different types of real-world processes. When modeling variations in the level of a process, three broad classes of practical importance are autoregressive (AR) models, integrated (I) models, and moving average (MA) models. Combinations of these ideas produce ARMA and ARIMA models.

5.1.1 Purposes of Modeling

As described in Chapter 2, biosurveillance data often have systematic effects (i.e., explainable trends and patterns). These can include day-of-the-week effects, where patient health-seeking behavior systematically varies according to the day of the week. It may also include seasonal effects where, for example, influenza-like illness (ILI) is generally higher in the winter months of the year than the summer months.

These trends and patterns can be used to build models, and the models can then be used both to better understand and to characterize historical trends, to assess how the current state compares to historical trends, and to forecast what is likely to occur in the near future. This latter point is important if biosurveillance systems are to facilitate achieving the third level of SA: projection. In statistical terms, projection is called *forecasting*.

Furthermore, many of the EED methods discussed in Chapters 6 to 8 are most effective when the systematic components of biosurveillance data are removed. This is best accomplished by first modeling the data, where the model is used to estimate the systematic effects, and then using the EED methods on the model *residuals*. The residuals are what remains after the modeled values (often referred to as the "fitted values") are subtracted from the raw data. This idea of subtracting the systematic effects from biosurveillance data is often referred to as *preprocessing*.

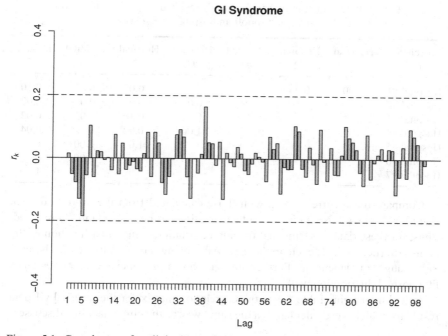

Figure 5.1. Correlogram for clinic GI syndrome *residuals* for various lags, $1 \leq k \leq 100$. When comparing this with Figure 4.1, it is apparent that the autocorrelation present in the first 20 days or so of the raw data has been reduced in the residuals.

5.1.2 Examples of Preprocessing

As originally demonstrated in Chapter 4, the clinic gastrointestinal (GI) and ILI data are relatively modestly autocorrelated (see the correlograms in Figs. 4.1 and 4.2 and associated discussion on page 83) because of the presence of systematic effects. To remove these effects, the data are preprocessed by fitting a model to the data and then taking the difference between the model estimates and the actual data. That is, for data $y_1, \ldots, y_n$ estimates are calculated via a model: $\hat{y}_1, \ldots, \hat{y}_n$. The residuals are then $\hat{\epsilon}_i = y_i - \hat{y}_i, i = 1, \ldots, n$.

Figures 5.1 and 5.2 are correlograms of clinic GI and ILI residuals, where the residuals are calculated as the difference between the lowess mean estimate (first discussed in Section 2.2.2 and shown in Figs. 2.4 and 2.5) and the actual observations. Using Equation 4.17 for the residuals, the autocorrelation for lag k is calculated as

$$r_k = \frac{\sum_{i=k+1}^{n} (\hat{\epsilon}_i - \bar{\epsilon})(\hat{\epsilon}_{i-k} - \bar{\epsilon})}{\sum_{i=1}^{n} (\hat{\epsilon}_i - \bar{\epsilon})^2}, \quad k = 1, 2, \ldots, 100, \tag{5.1}$$

where $\bar{\epsilon} = \frac{1}{n} \sum_{i=1}^{n} \hat{\epsilon}_i$.

Table 5.1. Correlation matrix for the GI residuals ($\hat{\epsilon}_{ij}$) from the seven
metropolitan hospitals

Correlation (r)	Hospital #1	Hospital #2	Hospital #3	Hospital #4	Hospital #5	Hospital #6	Hospital #7
Hospital #1	1.00	0.06	0.03	0.07	0.07	0.03	0.10
Hospital #2		1.00	−0.04	0.01	0.03	0.03	0.02
Hospital #3			1.00	0.02	0.10	0.03	0.02
Hospital #4				1.00	−0.02	0.02	0.04
Hospital #5					1.00	0.00	0.09
Hospital #6						1.00	0.07
Hospital #7							1.00

Compare these correlograms with those calculated from the original data in
Figures 4.1 and 4.2. Note how the autocorrelation has been substantially reduced.
Thus, for these data, it seems that the autocorrelation is mainly a function of the
long-term (i.e., annual) cycle in the data. After being removed, the residuals seem
to be roughly independent. Furthermore, as shown in Appendix B, the residuals
fit a normal distribution well.

In a similar vein, Table 5.1 is the correlation matrix for the hospital GI data
residuals, which were calculated in the same way as the clinic data just discussed.

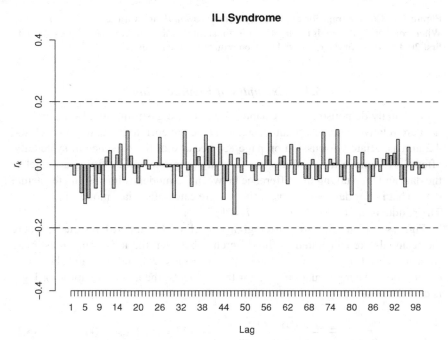

Figure 5.2. Correlogram for clinic ILI syndrome *residuals* for various lags, $1 \leq k \leq 100$.
Compared with Figure 4.2, the autocorrelation of the residuals is much less than the autocorrelation of the raw data.

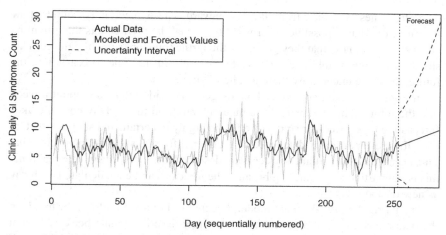

Figure 5.3. A "Holt-Winters" forecasting model (to be discussed in Section 5.2.2) to the clinic GI data. The black line in Figure 5.3 is the forecast for each day based on all of the previous days' data.

Compared with the original data (see Table 4.2 on page 79), Table 5.1 shows that the correlation between hospitals has been reduced substantially (although they were fairly modest to begin with). However, the data do still retain some small positive correlations, suggesting that the lowess model has not accounted for all the systematic effects in the data.

5.1.3 An Example of Forecasting

To illustrate the idea of forecasting, consider the clinic GI syndrome data, first depicted in Figure 2.4 with a lowess line overlaid. The lowess line shows some fairly pronounced trends in GI over the year, and as discussed in Chapter 2, the clinic data also have a weekly cycle in which people are more likely to come into the clinic on Thursdays (see Fig. 2.6 and associated discussion).

Figure 5.3 shows the results of fitting a "Holt-Winters" forecasting model (to be discussed in Section 5.2.2) to the clinic GI data. The black line in Figure 5.3 is the forecast for each day based on all of the previous days' data, where the reader will remember that there were 252 days of clinic data (which is the gray line in the figure).

Note how the forecasting model, similar to the lowess line in Figure 2.4, helps show the underlying trends in GI because it damps out some of the volatility in the raw data. However, also note that unlike the lowess, the forecasting model can be used to project what the GI trend is likely to be in the future. In Figure 5.3, a 30-day forecast is shown, where the model clearly carries the upward trend that occurred from day 225 to day 252 forward into the future.

A key point is that uncertainty bounds can (and should) be estimated and displayed around a forecast. In Figure 5.3, the uncertainty bounds are shown as the dotted lines extending from day 253 onward. These uncertainty bounds show the range of what is possible in terms of the actual daily GI counts that might be observed, where note that they get wider the farther one looks into the future. This should seem reasonable and intuitive because the further one forecasts into the future, the more uncertainty there is inherent in the forecast.

In Figure 5.3, the uncertainty bounds get very wide after only about a week into the future. This means that the inherent variation in the daily counts makes forecasting past a week or so into the future highly uncertain and suggests that, at least for these particular data, precise long-term forecasts are not possible. That said, because biosurveillance systems are designed to collect data in near real time, this is not particularly troubling because the forecast can be recalculated each day as new data are received.

The particular Holt-Winters model depicted in Figure 5.3 allows for trends in the data but not cycles. The rest of this chapter describes a number of different types of models, each with its pros and cons and that may be more or less suited to modeling any specific type of data.

5.2 Smoothing Models

The basic assumption behind moving average and other "smoothing" models is that the time series is "locally stationary," meaning that the process that generates the observed data is roughly constant over a short period of time, although perhaps with a mean that slowly varies over a longer period of time. Under these conditions, it is appropriate to take a moving (i.e., local) average to estimate the current value of the mean, and this value is then used as a short-term forecast.

Chapter 2 introduced one type of smoothing model, the lowess. Because the values estimated by the lowess depend on observations both before and after the time period in question, this type of smoothing model is useful for retrospective modeling but not for prospective modeling. As such, it will not be discussed further here. Instead, this section focuses on moving average models, both simple and exponentially weighted.

5.2.1 Simple Moving Average Models

The moving average is often called a smoothed version of the original data because averaging has the effect of smoothing out variation in the original time series. As discussed in Chapter 2 (see page 83), the amount of smoothing is adjusted by the size of the "window" of data used in the moving average calculation.

To illustrate the idea of moving average forecasting, consider the Hospital #7 GI syndrome data, first depicted using a lowess line in Figure 2.7. That figure shows a fairly regular and pronounced annual cycle in GI and, as discussed in Chapter 2, the hospital data also have a weekly cycle (similar to that shown on page 36 for respiratory syndrome).

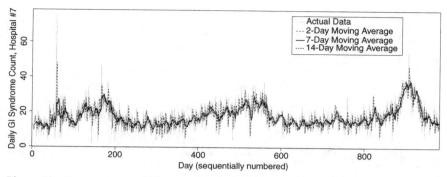

Figure 5.4. Two-, seven-, and fourteen-day moving average forecasts of GI syndrome daily counts for Hospital #7 superimposed over the raw time series data.

Figure 5.4 shows two-, seven-, and fourteen-day moving averages superimposed over the raw data. As forecasts, these moving averages differ slightly from the definition given in Equation 4.13. Here, the d-period moving average *forecast* for time $t + 1$, $\hat{y}_{t+1}$, is the moving average calculated from the d days prior to but *not including* day $t + 1$ (because at time t the results for time $t + 1$ have not been observed):

$$\hat{y}_{t+1} \triangleq \bar{y}_{t+1} = \frac{1}{d} \sum_{i=t-d+1}^{t} y_i. \qquad (5.2)$$

Now, in Figure 5.4, it is actually quite difficult to visually discern which of the moving averages best fit the data. This is partially because the graph is rather small, but even when enlarged it is difficult to tell "by eye" whether the two-, seven-, or fourteen-day moving average is best. For example, see Figure 5.5, which now plots only the last year of data; here the lines for all three moving averages seem to match the data fairly well.

To address this, three metrics are commonly used to judge time series model fit. The first is the *mean square error* (MSE) of the forecasts, defined as

$$\mathrm{MSE}\,(\hat{y}) = \frac{1}{n-d} \sum_{t=d+1}^{n} (y_t - \hat{y}_t)^2. \qquad (5.3)$$

The MSE of the forecasts is the average squared difference between the observations and their forecasted values where in Equation 5.3 $\hat{y}_t \triangleq \bar{y}_t$. Note that the summation in Equation 5.3 is over the entire set of data for which both an observation and its forecast exist. Here it starts at time $t = d + 1$ because the first d periods of data are required to calculate the first moving average forecast (and thus there can be no forecasts for time periods $t = 1, \ldots, d$).

For the Hospital #7 data, the MSE for the two-day moving average is 42.2; for the seven-day moving average, it is 32.8; and for the fourteen-day moving average, it is 33.4. In fact, looking over all possible d-day moving average forecasts, the MSE is minimized for $d = 7$, where the fact that it is a multiple of the shortest

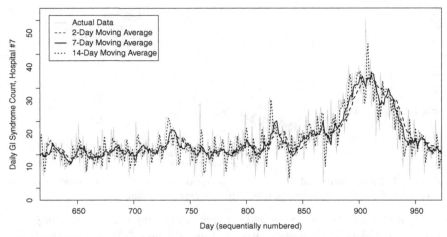

Figure 5.5. Two-, 7- and 14-day moving average forecasts of GI syndrome daily counts for the last year of hospital #7 data.

periodicity in the data should not be a surprise (cf. the discussion on page 83). Also, given that Figures 2.7 and 5.4 show these data have a fairly pronounced seasonal cycle, it is reasonable that the preferred averaging period is relatively short. By way of comparison, the MSE for Hospital #1 is minimized with a 35-day moving average, which is consistent with Figure 2.7, which shows the Hospital #1 data maintain a fairly constant level of GI over time with no pronounced cycles.

The other two metrics used to assess time series model fit are the *mean absolute error* (MAE) and the *mean absolute percent error* (MAPE). They are defined as

$$\text{MAE}\,(\hat{y}) = \frac{1}{n-d} \sum_{t=d+1}^{n} |y_t - \hat{y}_t|, \qquad (5.4)$$

and

$$\text{MAPE}\,(\hat{y}) = \frac{100}{n-d} \sum_{t=d+1}^{n} \left| \frac{y_t - \hat{y}_t}{y_t} \right|, \qquad (5.5)$$

where as in Equation 5.3 the summation starts at time $t = d + 1$ because the forecast is based on the d-period moving average. In general, as with the MSE, the MAE and MAPE are calculated over the set of data for which both an observation and its forecast exist. In terms of Hospital #7, the MAE and MAPE are consistent with the MSE results and indicate that a 7-day moving average is the preferred model for these data.

Figure 5.6 shows the last year of data and associated seven-day moving average, where it shows the the moving average visually follows the data quite well. Figure 5.6 also shows a thirty-day forecast into the future. With a moving average model, the forecast is rather simple; all it consists of is the forecast for the

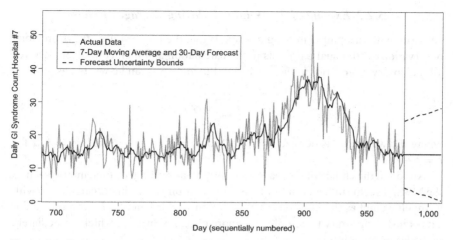

Figure 5.6. Seven-day moving average of hospital #7 GI data with a thirty-day forecast and uncertainty bounds around the forecast.

next period extended indefinitely into the future (as depicted by the horizontal line in the figure after day 980). More sophisticated models yet to be discussed can incorporate trends, cycles, and other systematic effects into the forecast, but not the moving average, and that is a significant limitation of this method for biosurveillance forecasting.

Now, as described in the opening to this chapter, it is important to quantify the uncertainty in any forecast. In Figure 5.6, the uncertainty is depicted as bounds around the forecast (denoted by the dotted lines). If the last observed value is at time t, the bounds are calculated at time $t + j$ as

$$\hat{y}_{t+j} \pm 2\hat{\sigma}_{t+j}, \quad j = 1, 2, 3, \ldots, \tag{5.6}$$

where $\hat{\sigma}_{t+j}$ is the estimated standard deviation of the observed data around the jth period ahead forecast. Unfortunately, there is no underlying statistical theory for how to calculate $\hat{\sigma}_{t+j}$ (Nau, 2012), so it is empirically estimated from the data by calculating

$$\hat{\sigma}_{t+j} = \sqrt{\frac{1}{n - d - j} \sum_{t=d+j+1}^{n} \left(y_t - \hat{y}_{t+j}\right)^2}, \tag{5.7}$$

where $d = 7$ in Figure 5.6.

Readers who have taken a statistics course will recognize the bounds as approximate 95 percent confidence intervals at each time period. They are calculated as the jth period ahead forecast value (which as previously discussed is a constant at value $\hat{y}_{t+j} = \bar{y}_{t+1}$, $j = 1, 2, \ldots$) plus or minus twice the estimated standard deviation for the jth period ahead forecast.

5.2.2 Exponentially Weighted Moving Average Models

An issue with the simple moving average is that the forecast uses the d previous observations with equal emphasis in the calculation and then completely ignores all the observations prior to them. That is, Equation 5.2 can be written as

$$\bar{y}_{t+1} = \sum_{i=1}^{t} w_i y_i, \tag{5.8}$$

where the weight w_i is defined as $w_i = 0$ for $i = 1, \ldots, t - d$ and $w_i = 1/d$ for $i = t - d + 1, \ldots, t$.

Although the choice of d is based on a best fit according to some metric such as the MSE, it seems rather arbitrary to use observation y_{t-d+1} in the calculation with as much weight as the most recent observation y_t, particularly if d is large, and it seems just as arbitrary to completely ignore observation y_{t-d}, which immediately precedes observation y_{t-d+1}.

5.2.2.1 Simple Exponentially Weighted Moving Average Models

An alternative is the *simple EWMA* model that gives successively less weight to observations further back in time according to a user-defined parameter λ, $0 < \lambda \leq 1$. The EWMA forecast is calculated as

$$\hat{y}_{t+1} \triangleq \bar{y}_{t+1} = \lambda y_t + \lambda(1 - \lambda)y_{t-1} + \lambda(1 - \lambda)^2 y_{t-2} + \cdots \tag{5.9}$$

$$= \sum_{i=1}^{t} \lambda(1 - \lambda)^{i-1} y_{t-i+1},$$

where now the weight for observation $t - i + 1$ is $w_i = \lambda(1 - \lambda)^{i-1}$. The forecast $\hat{y}_{t+1}$ is still an average of past observations; however, the more recent the observation, the greater its weight. Note that whereas smaller values of λ put relatively more emphasis on past observations, larger values put more emphasis on recent observations. For $\lambda = 1$, the EWMA forecast reduces to just the last observation: $\hat{y}_{t+1} = y_t$.

Equation 5.9 can be reduced to a simpler recursive equation in which the next forecast value is the weighted average of the current observation and the current forecast:

$$\bar{y}_{t+1} = \lambda y_t + (1 - \lambda)\bar{y}_t. \tag{5.10}$$

Thus, the forecast for the next time period can be calculated with just the value of the current observation y_t and its forecast $\bar{y}_t$. To use Equation 5.10, an initial forecast value $\hat{y}_1$ must be defined. A reasonable choice is $\hat{y}_1 = y_1$ where, because of the exponential smoothing, the effect of this initial choice diminishes rapidly.

The obvious question is how to choose the smoothing parameter λ. Generally speaking, for processes with shifts or short-run trends, larger values of λ are preferred because they put more weight on recent observations and thus make the forecasts more sensitive to shifts. On the other hand, smaller values of λ are better for stationary or nearly stationary data – meaning data that come from a process

Table 5.2. Forecasts for
Example 5.1, where
$\bar{y}_{t+1} = 0.3 \times y_t + 0.7 \times \bar{y}_t$

t	y_t	$\bar{y}_t$
1	7	7
2	13	7.00
3	7	8.80
4	12	8.26
5	11	9.38
6	9	9.87
7	8	9.61
8	9	9.13
9	5	9.09
10	14	7.86
11		9.70

that has few and small trends, cycles, or other changes, if any – because the more stationary the process, the more useful is older data.

The point is that the appropriate choice for λ depends on the specific data being modeled. Thus, a preferred method for choosing λ is by finding the value that minimizes the MSE (or MAE or MAPE, as preferred) on a set of historical data equivalent to what is to be expected in the future. That is essentially an empirical exercise, much like in the previous section with the selection of d.

As in the simple moving average, if the last observed value is at time t, the uncertainty bounds for time $t + j$, $j = 1, 2, 3, \ldots$, are calculated as

$$\bar{y}_{t+j} \pm 2\hat{\sigma}_{y_{t+j}} \tag{5.11}$$

but where

$$\hat{\sigma}_{y_{t+j}} = \hat{\sigma}_{y_t} \sqrt{\frac{\lambda}{2-\lambda}[1-(1-\lambda)^{2j}]}, \tag{5.12}$$

and where, as with the simple moving average, $\bar{y}_{t+j} = \bar{y}_{t+1}$ for $j = 2, 3, 4, \ldots$. What is required, then, is an estimate of the standard deviation of the observations at time t, $\hat{\sigma}_{y_t}$, which is calculated in the usual way (i.e., Equation 4.6 on page 75) from a recent window of the data, $y_{t-d}, y_{t-d+1}, \ldots, y_t$.

Example 5.1. Calculate the EWMA forecasts for times $t = 1, \ldots, 11$, using $\lambda = 0.3$, for the following data:

t	1	2	3	4	5	6	7	8	9	10
y_t	7	13	7	12	11	9	8	9	5	14

Solution: Table 5.2 gives the forecasts, calculated as $\bar{y}_{t+1} = 0.3 \times y_t + 0.7 \times \bar{y}_t$. The forecast for time $t = 11$ is $\bar{y}_{11} = 9.7$. Given that the data were randomly generated from a Poisson distribution with mean $\mu = 10$, the forecast at time 11 is actually quite close to the true value.

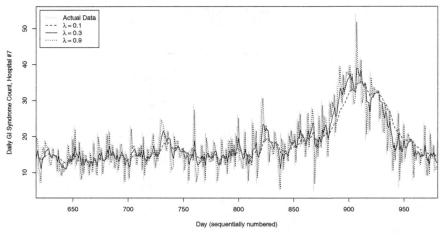

Figure 5.7. A plot of the EWMAs for $\lambda = 0.1, 0.3$, and 0.9 versus the Hospital #7 GI data.

Example 5.2. Returning to the Hospital #7 GI data, calculate the EWMA using $\lambda = 0.1, 0.3$, and 0.9. Plot the moving averages over the data to visually show how they fit to the data. Then determine the value of λ that minimizes the MSE. Compare and contrast the results with the 7-day moving average forecast shown in Figure 5.6.

Solution: Figure 5.7 is a plot of the EWMAs for $\lambda = 0.1, 0.3$, and 0.9 versus the data. As with the moving averages in Figure 5.4, it is difficult to visually discern which of the forecasts best fit the data.

However, looking carefully at Figure 5.7, it does seem that although the forecasts for $\lambda = 0.9$ match quite closely to the prior period, they are often quite a bit off from the data of the forecasted period. For data such as these, where there is quite a bit of volatility in the GI count from day to day, this suggests that smaller values of λ are likely to perform better for forecasting. That said, for $\lambda = 0.1$, it also seems like the forecasts during the spike in GI around day 900 seem to lag behind the actual data. This suggests that values for λ that are excessively small may result in degraded forecasts as well

Figure 5.8 is a plot of MSE versus λ for $0.01 \le \lambda \le 0.99$. It shows that the MSE is minimized at $\lambda = 0.16$ with a value of 32.17. This is slightly less than the MSE for the 7-day moving average (32.8). This suggests the EWMA is a slightly better model for these data than a simple moving average. However, it is important to remember that neither of these models can incorporate trends or cycles into their forecasts, which is a significant impediment to their application to biosurveillance.

Figure 5.9 is the final EWMA model with $\lambda = 0.16$, showing a 90-day forecast and uncertainty bounds.

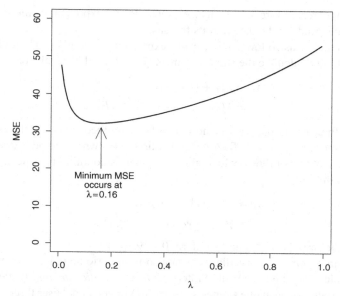

Figure 5.8. A plot of MSE versus λ for an EWMA model of Hospital #7 GI data. MSE is minimized at λ = 0.16, suggesting that this is the preferred choice of the smoothing parameter for these data.

5.2.2.2 More Complex Exponentially Weighted Moving Average Models

For biosurveillance data with trends, a better alternative is *double exponential smoothing*, also referred to as Brown linear exponential smoothing (Brown, 1963, 1959), which not only takes a weighted average of the most recent observation and the most recent forecast but also takes a weighted average of the most recent change

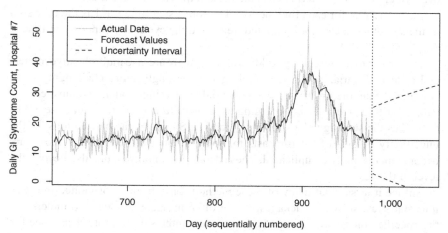

Figure 5.9. A plot of the EWMAs for λ = 0.16 for the hospital #7 GI data with a 90-day forecast and uncertainty bounds. The MSE for this model is 32.206.

and the most recent forecast change. As such, double exponential smoothing can incorporate trends in the data into its forecast.

The model is as follows. First, using exponential smoothing for a chosen λ value, at time t calculate the smoothed mean $\bar{y}_t$ and trend T_t for the data:

$$\bar{y}_t = \lambda y_t + (1 - \lambda)\bar{y}_{t-1},$$
$$T_t = \lambda(\bar{y}_t - \bar{y}_{t-1}) + (1 - \lambda)T_{t-1}. \tag{5.13}$$

Then the forecast at time $t + 1$ is the sum of the smoothed mean and the estimated trend at time t: $\hat{y}_{t+1} = \bar{y}_t + T_t$. A generalization to Brown's method is due to Holt (1957) and Winters (1960), which allows separate smoothing parameters for the mean and the trend:

$$\bar{y}_t = \lambda y_t + (1 - \lambda)\bar{y}_{t-1},$$
$$T_t = \gamma(\bar{y}_t - \bar{y}_{t-1}) + (1 - \gamma)T_{t-1}, \tag{5.14}$$

where as before $0 < \lambda \leq 1$ and similarly $0 < \gamma \leq 1$.

Of course, some biosurveillance data also have periodic (e.g., weekly or seasonal) cycles, for which the Holt-Winters *triple exponential smoothing* model may be appropriate. As the name suggests, the Holt-Winters model uses three weighted averages: the most recent observation and forecast, the most recent change and forecast change, and the most recent cyclical deviation and forecast cycle value.

The triple exponential smoothing model is:

$$\bar{y}_t = \lambda y_t + (1 - \lambda)\bar{y}_{t-1},$$
$$T_t = \gamma(\bar{y}_t - \bar{y}_{t-1}) + (1 - \gamma)T_{t-1},$$
$$S_t = \delta(y_t - \bar{y}_t) + (1 - \delta)S_{t-s}, \tag{5.15}$$

where, as with λ and γ, $0 < \delta \leq 1$. The user chooses s, which is the periodicity over which the cyclical term is calculated, and the calculations must keep track of s S_{t-s} terms, one for each time period. The forecast at time $t + 1$ is then the sum of the smoothed mean, the estimated trend, and the cyclical component at time t: $\hat{y}_{t+1} = \bar{y}_t + T_t + S_t$.

In addition to the foregoing additive models, there are also multiplicative models and a host of variants. These models get increasingly more challenging to fit where, for example, in the triple exponential smoothing model, one must choose values for three parameters according to some criteria (e.g., minimize the MSE) as well as the starting values for $\bar{y}_1$, T_1, and S. Similarly, the calculations for the uncertainty bounds of the forecasts for some number of periods into the future become increasingly complicated. These details are important but also beyond the level of this text.

Suffice it to say that many of these methods have been incorporated into various statistical software packages, which often mitigates the need to understand the specific computational details. For readers interested in more detail, see the Additional Reading section at the end of this chapter. What is most important is that a model is fit to the data that gives both appropriate forecasts, meaning

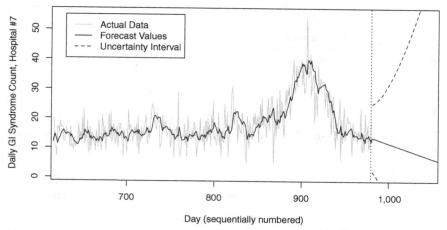

Figure 5.10. A plot of the Holt double exponential model with $\lambda = 0.2$ and $\gamma = 0.06$ for the Hospital #7 GI data with a 90-day forecast and uncertainty bounds.

forecasts that incorporate both trends and cycles as necessary, and that provides correct uncertainty bounds for the forecasts.

Example 5.3. Compare and contrast the EWMA model of the previous example with Holt-Winters double and triple exponential smoothing applied to the Hospital #7 GI data. Use the models to generate ninety-day forecasts and associated uncertainty bounds. Which one of the models is most appropriate for these data?

Solution: Figures 5.10, 5.11, and 5.12 plot the results from fitting a Holt double exponential model, Holt-Winters triple exponential model with $s = 7$, and Holt-Winters triple exponential model with $s = 365$, respectively.[2] For the triple exponential models, $s = 7$ and $s = 365$ were chosen because there is some evidence of a weekly cycle in the data and it is also reasonable to assume that an annual cycle may be present. For comparison, Figure 5.9 plots the results from fitting an EWMA.

Visually, all four models have pros and cons. The simple exponential smoothing model in Figure 5.9 has the desirable feature of being the most simple and visually looks like the forecast is reasonable compared with the past. On the other hand, during the outbreak around day 900, this model would not be able to incorporate the upward and downward trends. In comparison, the double exponential model in Figure 5.10 picks up the trend in the data, but clearly extending the trend out 90 days is unrealistic.

[2] These models were fit using the *R* statistical software package using the `HoltWinters` function to fit the models and the `forecast` library to calculate the forecasts and associated uncertainty bounds.

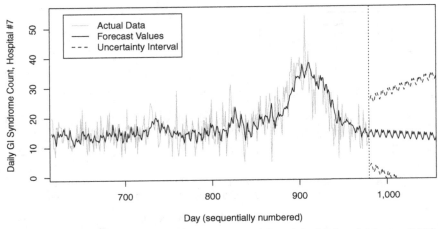

Figure 5.11. A plot of Holt-Winters triple exponential model with $\lambda = 0.16$, $\gamma = 0.003$, $\delta = 0.05$, and $s = 7$ for the Hospital #7 GI data with a 90-day forecast and uncertainty bounds.

Now, the triple exponential model in Figure 5.11 with $s = 7$ can model both trends in the data and a weekly cycle, and the latter is evident in the prediction (and incorporated into the uncertainty bounds). However, the forecast weekly cycle seems to strongly reflect the cycle in the last few weeks of the data, which does not seem to be as visually present in the earlier part of the data. Finally, the triple exponential model in Figure 5.12 with $s = 365$ can model both trends in the data and annual cycles in the data. Here the forecast is much noisier than any of the other models, but in some ways it looks much more realistic. However, it is not clear visually whether this model is or is not modeling the data particularly well.

To quantitatively compare the model fits, Table 5.3 gives the MSE, MAE, and MAPE for each. The table shows that the double exponential model fits least well followed by the triple exponential model with $s = 7$. In terms of the simple exponential model and the triple exponential model with $s = 365$, the simple exponential model has the smallest MSE, and the triple exponential model has the smallest MAE and MAPE. The former suggests that the triple exponential model can result in large deviations from the actual counts, which when squared results in an inflated MSE, but that the deviations on average are smaller than those with the simple exponential model.

It is interesting to note that the two triple exponential models achieve essentially the same MSE, which suggests that there is benefit to incorporating both a weekly and annual cycle into a forecast model. Unfortunately, the standard Holt-Winters triple exponential model, as defined in Equation 5.15, can only explicitly incorporate the period of one cycle.

Table 5.3. MSE, MAE, and MAPE for exponential models fit to Hospital #7 data

Model	λ	γ	δ	s	MSE	MAE	MAPE
Simple Exponential	0.16	–	–	–	32.206	4.163	0.314
Double Exponential	0.2	0.06	–	–	34.267	4.364	0.322
Triple Exponential	0.16	0.003	0.05	7	33.035	4.219	0.311
Triple Exponential	0.14	0.0	0.63	365	32.995	3.820	0.249

5.3 Regression-Based Models

Linear regression is a statistical methodology typically used for modeling the relationship between a "dependent variable" (usually denoted as y) and one or more "independent" or explanatory variables (usually denoted as $x_1, \ldots, x_p, p \geq 1$). With only one independent variable, the model is often referred to as simple linear regression; when there is more than one independent variable, it is referred to as multiple regression.

Linear regression is typically applied to cross-sectional data, where the dependent variable is modeled as a linear function of the independent variables. The unknown model parameters (intercept and slope or partial slopes) are estimated from the data. This section begins with an explanation of linear regression in the standard cross-sectional data context and then proceeds to describe approaches to applying linear regression to time series data and particularly biosurveillance data.

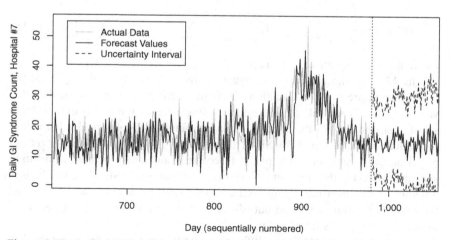

Figure 5.12. A plot of Holt-Winters triple exponential model with $\lambda = 0.14$, $\gamma = 0.0$, $\delta = 0.63$, and $s = 365$ for the Hospital #7 GI data with a ninety-day forecast and uncertainty bounds.

5.3.1 Linear Regression

Simple linear regression models a dependent variable as a linear function of a single independent variable. Mathematically, the model is

$$y = \beta_0 + \beta_1 x + \epsilon, \tag{5.16}$$

where β_0 and β_1 are the true (and unobserved) intercept and slope, and ϵ is the error term that can be interpreted as random noise. The standard assumptions for a linear regression model are:

- There is a linear relationship between y and x.
- The error term is a random variable from a symmetric distribution with mean zero and constant variance. Often it is assumed that the error term is normally distributed, and then the assumption can be expressed as $\epsilon \sim N(0, \sigma_\epsilon^2)$.

Note that from these assumptions it follows that for a given value of x, the dependent variable has a normal distribution with mean $\beta_0 + \beta_1 x$ and variance σ_ϵ^2. Often this is written as $Y_x \sim N(\beta_0 + \beta_1 x, \sigma_\epsilon^2)$. The key take-away of this result is that the dependent variable must be continuous for linear regression modeling to be appropriate.

When fitting a linear regression model, the slope and intercept are estimated from data, $\{(y_1, x_1), (y_2, x_2), \ldots, (y_n, x_n)\}$, so that they minimize the mean square error. This is often referred to as *least squares* or *ordinary least squares*. Denoting the estimated intercept and slope as $\hat{\beta}_0$ and $\hat{\beta}_1$, the fitted model is

$$\hat{y}_i = \hat{\beta}_0 + \hat{\beta}_1 x_i, i = 1, \ldots, n, \tag{5.17}$$

and the chosen values of $\hat{\beta}_0$ and $\hat{\beta}_1$ minimize the mean square error *of the residuals*

$$\text{MSE}(\hat{\epsilon}) = \frac{1}{n-2} \sum_{i=1}^{n} (y_i - \hat{y}_i)^2 = \frac{1}{n-2} \sum_{i=1}^{n} \left(y_i - (\hat{\beta}_0 + \hat{\beta}_1 x_i) \right)^2, \tag{5.18}$$

where the residuals are defined as $\hat{\epsilon}_i = y_i - \hat{y}_i, i = 1, \ldots, n$.

The MSE of the residuals is fundamentally different from the MSE of the forecasts first presented in Equation 5.3. With the MSE of the residuals, the fitted values $\hat{y}_1, \ldots, \hat{y}_n$ are calculated based on a single regression model fit to a single set of data, and each of the fitted values corresponds to an observed value within the sample of data. For the MSE of the forecast, the $\hat{y}_{t+1}$ values are forecasts based on prior data, and each of the forecasted values may be based on fitting separate models to different sets of prior data. Hence, the MSE of the residuals is a within-sample measure of how well a single model fits a single set of data, and the MSE of the forecasts is an out-of-sample measure of how well a forecasting methodology predicts future values.

Given that the two MSEs are different, it should not be a surprise that the 2 in the denominator in Equation 5.18 is not equivalent to the d in Equation 5.3. The reason for subtracting 2 from n in Equation 5.18 is that the MSE is an unbiased estimate of σ_ϵ^2.

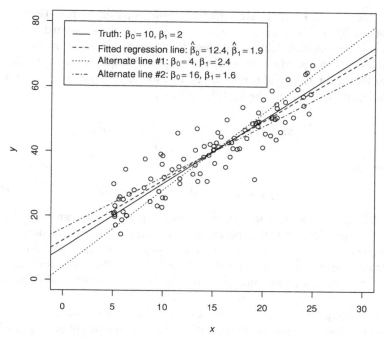

Figure 5.13. A regression line fit to a simulated set of data, for $n = 100$ simulated paired observations of dependent and independent variables, with $\hat{\beta}_0 = 12.4$ and $\hat{\beta}_1 = 1.9$. Also shown is the "true" line ($\beta_0 = 10$ and $\beta_1 = 2$), from which the data were simulated, and two other lines for comparison.

Figure 5.13 illustrates a regression line fit to a simulated set of data, where in the simulation $\beta_0 = 10$ and $\beta_1 = 2$. For the $n = 100$ simulated paired observations of dependent and independent variables shown, the fitted regression line has an estimated intercept $\hat{\beta}_0 = 12.4$ and estimated slope $\hat{\beta}_1 = 1.9$. Also shown are two other lines for visual comparison.

The fitted regression line differs from the true line because of randomness in the data, which occurs because of the error term in Equation 5.16. For the simulated data, $\epsilon \sim N(0, \sqrt{5})$. The randomness arising from the error term is evident in Figure 5.13 because of the way data are distributed around the line.

As previously discussed, the fitted regression line achieves the smallest MSE for this set of data, even when compared with the MSE for the true line. It is literally the line that "best fits" the data according to the criteria of minimizing the mean square error.

Multiple linear regression is similar to simple linear regression but with more independent variables. For p independent variables, the model is

$$y = \beta_0 + \beta_1 x_1 + \beta_2 x_2 + \cdots + \beta_p x_p + \epsilon$$

$$= \beta_0 + \sum_{i=1}^{p} \beta_i x_i + \epsilon, \tag{5.19}$$

where the β_i, $i = 1, \ldots, p$, are referred to now as partial slopes. The same assumptions from simple linear regression apply, with the additional assumption that the independent variables (and linear functions of subsets of the independent variables) are independent, or nearly so. As with simple linear regression, the values for the intercept and partial slopes are estimated from the data so that they minimize the MSE, where the MSE is defined as

$$\text{MSE}\,(\hat{y}) = \frac{1}{n - p - 1} \sum_{i=1}^{n} (y_i - \hat{y}_i)^2, \tag{5.20}$$

and where

$$\hat{y}_i = \hat{\beta}_0 + \hat{\beta}_1 x_{i,1} + \hat{\beta}_2 x_{i,2} + \cdots + \hat{\beta}_p x_{i,p}. \tag{5.21}$$

This definition for MSE is actually the general expression for regression, and that given in Equation 5.18 is the specific form for simple linear regression. That is, in simple linear regression, $p = 1$ and thus $n - p - 1$ in Equation 5.20 becomes $n - 2$ for simple linear regression. As in Equation 5.18, the reason for subtracting $p + 1$ from n in the denominator is that the MSE is an unbiased estimator of σ_ϵ^2.

Multiple regression allows for fitting more complicated models, not only in the sense of adding more independent variables but also in terms of adding quadratic and higher order terms, which then allows for a nonlinear relationship between the dependent variable and the independent variable or variables. For example, consider the case of just one independent variable x but for which there is a quadratic relationship between y and x. This can be modeled as

$$y = \beta_0 + \beta_1 x + \beta_2 x^2 + \epsilon. \tag{5.22}$$

Now, although the dependent variable must be continuous, independent variables can be either continuous or discrete. For example, consider a multiple regression model where y is patient weight and the goal is to model weight as a function of age and gender. Denote age, a continuous variable, by x and denote gender, a binary variable, by I. The use of the I notation is to emphasize that this is an *indicator* variable, where $I = 0$ means the patient is female and $I = 1$ means the patient is male. The model, then, is

$$y = \beta_0 + \beta_1 x + \beta_2 I + \epsilon. \tag{5.23}$$

The resulting model assumes that the lines fitted for men and women have the same slopes but different intercepts. That is, with a little algebra, Equation 5.23 reduces to

$$y = \begin{cases} \beta_0 + \beta_1 x + \epsilon, & \text{for female patients (i.e., } I = 0) \\ (\beta_0 + \beta_2) + \beta_1 x + \epsilon, & \text{for male patients (i.e., } I = 1), \end{cases} \tag{5.24}$$

where the slopes for both males and females is β_1, and the intercept is β_0 for females and $\beta_0 + \beta_2$ for males.

For a categorical variable with m levels, $m - 1$ indicator variables are required in the linear regression model. Furthermore, if m indicator variables are used, a regression model cannot be fit because the model violates the assumption of independence (because membership in any category is completely defined by knowledge of the other $m - 1$ categories). Thus, for example, six indicator variables are used in a regression model to account for day-of-the-week effects in biosurveillance data (for a 7-day week).

Now, the assumption of equal slope for males and females in Equations 5.23 and 5.24 may not be realistic. Different slopes can be accommodated with *interaction terms*. For example, consider the model

$$y = \beta_0 + \beta_1 x + \beta_2 I + \beta_3 x I + \epsilon, \tag{5.25}$$

where x and I are defined as before. The model can be restated as

$$y = \begin{cases} \beta_0 + \beta_1 x + \epsilon, & \text{for female patients} \\ (\beta_0 + \beta_2) + (\beta_1 + \beta_3)x + \epsilon, & \text{for male patients,} \end{cases} \tag{5.26}$$

where the intercepts by gender are the same as before, and so is the slope of the line for females, but the slope for males is now $\beta_1 + \beta_3$.

Depending on the complexity of the data and the phenomenon being modeled, even more complicated models can be fit. For example, quadratic terms could be added to Equation 5.25 to allow for nonlinearities. However, all of the regression models described thus far are cross-sectional in nature and thus of limited use for biosurveillance forecasting. That said, as the next section shows, regression can be adapted for use with time series data.

5.3.2 Autoregression

An *autoregressive (AR) model* is similar to the regression models of the previous section, but they are applied to time series data and use previous values of the dependent variable for predicting the current value of the dependent variable. An autoregression model of order p, denoted AR(p), is

$$y_t = \beta_0 + \sum_{i=1}^{p} \beta_i y_{t-i} + \epsilon, \tag{5.27}$$

where the term *order* refers to the maximum time lag used in the model. The simplest model is an AR(1), where the current value of y only depends on the last value:

$$y_t = \beta_0 + \beta_1 y_{t-1} + \epsilon. \tag{5.28}$$

As with the exponential models, autoregressive models can be challenging to fit where, for example, the choice of p requires fitting multiple models, and the appropriate calculations for the uncertainty bounds of the forecasts can be quite complicated. These details are important but, as with the exponential models, the

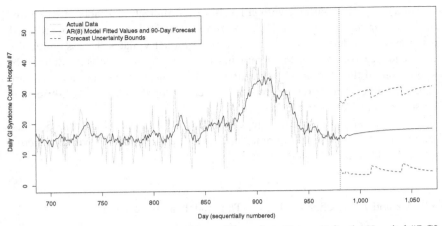

Figure 5.14. A plot of the autoregression model results with $p = 8$ for the Hospital #7 GI data with a ninety-day forecast and uncertainty bounds.

use of a good statistical software package will take care of the computational intricacies.

Example 5.4. Fit an autoregressive model to the Hospital #7 GI data, determining the order and coefficients that result in a "best fit." Compare and contrast this model with the exponential models in Example 5.3. Is the autoregressive model more or less appropriate for these data?

Solution: Figure 5.14 shows the best fit autoregressive model,[3] for order $p = 8$, which is

$$y_t = \beta_0 + 0.178y_{t-1} + 0.099y_{t-2} + 0.067y_{t-3} + 0.108y_{t-4}$$
$$+ 0.090y_{t-5} + 0.153y_{t-6} + 0.085y_{t-7} + 0.081y_{t-8}.$$

Note how the forecast quickly smooths out after it has extended just a couple of multiples of the order into the future. Also note that the figure shows an interesting pattern in the uncertainty bounds that occurs about every thirty days or so. Why this is occurring is not clear, but it is also not particularly important because, for biosurveillance, forecasts of a week or two into the future are of primary interest, and the forecasts will be refit each day anyway.

For the autoregressive model, MSE = 31.753, MAE = 4.179, and MAPE = 0.314. Comparing these with those from the exponential models in Table 5.3, the autoregressive model metrics are equal to or less than the minimum values across all of the exponential models. This suggests that the autoregressive model is a better model to use with the Hospital #7 data.

---

[3] The model was fit using the `ar` function in R.

5.3.3 Adaptive Regression

Burkom *et al.* (2006) first proposed the *adaptive regression model with sliding baseline* to model the systematic component of syndromic surveillance data. The idea is as follows. At time t, fit a linear regression of the observations from the past n days, $\{y_t, y_{t-1}, \ldots, y_{t-n+1}\}$, on time relative to the current period as represented by the set of integers $\{n, n-1, \ldots, 1\}$. That is, the data for the regression are $\{(y_t, n), (y_{t-1}, n-1), \ldots, (y_{t-n+1}, 1)\}$, where the integers are the "independent variables" and where it is assumed that $t \geq n$.

The model for day i, $t \geq i \geq t - n + 1$, is

$$y_i = \beta_0 + \beta_1 \times (i - t + n) + \epsilon, \tag{5.29}$$

where the model is fit using ordinary least squares and, as with other linear regression models, ϵ is the error term that is assumed to follow a symmetric distribution with mean 0 and standard deviation σ_ϵ.

The "with sliding baseline" in the name means to repeat this process each day, always using the most recent n observations as the sliding baseline in the regression to calculate the forecast for time $t + 1$. That is, having fit the regression at time t, use the slope and intercept from the data, $\hat{\beta}_0(t)$ and $\hat{\beta}_1(t)$, where the t in parentheses is intended to stress that the slope and intercept will be re-estimated at each time period, to forecast the observation for the next time period as

$$\hat{y}_{t+1} = \hat{\beta}_0(t) + (n+1) \times \beta_1(t). \tag{5.30}$$

When using regression to predict future observations, the question naturally arises as to how much historical data should be used for the regression's sliding baseline. Burkom *et al.* (2006) recommended an eight-week sliding baseline ($n = 56$ for a seven-day week). In a simulation study, Fricker *et al.* (2008a) found that the optimal n varied depending on the data, ranging from $n = 15$ to $n = 56$ time periods, where the optimal choice was based on minimizing the MSE of the forecast.

All other factors being equal, regressions based on a shorter sliding baseline will less accurately model the underlying systematic effects in the data than those based on longer sliding baselines. However, although a longer sliding baseline theoretically should allow for fitting a more detailed regression model, the longer sliding baseline will also make the resulting forecasts less responsive to quick changes in disease incidence. Furthermore, in syndromic surveillance, the amount of available data may be limited, and older data may be of less relevance because of changing trends or phenomena. Hence, there is a trade-off to be made between the amount of historical data used in a particular model and the predictive accuracy of that model.

As shown in Fricker *et al.* (2008a), the standard deviation of the forecast error at time $t + 1$ for a simple linear adaptive regression is

$$\sigma_{t+1} = \sigma_\epsilon \sqrt{\frac{(n+2)(n+1)}{n(n-1)}}, \tag{5.31}$$

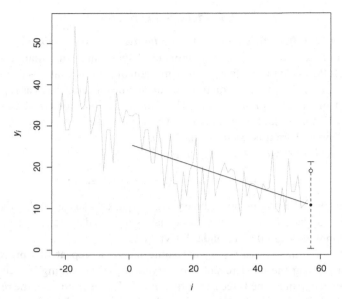

Figure 5.15. An adaptive regression line fit to Hospital #7 daily GI syndrome counts for days 924 to 979. The dark dot is the predicted value, the dotted line shows the uncertainty bounds for the predicted value, and the white dot is the actual value for day 980.

where σ_ϵ is the standard deviation of ϵ in Equation 5.30 and σ_{t+1} is the standard deviation of the prediction error at time $t + 1$. Because σ_ϵ will not be known, it is estimated from the data as the square root of the MSE (often referred to as the *root mean square error* or RMSE) in Equation 5.20 and then used in Equation 5.33 to estimate σ_{t+1}.

Figures 5.15 and 5.16 illustrate the application of the adaptive regression method to the Hospital #7 GI data. Specifically, Figure 5.15 shows the adaptive regression line with $n = 56$ fit to the daily counts, for days 924 to 979. The dark dot is the forecast for day 980 ($\hat{y}_{980} = 10.78$), the white dot is the actual value for day 980 ($y_{980} = 19$), and the dotted line denotes the uncertainty bounds around $\hat{y}_{980}$.

To calculate the uncertainty bounds, σ_ϵ is estimated from the data (using Equation 5.20) as $\hat{\sigma}_\epsilon = 5.14$. Then the uncertainty bounds for $\hat{y}_{980}$, calculated as a 95% prediction interval, is

$$\hat{y}_{980} \pm 1.96\sigma_{980} = \hat{y}_{980} \pm 1.96 \times 5.14\sqrt{\frac{(58)(57)}{(56)(55)}} = 10.78 \pm 10.44.$$

As Figure 5.15 shows, the actual observed count for day 980 falls within the uncertainty bounds.

Figure 5.16 illustrates how the adaptive regression adjusts to the sliding baseline of the most recent n observations. In the figure, the lines are the adaptive regressions for the last month of Hospital #7 daily GI syndrome counts, and the

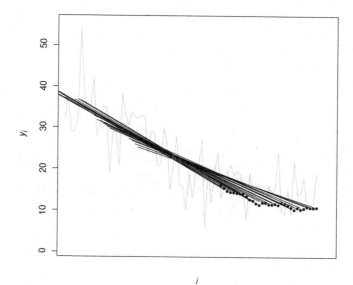

i

Figure 5.16. Adaptive regression lines used to predict the last month of Hospital #7 daily GI syndrome counts.

dots are their associated predicted values for the next day, where each regression line is based on the previous $n = 56$ observations. The figure shows how regression lines change over time, conforming to "best fit" the sliding baseline of data. As a result, the predictions follow the trends in the data.

As with other regression models, Equation 5.30 can also be adapted to allow for nonlinearities and other effects by adding additional terms into the equation. For example, a model that also includes day-of-the-week effects (for a seven-day week) is

$$y_i = \beta_0 + \beta_1 \times (i - t + n) + \beta_2 I_{\text{Mon}} + \beta_3 I_{\text{Tues}} \\ + \beta_4 I_{\text{Wed}} + \beta_5 I_{\text{Thurs}} + \beta_6 I_{\text{Fri}} + \beta_7 I_{\text{Sat}} + \epsilon, \qquad (5.32)$$

where the Is are indicator variables – $I = 1$ on the relevant day of the week and $I = 0$ otherwise – and ϵ is the error term, which is assumed to follow a symmetric distribution with mean 0 and standard deviation σ_ϵ.

It is important to note that the appropriate calculations for the standard deviation of the forecast error at time $t + 1$ depend on the form of the regression, where for the model in Equation 5.32, Fricker *et al.* (2008a) showed

$$\sigma_{t+1} = \sigma_\epsilon \sqrt{\frac{(n + 7)(n - 4)}{n(n - 7)}}. \qquad (5.33)$$

Also, although the data may contain nonlinearities, a linear model may still provide good predictions. See Fricker *et al.* (2008a) for additional details.

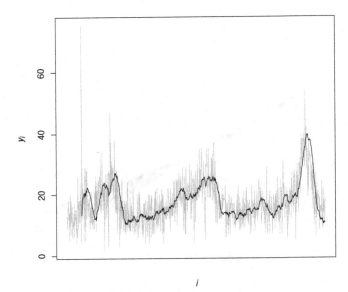

Figure 5.17. Forecasts from a simple linear adaptive regression model with a sliding base-line of size $n = 56$. The gray line shows the actual data, and the black line shows the forecasts. Visually, the forecasts have a noticeable delay in reflecting the trends in the data.

Example 5.5. For the hospital #7 GI syndromic surveillance data, determine the optimal value of n, where "optimal" means minimizing the MSE of the forecast.

Solution: Figure 5.17 shows the forecasts from a simple linear adaptive regression model with a sliding baseline of size $n = 56$. The gray line shows the actual data, and the black line shows the forecasts, and visually it looks like the forecasts have a noticeable delay in reflecting the trends in the data. In fact, the forecast MSE is 36.903, which is substantially worse than the EWMA and autoregressive models of Examples 5.3 and 5.4.

Figure 5.18 shows the forecast values for the optimal simple linear adaptive regression model which, for the Hospital #7 GI data, is $n = 30$. Using a sliding baseline of size $n = 30$ results in a forecast MSE of 34.919, which is a substantial improvement, and a visual comparison of the two figures shows the fit is better. However, for these data, it seems adaptive regression does not perform nearly as well as either autoregressive or exponential smoothing models. This result is consistent with that of Burkom *et al.* (2006).

5.4 ARMA and ARIMA Models

ARMA and ARIMA models are a general class of models useful for forecasting many different types of time series data. The acronyms stand for *autoregressive*

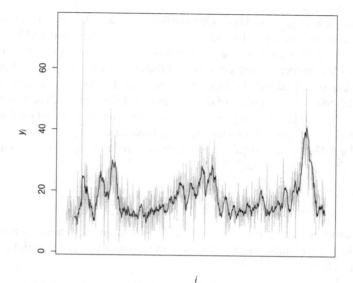

Figure 5.18. Forecasts from a simple linear adaptive regression model with a sliding baseline of size $n = 30$. The gray line shows the actual data, and the black line shows the forecasts. Compared with Figure 5.17, the forecasts more closely track with the actual data.

moving average and *autoregressive integrated moving average* models. Along with the smoothing and regression-based models of the previous sections, ARMA and ARIMA models are useful for modeling autocorrelated time series data.

5.4.1 Autoregressive Moving Average Models

Given time series data $\{y_1, y_2, \ldots, y_t\}$, an ARMA($p,q$) model consists of two parts, an autoregressive part and a moving average part, where p is the order of the autoregressive part of the model and q is the order of the moving average part.

The autoregressive part of the model is just as described in Section 5.3.2. However, in this section, so that the notation is consistent with conventions in the literature, the coefficients for an AR(p) model will be denoted by $\phi_0, \phi_1, \ldots, \phi_p$.

On the other hand, the moving average part of the model is *not* the same as the moving average models presented in Section 5.2.1. Rather, in the context of ARMA models (and ARIMA models in the next section), a first-order moving average model, MA(1), is

$$\hat{y}_t = \theta_0 + \epsilon_t - \theta_1 \epsilon_{t-1}, \tag{5.34}$$

where the ϵ's are assumed to have a normal distribution with mean zero and constant variance. For a qth-order moving average model, MA(q), the model is

$$\hat{y}_t = \theta_0 + \epsilon_t - \sum_{i=1}^{q} \theta_i \epsilon_{t-i}. \tag{5.35}$$

A moving average model is similar to a linear regression of the current value of the series against the q previous error terms. The distinction in the MA(q) model is that the error terms are propagated forward into future values of the time series. Fitting an MA model is more complicated than the AR models because the error terms are unobserved and the MA models are also harder to interpret compared with AR models. As with some of the previous modeling approaches, the details of model fitting will be left to a good statistical software package, and interpretation of the model is of less interest than accurate forecasts.

For the ARMA(p,q) model, the autoregressive and moving average components are combined into one model:

$$\hat{y}_t = \phi_0 + \sum_{i=1}^{p} \phi_i y_{t-i} + \epsilon_t - \sum_{i=1}^{q} \theta_i \epsilon_{t-i}. \tag{5.36}$$

Quite complex models can result if p and q are large. A standard strategy is to try to identify parsimonious models, meaning models with small p and q, that fit the data well.

Example 5.6. Fit an ARMA model to the Hospital #7 GI data, determining p and q that minimize the forecast MSE. Compare and contrast this model with the previous models. Is the ARMA model to be preferred for these data?

Solution: The optimal model is ARMA(8,6),[4] which achieves a forecast MSE of 30.516. Thus, the addition of the moving average portion of the ARMA model improves the fit over the pure autoregressive model of Example 5.4 and is better than the EWMA models fit in Example 5.3. Hence, the ARMA(8,6) model is the preferred model for the Hospital #7 GI syndromic surveillance data.

5.4.2 Autoregressive Integrated Moving Average Models

An ARIMA model is a generalization of the ARMA model that is used for longitudinal data with long-term trends. An initial differencing step (which is the "integrated" part of the model) is used to first remove the trend prior to fitting the autoregressive and/or moving average coefficients.

The model is generally denoted as ARIMA(p,d,q), where p, d, and q are the order values of the autoregressive, integrated, and moving average parts of the model. When one or more of the terms is zero, the ARIMA model reduces to a simpler form, many of which have already been discussed. For example, an ARIMA(1,0,0) is a pure first-order autoregressive model, and an ARIMA(8,0,6) model is the ARMA(8,6) model that gave the optimal fit in Example 5.6.

To fit an ARIMA model, the first step is to identify the order of differencing (i.e., d) needed to remove the long-term trend or trends in the data. No trend in the data is modeled by setting $d = 0$, a linear trend is modeled by setting $d = 1$, and

---

[4] The model was fit in R using the `arima` function.

a quadratic trend is modeled by $d = 2$. In terms of biosurveillance, these types of trends might arise if the population being monitored is either growing or shrinking over time, and that change is reflected in the rate of patients presenting.

Example 5.7. Fit an ARIMA model to the Hospital #7 GI data, determining the p, d, and q that minimize the forecast MSE. Compare and contrast this model with the optimal ARMA model of Example 5.6. Is the optimal ARIMA model to be preferred over the optimal ARMA for these data?

Solution: The optimal model is of order $d = 0$, so the ARMA(8,6) of Example 5.6 is the best model. This should actually be intuitive from the plot of the Hospital #7 data where there are short-term fluctuations in the data, corresponding to seasonal outbreaks and day-to-day noise, but the plots do not show any sort of sustained long-term trends. That is, after each outbreak, the time series returns to a non-outbreak state that is characterized by a very constant average of about 14 patients per day presenting with GI syndrome symptoms.

5.5 Change Point Analysis

Change point analysis (Taylor, 2012a) is a retrospective analytical approach useful for identifying discrete points in time at which the mean of a time series has changed. Although not a forecasting method, when it is applied to non-stationary biosurveillance data, it is useful for helping to determine when changes, such as outbreaks, start and end.

The idea of change point analysis (CPA) is to model time series data with a set of sample means calculated from contiguous sequences of the data. The time periods immediately after the end of each contiguous sequence are the "change points," where they represent the times at which the mean of the time series has changed. CPA is a computationally intensive method that uses a number of statistical techniques beyond the scope of this book (particularly the bootstrap) and some that are discussed in later chapters (namely a variant of the cumulative sum [CUSUM] described in Chapter 7).

The idea of CPA, however, is straightforward to describe. It works as follows. CPA begins by modeling time series simply using the sample mean calculated from all the data, which is the same as assuming there are no change points. That is, for a set of data $y_1, \ldots, y_t$, the sample mean is

$$\bar{y} = \frac{1}{t} \sum_{i=1}^{t} y_i \tag{5.37}$$

and using MSE as a measure of fit,

$$\text{MSE}_0 = \frac{1}{t} \sum_{i=1}^{t} (y_i - \bar{y})^2 . \tag{5.38}$$

That is, in the first stage, the model assumes that the fitted values for the data are all equal to the sample mean: $\hat{y}_i = \bar{y}, i = 1, \ldots, t$.

Next, a change point k is identified, $1 < k \leq t$, and the model is redefined so that each part of the data is now modeled by its associated sample mean. Thus, given a change point is identified, there are now two sample means,

$$\bar{y}_1 = \frac{1}{k-1} \sum_{i=1}^{k-1} y_i \text{ and } \bar{y}_2 = \frac{1}{t-k+1} \sum_{i=k}^{t} y_i, \tag{5.39}$$

and the MSE is calculated as

$$\text{MSE}_1 = \frac{1}{k-1} \sum_{i=1}^{k-1} (y_i - \bar{y}_1)^2 + \frac{1}{t-k+1} \sum_{i=k}^{t} (y_i - \bar{y}_2)^2 . \tag{5.40}$$

Now the model is $\hat{y}_i = \bar{y}_1$ for $i = 1, \ldots, k-1$ and $\hat{y}_i = \bar{y}_2$ for $i = k, \ldots, t$ and, if this model fits better than the previous one, $\text{MSE}_1 < \text{MSE}_0$.

In the next step, each of of the two segments of the data is examined for change points. For each segment, if a change point is identified, then the method proceeds as in the previous step.

For example, imagine that change points j and l are identified, one in each segment of the data, so that there are now three change points: $1 < j < k < l \leq t$. Then there are four sample means,

$$\bar{y}_1 = \frac{1}{j-1} \sum_{i=1}^{j-1} y_i, \bar{y}_2 = \frac{1}{k-j} \sum_{i=j}^{k-1} y_i,$$

$$\bar{y}_3 = \frac{1}{l-k} \sum_{i=k}^{l-1} y_i, \quad \text{and} \quad \bar{y}_4 = \frac{1}{t-l+1} \sum_{i=l}^{t} y_i, \tag{5.41}$$

and the MSE is

$$\text{MSE}_2 = \frac{1}{j-1} \sum_{i=1}^{j-1} (y_i - \bar{y}_1)^2 + \frac{1}{k-j} \sum_{i=j}^{k-1} (y_i - \bar{y}_2)^2$$

$$+ \frac{1}{l-k} \sum_{i=k}^{l-1} (y_i - \bar{y}_3)^2 + \frac{1}{t-l+1} \sum_{i=l}^{t} (y_i - \bar{y}_4)^2 . \tag{5.42}$$

The model at this stage is $\hat{y}_i = \bar{y}_1$ for $i = 1, \ldots, j-1, \hat{y}_i = \bar{y}_2$ for $i = j, \ldots, k-1$, $\hat{y}_i = \bar{y}_3$ for $i = k, \ldots, l-1$, and $\hat{y}_i = \bar{y}_4$ for $i = l, \ldots, t$, and the method continues to iterate until no more change points are found.

Figure 5.19 shows the results of applying CPA to the Hospital #7 GI syndrome data, where CPA identified 19 change points. The sample means seem to visually well describe the data, although in the last outbreak period around day 900, the discrete steps of the sample means look to be a bit artificial.

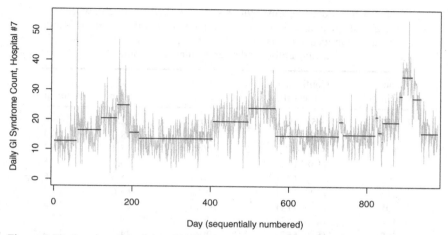

Figure 5.19. Results of applying CPA to the Hospital #7 GI syndrome data, where CPA identified 19 change points. The sample means seem to visually well describe the data, although in the last outbreak period around day 900, the discrete steps of the sample means look to be a bit artificial.

Table 5.4 shows the results output from Taylor's software (Taylor, 2012b), where the specific change points are identified along with confidence intervals and associated confidence levels for each change point, as well as the sample means before and after each change point.

Now, the previous description of CPA is not quite accurate as reduction in MSE is not the criteria for determining either whether to include a change point or when to stop the procedure. Indeed, if that was the stopping criterion, the procedure would not stop until the time series was divided up into t segments each composed only of one point (because then the MSE is zero). Rather, the CPA uses a cumulative sum (CUSUM) method to identify candidate change points and the bootstrap to determine if candidate change points are statistically significant (and thus should be kept). In addition, Taylor (2012a) recommends using a backward elimination procedure to ensure that as candidate change points are added that the previously identified change points remain statistically significant (and, if not, are removed). Readers interested in the details should consult Taylor (2012a) and Kass-Hout *et al.* (2012).

It is important to mention that the bootstrap methodology as implemented in the software used to find the change points in the Hospital #7 GI data and as posted on the collaborative site assumes the data are not autocorrelated. That is clearly not true in general for biosurveillance data, although the results as shown in Figure 5.19 look reasonable. Nonetheless, additional research is required to modify

---

[5] In addition to Taylor's software, a collaborative site has been established with open source software developed specifically for biosurveillance: https://sites.google.com/site/changepointanalysis/.

Table 5.4. CPA output from Taylor's software (Taylor, 2012b), where the specific change points are identified along with confidence intervals and associated confidence levels for each change point, as well as the sample means before and after each change point

Change point	Confidence interval	Confidence level	From mean	To mean
57	(57, 58)	100%	12.6	48.0
59	(58, 59)	94%	48.0	16.4
119	(94, 141)	100%	16.4	20.3
160	(138, 190)	99%	20.3	25.6
192	(187, 195)	100%	25.6	15.6
216	(193, 395)	92%	15.6	13.5
405	(399, 414)	100%	13.5	19.4
496	(485, 515)	100%	19.4	24.3
565	(560, 567)	100%	24.3	14.7
727	(718, 730)	100%	14.7	20.3
738	(735, 752)	93%	20.3	14.9
820	(815, 822)	91%	14.9	23.7
827	(822, 828)	96%	23.7	16.4
836	(835, 836)	96%	16.4	6.5
838	(838, 845)	93%	6.5	19.3
881	(870, 883)	93%	19.3	27.0
889	(887, 896)	100%	27.0	35.4
915	(911, 921)	100%	35.4	27.6
937	(934, 938)	99%	27.6	15.8

the software so that it appropriately handles autocorrelated data. One possibility is to first preprocess the data by modeling the systematic components in the data using one of the methods in this chapter and then use CPA on the residuals that remain after the systematic effects are subtracted.

Returning to the application of CPA to biosurveillance, CPA is most relevant for establishing situational awareness level 2 (comprehension) and technically it belongs in Chapter 4. However, it is included here because it is also closely related to the problem of early event detection and thus is something of a bridge to Chapters 6 to 8. CPA is included here with the other methods for situational awareness because it is most useful for retrospective analyses of time series data. In comparison, EED is focused on prospectively identifying changes.

Indeed, CPA has been implemented in BioSense 2.0 expressly for the purpose of improving SA and augmenting the early event detection methods. As the current director of the Centers for Disease Control and Prevention's (CDC's) Division of Informatics Solutions and Operations said,

When we combined forecasting with CPA, we were actually able to get timely picture of the situation and to answer questions; such as, is the incidence going up, down or is stable and when combined with EARS [Early Aberration Reporting System] we were able to make sure not to miss sudden or subtle changes. (Kass-Hout, 2012a)

5.6 Discussion and Summary

This chapter began with the use of statistical models for preprocessing biosurveillance data and then came full circle back to the application of preprocessing when CPA is used for autocorrelated biosurveillance data. Preprocessing is also important for the proper application of many of the EED methods discussed in Chapters 6 to 8. As with CPA, most of these methods are designed for data that are not autocorrelated. Given that autocorrelation is inherent in biosurveillance data, preprocessing can be used to eliminate, or at least mitigate, autocorrelation by first modeling and removing the systematic effects in the data and then using CPA and the EED methods on the residuals.

The main focus of this chapter is on statistical models useful for the projection step of SA, including smoothing, regression-based, and time series models. The examples in this chapter were almost all centered around one set of data, for which it turned out that an ARMA model gave the best forecasts. However, this is not a general result, and it is almost surely true that other models will be better for other types and sets of data. What is generally true is that no one method will be universally applicable or optimal. Biosurveillance system designers and operators should allow for and apply a suite of modeling tools to find and then use the best model.

Despite its length, this chapter has really only scratched the surface of smoothing, regression, and time series modeling. Each of these topics is worthy of, and indeed is the subject of, numerous textbooks. This chapter has mainly introduced the general ideas of each of the types of models and illustrated their application to biosurveillance data via the examples. Not mentioned in this chapter are the details and and intricacies of model fitting, including model diagnostics for checking whether assumptions are violated and numerous model variants and extensions. Readers interested in learning more about a particular methodology should consult one or more of the references in the Additional Reading section.

Additional Reading

For those who would like to delve more deeply into the material consider:

- For additional reading on preprocessing, including other methods and applications, see Hagen *et al.* (2011), Shmueli and Burkom (2010), Lotze *et al.* (2008), Fricker *et al.* (2008a), Fricker *et al.* (2008b), and Burkom *et al.* (2006).
- Although almost any statistics textbook will provide at least a brief introduction to linear regression, an excellent text focused just on regression is *Introduction to Linear Regression Analysis* (Montgomery *et al.*, 2012). In addition, *Time Series Analysis: Regression Techniques* by (Ostrom, 1990) is a good introduction to the application of regression to modeling time series data.
- In terms of time series modeling, a good introduction to smoothing and ARIMA models is *Introduction to Time Series Analysis and Forecasting*

(Montgomery *et al.*, 2008). *Introduction to Time Series and Forecasting* (Brockwell & Davis, 2002) is a more advanced treatment with a focus on ARMA and ARIMA models. A good advanced text is *Time Series Analysis: Forecasting and Control* (Box *et al.*, 2008).

- For other examples of the application of models to biosurveillance data, see Hagen *et al.* (2011), who applied adaptive regression to syndromic surveillance data; Burkom *et al.* (2006), who compared a loglinear regression model, an adaptive regression model with sliding baseline, and a Holt-Winters method for generalized exponential smoothing; the CDC's cyclical regression models discussed in Hutwagner *et al.* (2003b); log-linear regression models in Farrington *et al.* (1996); and time series models in Reis and Mandl (2003). Also see Fricker *et al.* (2008a) and Fricker *et al.* (2008b) for the use of adaptive regression on simulated biosurveillance data and Shmueli and Burkom (2010) for additional discussion of the use of regression and time series methods for syndromic surveillance.

- For more on CPA applied to biosurveillance data, see Kass-Hout *et al.* (2012), where they compare Taylor's method to two alternative methods. Readers interested in collaborating on developing CPA software or downloading open source programs should see Kass-Hout (2012b).

Part III

Early Event Detection

6

Early Event Detection Design and Performance Evaluation

... a general challenge for all biosurveillance research is to develop improved methods for evaluating detection algorithms in light of the fact that we have little data about outbreaks of many potential diseases that are of concern.

Henry Rolka *et al.* (2007)

Early event detection (EED) is one of the two main functions of a biosurveillance system. Per Homeland Security Presidential Directive 21 (HSPD-21), biosurveillance is "the process of active data-gathering with appropriate analysis and interpretation of biosphere data that might relate to disease activity and threats to human or animal health . . . in order to achieve *early warning of health threats, early detection of health events*, and overall situational awareness of disease activity" [emphasis added] (US Government, 2007).

This chapter opens by describing the mathematical notation and the assumptions that are used followed by a discussion of some important principles for good EED methods design. It then compares and contrasts EED to statistical methods commonly used in public health and epidemiological practice: binary classification and hypothesis testing. The chapter concludes with a discussion of EED performance metrics with a focus on a set of useful metrics and procedures for appropriately evaluating EED performance, either as part of a fielded biosurveillance system or as part of a research effort. This chapter lays the foundation for the specific early event detection methods – univariate and multivariate, temporal and spatio-temporal – described in Chapters 7 and 8.

Many of the methods used in biosurveillance EED have been drawn from the statistical process control (SPC) literature. As discussed in Chapter 1 and as summarized in Table 6.1, there are important differences between the typical SPC problem and the biosurveillance problem, which means that the standard SPC methods usually must be modified before being applied to biosurveillance. To distinguish between the two different uses, methods designed for or discussed within an SPC context are referred to as *control charts*, and methods designed for or discussed within a biosurveillance context are referred to as *detection methods*, *EED methods*, or just *methods* for short.

149

Chapter Objectives

Upon completion of this chapter, the reader should be able to:

- Compare and contrast how typical biosurveillance data differ from classical SPC data.
- Discuss important EED method design principles and, in particular, explain why it is important that:
  - Biosurveillance system design should be based on the purpose of the system.
  - Design and operation should use the KISS principle.
  - The main goal of EED is fast and accurate detection.
- Explain how EED methods differ from:
  - Binary classification tests
  - Hypothesis tests
  - Sequential probability ratio tests
- Define and describe the temporal EED method metrics average time between false signals (ATFS), conditional expected delay (CED), and probablity of successful detection (PSD), including:
  - Describe how these metrics are measures of sensitivity, specificity, and timeliness.
  - Discuss why these measures will help biosurveillance system designers and operators characterize performance.
  - Explain why having a common set of metrics is important for advancing the effective practice of biosurveillance.
- Compare and contrast the ATFS, CED, and PSD metrics with alternate metrics.

Mathematical Notation

A	Sequential probability ratio test (SPRT) upper boundary
ARL_0	In-control average run length
ARL_1	Out-of-control average run length
B	SPRT lower boundary
$\mathbb{E}(Y)$	Expected value of Y
$f(x; \theta)$	Probability density function (pdf) of random variable x with parameter θ
F_0	In-control or non-outbreak cumulative distribution function (cdf)
F_1	Out-of-control cumulative distribution function (cdf)
F_τ	Outbreak cumulative distribution function (cdf)
H_0	Null hypothesis
H_a	Alternative hypothesis
I_t	SPRT increment at time t
t^*	Time of first signal from an EED method
t^{**}	Time of next signal from an EED method
S_t	Value of SPRT at time t
T_t	Generic EED statistic at time t
X	Model covariate data
Y	Biosurveillance data
$\hat{Y}_t$	Predicted value of Y for day t
Z	Standardized biosurveillance data or residual
α	Probability of a type I error
β	Probability of a type II error
μ_0	Expected value of random variable with distribution F_0
$\hat{\mu}_0$	Estimated mean of random variable with distribution F_0
θ	Generic parameter
θ_0	Value of generic parameter given H_0 true
θ_1	Value of generic parameter given H_a true
σ_0^2	Variance of random variable with distribution F_0
$\hat{\sigma}_0^2$	Estimated variance of random variable with distribution F_0
τ	(Unknown) time of change from F_0 to F_1
τ_l	Last time period of outbreak
τ_s	Start time period of outbreak
$\hat{Y}_t$	Predicted value of Y for day t

6.1 Notation and Assumptions

Starting in this chapter, biosurveillance data taken sequentially over time will be denoted as $Y_1, Y_2, Y_3, \ldots$. The switch from lowercase letters ($y_1, y_2, y_3, \ldots$) used in the previous chapters to uppercase letters follows the standard convention used in probability and statistics where the lowercase letters represent specific values of observed data while uppercase letters represent the data as random observations from some distribution. Thus, y_i is a number, and Y_i is a random variable. Using this notation, the mathematical statement $Y_i = y_i$ means that the observed value of random variable Y at time i is y_i. (For a brief review of some of the fundamental concepts from probability and statistics, see Appendix A.)

The additional notation is necessary because EED methods are designed using information about how future data are characterized probabilistically. That is, prior to observing future observations, information (perhaps from past observations) will be used to define how biosurveillance data (or the residuals from modeling such data, say using one of the methods described in Chapter 5) behave probabilistically, and this information will then be used to choose and parameterize a particular EED method. Notationally, Y is a random variable representing an unknown observation that has probability distribution function F (also referred to as a cumulative distribution function). The notation $Y \sim F$ means the random variable has (or follows) distribution function F.

As in Chapter 5, $\hat{Y}_t$ denotes the predicted value for time t from some type of model, perhaps based on prior biosurveillance data, $Y_{t-1}, Y_{t-2}, Y_{t-3}, \ldots$, or other types of covariate information, $X_1, X_2, X_3, \ldots$, such as population demographics, or both. The notation $Z_1, Z_2, Z_3, \ldots$ generically denotes the residuals from a model,

$$Z_t = Y_t - \hat{Y}_t, t = 1, 2, 3, \ldots,$$

or the standardized residuals,

$$Z_t = \frac{Y_t - \hat{Y}_t}{\sigma_{Y_t - \hat{Y}_t}}, t = 1, 2, 3, \ldots.$$

As discussed in Chapter 5, residuals are relevant when the biosurveillance data are autocorrelated, say as a result of systematic effects such as seasonality. In these situations, a model may be used to remove (or at least mitigate) the systematic effects, and then the residuals are monitored. The advantage of this approach is that the residuals should have less autocorrelation and thus be more appropriate for methods that assume temporal independence. Because autocorrelated data are typical in biosurveillance, monitoring residuals is the general and more likely case. And under certain circumstances, the model residuals may be normally distributed, hence the use of Z to denote the residuals.

In the absence of a disease outbreak or bioterrorism attack, assume that Y_t or $Z_t \sim F_0$ for all $t < \tau$, where τ is the first time of an outbreak. (In the SPC literature, F_0 is usually referred to as the "in-control" distribution.) Of course, there may have been outbreaks sometime prior to τ but assume those outbreaks are sufficiently far in the past that they can be ignored or, if not, the data associated with the past outbreaks can be identified and removed.

The key idea is to assume the biosurveillance data or residuals are stochastic (i.e., they are random variables), and when there is no outbreak, they are independent and identically distributed (*iid*) according to a specific distribution denoted F_0. For observations or residuals distributed according to F_0, denote the expected value as μ_0 and the variance as σ_0^2. Denote the expected value and variance estimated using some historical data distributed according to F_0 as $\hat{\mu}_0$ and $\hat{\sigma}_0^2$.

The *iid* assumption is important to emphasize. In the application of SPC to industrial quality control problems, with appropriate implementation of the procedures this assumption can often be met with the raw data. But this is generally not the case for biosurveillance data. There are two main reasons for the difference.

- First, although both industrial quality control and biosurveillance are time series data, in industrial quality control, the process is explicitly controlled, and thus the raw data is the noise resulting from the process when it is in control. As such, the data can reasonably be assumed to be identically distributed. In contrast, background disease incidence process in biosurveillance is inherently uncontrollable, and thus the data themselves are usually autocorrelated, so they cannot be identically distributed.
- Second, industrial quality control data are typically samples from a process, and the sampling times are controlled with the data taken far enough apart in time so that the resulting data are at least approximately independent from one sample to the next. In contrast, in the interest of making EED as fast as possible, biosurveillance uses all the available data so that autocorrelation is virtually unavoidable.

Thus, biosurveillance data generally violate the *iid* assumption underlying most SPC procedures. However, it is often reasonable to assume that the residuals from a model that removes the systematic effects from biosurveillance data *are iid*.

The lack of independence between observations is only one way that biosurveillance differs from the typical SPC data assumptions. As shown in Table 6.1, other differences include a lack of time series stationarity (cf. Chapter 5), what types of statistics to monitor in order to most effectively detect outbreaks, and how the transient nature of outbreaks affects EED performance. For best performance, EED methods should be designed to accommodate these and other biosurveillance data characteristics. Conversely, the blind application of traditional SPC or other methods that ignore the inherent characteristics of biosurveillance data will likely result in suboptimal detection performance, which could include poor detection of outbreaks, excessive false positives, or both.

When an outbreak occurs, the assumption is that the distribution of the data changes in some way. In classical SPC problems, the change is often assumed to be a jump in the mean of the distribution. Denoting this "out-of-control" distribution as F_1, SPC assumes that $Y_\tau, Y_{\tau+1}, Y_{\tau+2}, \ldots \sim F_1$, where $\mathbb{E}(Y_\tau) = \mu_1 = \mu_0 + \delta$

Table 6.1. Characteristics of typical SPC data compared to biosurveillance data

Typical SPC Data Characteristics	Typical Biosurveillance Data Characteristics
1. The in-control distribution (F_0) is (or can reasonably be assumed to be) stationary.	1. There is little to no control over disease incidence, and the disease incidence distribution is usually nonstationary.
2. Observations can be drawn from the process so they are independent (or nearly so).	2. Autocorrelation and the need to monitor all the data result in dependence.
3. The asymptotic distributions of the statistics being monitored are known and thus can be used to design control charts.	3. Individual observations are being monitored, so asymptotic sampling distributions are not relevant.
4. Monitoring the process mean and standard deviation is usually sufficient.	4. Little is known about which statistics are useful, often looking for anything unusual.
5. Out-of-control condition remains until it is detected and corrective action is taken.	5. Outbreaks are transient, with disease incidence returning to its original state when the outbreak has run its course.
6. Temporal detection is the critical problem.	6. Detecting both temporal and spatial anomalies are critical.

for $\delta \neq 0$. The jump change in the mean is an idealization of what likely happens in practice, but it has served as a reasonable and appropriate approximation for many quality control problems. Note that this formulation assumes the process remains in the out-of-control state indefinitely until a signal is generated. The biosurveillance problem is not this simple for two reasons: (1) the outbreak distribution likely changes over time as the disease or bio-agent spreads through a population and (2) the outbreak is transient so that, at some time in the future, even without intervention, the process will return to its non-outbreak state with the data or residuals distributed according to F_0.

Denoting the duration of the outbreak as D, the general biosurveillance problem is to detect as quickly as possible an outbreak that starts at time τ, where $\ldots, Z_{\tau-3}, Z_{\tau-2}, Z_{\tau-1} \sim F_0$ followed by $Z_\tau \sim F_\tau$, $Z_{\tau+1} \sim F_{\tau+1}, \ldots, Z_{\tau+D-1} \sim F_{\tau+D-1}$ and then followed by $Z_{\tau+D}, Z_{\tau+D+1}, \ldots \sim F_0$. Most generally, the distributions $F_\tau, F_{\tau+1}, \ldots, F_{\tau+D-1}$ are simply assumed to be not the same as F_0, although it will frequently be useful to further assume some relationship between F_0 and the outbreak distributions.

6.2 Design Points and Principles

This section describes some principles for the effective design and implementation of EED methods.

6.2.1 Principle # 1: Design Should Flow from Purpose

Most fundamentally, the goal of EED is finding a signal amid background noise, but what is considered signal and what is considered noise depends on the purpose of biosurveillance. For example, when monitoring for natural disease outbreaks, a flu outbreak is a signal. On the other hand, when monitoring for bioterrorism, a flu outbreak is part of the background noise. Thus, the design of EED methods should flow from their intended purpose. This may seem like an obvious point, but there are a number of ways to classify the purpose of biosurveillance, including:

- Natural disease versus bioterrorism detection
- Retrospective analysis versus prospective outbreak monitoring
- Temporal trends versus spatial (cluster) identification
- General anomaly versus specific event detection

Specifying the purpose of biosurveillance is important because it does not follow that a biosurveillance system optimized for one purpose will serve other purposes well. Similarly, systems that try to accommodate all purposes may not serve any particular purpose well. As Stroup *et al.* (1993, p. 377) say, "Since a single method cannot be expected to distinguish between a change in historical trend and a one-time outbreak with an unsustained level, the analyst must identify the purpose of the analysis before choosing an analytic method."

To most efficiently and effectively conduct EED, the events to be detected should be defined as precisely as possible. In so doing, methods can be designed and employed that are most sensitive for detecting those events. For example, in industrial quality control, changes in the mean of the distribution are often of interest, and thus most SPC methods are designed to detect changes in the mean of F_0. In general, these methods are *not* designed to detect:

- Individual outliers or unusual observations
- Groupings or clusters of observations
- General changes in F_0

Control charts may produce signals under such conditions, but they are not designed to do so. This is an important point for biosurveillance: *Applying classical SPC methods to biosurveillance implicitly assumes that detecting changes in average disease incidence is what is most important.* Detecting changes in the average disease incidence is important, but it is probably not the only measure of interest.

This leads to a conundrum for biosurveillance: Narrowly defining the events to be detected leads to greater sensitivity, but little is known in advance about how an outbreak might manifest in the data. However, a few points are clear. First, EED methods designed to detect increases in average disease incidence combined with other EED methods designed to detect clusters likely cover many of the outbreak manifestations of interest. Second, EED methods designed to (effectively) detect specific events but that are also robust at detecting other types of events are to be preferred over less robust methods. And, third, methods designed to be overly general, meaning methods capable of detecting any type of change in F_0, are likely to be less sensitive to the changes most likely to occur and thus are less effective.

6.2.2 Principle # 2: Keep It Scientific But Simple

In biosurveillance, the underlying disease incidence phenomena are often very complicated, and there is sometimes quite a bit of data available. This can lead to the temptation to create and implement some very complicated EED methods. However, such temptations should be tempered by the fact that:

- Data availability or precision or other real-world constraints may not support some methods.
- Simpler methods are more likely to be correctly implemented in the field and thus widely used.

The latter point is supported by evidence in industrial quality control where simple univariate control charts are predominantly used in spite of many advances in the literature on multivariate control charts. As Stroup *et al.* (1993, p. 379) say, "For any analytic method to be useful, it must be easily implemented in the routine work of the practicing epidemiologist." Besides ease of implementation,

- Biosurveillance system operators must be able to diagnose signals to determine their origin.
- Signals determined to be true must be explainable to decision makers.

Overly complex methods viewed as "black boxes" by system operators, managers, or decision makers are likely to fail to meet both of these requirements. This leads to the principle that, all else being equal, simpler EED methods are preferred because they are usually easier to understand, implement, and diagnose. This principle is really just a variant of Occam's razor and the law of parsimony: If there are two equally likely solutions to a problem, choose the simplest.

In addition, given nonstationarity in the background incidence data, it may be the case that historical data further back in time are less relevant, and it also may be that other data limitations or weaknesses should limit the complexity of any method. This is not meant to suggest that an analysis should be unnecessarily or inappropriately oversimplified but rather that an EED method should only be as complex as the data will appropriately support.

Furthermore, a focus on simplicity does not mean scientifically and statistically sound methods should be abandoned for overly simple *ad hoc* methods. The phrase "all else being equal" is critical, and *ad hoc* methods often do not perform as well as those based on sound statistical and scientific theory. Thus, the principle can be summed up with the acronym KISS: *Keep It Scientific but Simple.*

Note that simpler EED methods do not necessarily compromise detection performance nor does it follow that more complex EED methods result in better detection performance. A good example of such a counterintuitive result was published by Chang and Fricker (1999), who compared a generalized likelihood ratio test designed explicitly for the problem of detecting a monotonically increasing mean of a distribution to simpler methods such as the cumulative sum (CUSUM) and exponentially weighted moving average (EWMA) control charts. It turned out that the simpler methods (appropriately applied to the problem) frequently out performed the more complicated generalized likelihood ratio test.

6.2.3 Goal: Fast and Accurate Detection

In biosurveillance, the whole point of EED is quick detection of outbreaks, and this in turn implies that speed of outbreak detection is an important system performance measure. This has long been recognized in the design and implementation of control charts, where the standard measures are based on the time to signal. However, as illustrated in Table 6.1, biosurveillance differs in significant ways from the typical statistical process control problem, making the measures used in SPC not directly applicable to biosurveillance EED.

A challenge in biosurveillance is that outbreaks are transient, which implies that accuracy is also an important metric. That is, not only is it important to signal quickly, but it is also important to signal accurately, meaning EED methods should be designed and implemented so they are highly likely to signal during an outbreak. However, the focus on speed and accuracy must be tempered so that the rate of false-positive signals inherent in any implementation is managed to be within resource constraints.

6.3 Early Event Detection Methods Differ from Other Statistical Tests

Although the detection methods described in Chapters 7 and 8 are similar to hypothesis testing in some ways, they are also quite different in other ways. Clearly understanding the similarities and differences is helpful when thinking about how best to employ the EED methods. To compare and contrast them, this section begins with a short review.

6.3.1 Binary Classification Tests

Consider a new medical device to be used to screen for a disease. To assess how well the device performs, a sample of n subjects on whom the screening test will be applied are recruited. Within the sample, each subject is known either to have the disease or not, and the screening test (without knowledge of an individual's actual status) classifies each individual as either sick or healthy. Thus, after administering the test, an individual can be in one of four possible states:

- *True positive* (TP): a sick individual correctly diagnosed by the test
- *False positive* (FP): a healthy individual wrongly diagnosed by the test
- *True negative* (TN): a healthy individual correctly diagnosed by the test
- *False negative* (FN): a sick individual wrongly diagnosed by the test

Test Outcome

		Positive	Negative
Actual Status	Sick	TP	FN
	Healthy	FP	TN

Figure 6.1. In a binary classification test, a subject ends up in one of four possible states: TP, FP, TN, and FN.

Figure 6.1 illustrates the four possible states an individual can be in after being classified by the screening test.

Two metrics commonly used for assessing the performance of these types of binary classification tests are:

- *Sensitivity*: the probability a test correctly classifies a sick person as sick
- *Specificity*: the probability a test correctly classifies a healthy person as healthy

Sensitivity and specificity are estimated from the test data as

$$\widehat{\text{sensitivity}} = \frac{\#TP}{\#TP + \#FN} \tag{6.1}$$

and

$$\widehat{\text{specificity}} = \frac{\#TN}{\#TN + \#FP}, \tag{6.2}$$

where the notation #TP, for example, stands for the number of true positive individuals out of all n individuals and the "hat" (^) indicates that the quantities are estimates of the unobserved true sensitivity and true specificity.

In Equation 6.1, sensitivity is an estimate of the probability that a sick person is correctly classified by the screening test as being sick. Similarly, in Equation 6.2, specificity is an estimate of the probability that a healthy person is correctly classified by the test as not being sick. For the calculations in Equations 6.1 and 6.2 to be correct estimates of the true probabilities, the test of each individual must be mathematically independent of all other tests. That is, the classification of one individual cannot use information from the classification of others. And for the probabilities to be used as estimates of how the screening test would perform in a larger population, the sample must be representative of that larger population.

For an ideal test, sensitivity = specificity = 1. However, in the real world, tests are subject to error: failing to classify a sick person as sick (false negative) and incorrectly classifying a healthy person as sick (false positive). Thus, in a real-world test, it is generally the case that $0 <$ sensitivity < 1 and $0 <$ specificity < 1. Furthermore, sensitivity and specificity trade off. Setting up a test to achieve higher sensitivity results in lower specificity (as well as a higher number of false positives), and setting the test for higher specificity results in lower sensitivity.

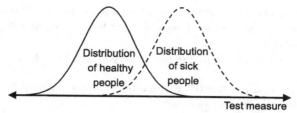

Figure 6.2. Hypothetical distributions of the test measure for two populations: sick and healthy.

The way to think about it is that the test measures each person, perhaps via some type of continuous measure but ultimately must make a binary classification: sick or healthy. The binary classification is made by specifying a threshold, where perhaps those with test measures below the threshold are classified as healthy and those with test measures above the threshold are classified as sick. However, people vary in whether and how the measure corresponds to being healthy or sick, and there is generally no one threshold that definitively splits that population perfectly into two groups that are all correctly classified as sick and healthy.

Figure 6.2 illustrates this idea, where those in the population who are healthy come from one distribution of the test measure and those who are sick come from another distribution. However, these distributions overlap, so any specific choice of test measure level used to distinguish between the two groups will result in some number false positives, false negatives, or both.

A *receiver operating characteristic* (ROC) curve is a plot of sensitivity versus one minus specificity for all possible values of the threshold. Figure 6.3 is an illustration of an ROC curve, where the closer the curve is to the upper left corner in the plot, the more effective the test. That is, the closer the curve is to the upper left corner, the higher the sensitivity and specificity are over a range of thresholds. Sometimes the area under the ROC curve is used as a measure of test effectiveness,

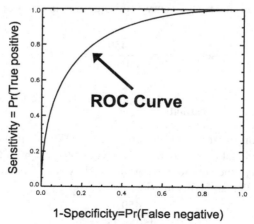

Figure 6.3. An illustrative ROC curve for a binary classification test.

where an area of one corresponds to a perfect test and an area of one-half means the test is, on average across all possible thresholds, no better than randomly classifying individuals.

Other metrics sometimes used in binary classification problems are:

- *Predictive value positive* (PVP): an estimate of the probability that a person who tests positive actually is sick
- *Predictive value negative* (PVN): an estimate of the probability that a person who tests negative actually is healthy,

where

$$\widehat{PVP} = \frac{\#TP}{\#TP + \#FP}$$

and

$$\widehat{PVN} = \frac{\#TN}{\#TN + \#FN}.$$

Example 6.1. The Centers for Disease Control and Previation is evaluating the performance of a newly proposed Rapid Influenza Diagnostic Test (RIDT) to screen for the H1N1 (swine flu) virus at the point of care. As a point-of-care screening test, the RIDT is subject to error, but its results can be compared against a laboratory-based "gold standard" test that can determine definitively whether someone has H1N1 or not. The purpose of this evaluation is to assess the proposed test's sensitivity and specificity to determine whether it should be used or not.

Table 6.2 shows the results of applying the screening test to $n = 1,000$ individuals, 500 of whom had the H1N1 virus and 500 who did not.

How effective is the test? To answer this question in terms of sensitivity and specificity:

$$\widehat{\text{sensitivity}} = \frac{450}{450 + 50} = 0.900$$

and

$$\widehat{\text{specificity}} = \frac{475}{475 + 25} = 0.950.$$

That is, based on the test data, the proposed RIDT is estimated to correctly classify an individual as having the H1N1 virus 90 percent of the time and to correctly classify a person not having the H1N1 virus 95 percent of the time. In terms of the PVP and PVN metrics:

$$\widehat{PVP} = \frac{450}{450 + 25} = 0.947$$

Table 6.2. Results of testing a (hypothetical) RIDT for H1N1

	RIDT Outcome	
	Positive (for H1N1)	Negative (for H1N1)
Lab test positive	450	50
Lab test negative	25	475

and

$$\widehat{PVN} = \frac{475}{475 + 50} = 0.905.$$

Thus, it is estimated that 94.7 percent of those classified by the proposed RIDT test as having the H1N1 virus actually do have it and 90.5 percent of those classified as well do not have the H1N1 virus.

6.3.2 Hypothesis Tests

Classical hypothesis tests are another type of binary classification test. As with the medical test just described, the classification is based on a random sample drawn from a population. However, in hypothesis testing, the goal is not to classify each observation in the sample but rather to use the sample to make a binary decision about a parameter of a probability distribution.

This binary choice is typically written in a formal way, such as $H_0 : \theta \leq \theta_0$ versus $H_a : \theta > \theta_0$. The former is referred to as the *null hypothesis*, and, in this example, it says that the parameter θ of a probability distribution is less than some value θ_0. The latter statement is the *alternative hypothesis*, and in this example, it says that the parameter θ is greater than some value θ_0.

The equivalent of Figure 6.2 in a hypothesis testing framework is Figure 6.4, where the two curves are now the probability densities of a random variable when the null hypothesis is true with $\theta = \theta_0$ and when the alternative hypothesis is true for $\theta = \theta_1 > \theta_0$. The outcome of a hypothesis test is the binary statement that either the null or alternative hypothesis is true (and thus the other is false).

Just as errors can be made in binary classification tests, so can they be made in hypothesis testing. Formally called *Type I* and *Type II* errors, a Type I error occurs

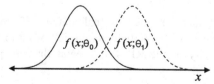

Figure 6.4. Sampling distributions for $\theta = \theta_0$, the parameter under the null hypothesis, and $\theta = \theta_1$, a specific parameter value under the alternative hypothesis.

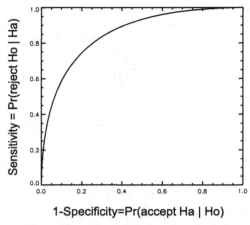

Figure 6.5. An illustrative ROC curve for a hypothesis test.

when the null hypothesis is rejected when it is true, and a Type II error is failing to reject the null hypothesis when it is false. The probabilities of these types of errors are denoted α and β, respectively, and can be written as $\mathbb{P}(\text{reject } H_0 | H_0 \text{ is true}) = \alpha$ and $\mathbb{P}(\text{accept } H_0 | H_a \text{ is true}) = \beta$.

The concepts of sensitivity and specificity apply to hypothesis testing, but now they are explicitly probabilities. Descriptively, sensitivity is the probability of rejecting the null hypothesis when the alternative hypothesis is true, and specificity is the probability of accepting the null hypothesis when it is true. Mathematically,

$$\text{sensitivity} = 1 - \mathbb{P}(\text{Type II error}) = \mathbb{P}(\text{reject } H_0 | H_a \text{ is true}) = 1 - \beta$$

and

$$\text{specificity} = 1 - \mathbb{P}(\text{Type I error}) = \mathbb{P}(\text{accept } H_0 | H_0 \text{ is true}) = 1 - \alpha.$$

In classical hypothesis testing terminology, α is referred to as the *significance level* of the test, and $1 - \beta$ is referred to as the *power* of the test.

Similarly, the concept and interpretation of the ROC curve applies to hypothesis testing. For example, Figure 6.5 is the same as the previous ROC curve in Figure 6.3 with the exception of the axes labels that now reflect the appropriate definitions of sensitivity and specificity for hypothesis testing.

Example 6.2. Given that the specificity calculated in Example 6.1 is an estimate of the true, unobserved specificity, one might want to test the hypothesis that the true specificity of the RIDT is greater than 90 percent. Write the hypotheses as

$$H_0 : p \leq 0.90$$
$$H_a : p > 0.90$$

where

p = specificity of the H1N1 RIDT

$\quad$ = $\mathbb{P}$(RIDT classifies a person as healthy|person does not have H1N1).

For a significance level of $\alpha = 0.01$ and a random sample of size $n = 500$, the rejection region of the hypothesis test is $\hat{p} \geq 0.93$, where $\hat{p} = \#\text{TN}/500$, which corresponds to observing $\#\text{TN} \geq 465$. Using the data in the second row of Table 6.2 of Example 6.1 (assuming it had been collected *after* the hypotheses were generated) gives $\hat{p} = 475/500 = 0.95$. Alternatively, for $\hat{p} = 0.95$ (equivalently, $\#\text{TN} = 475$) the p-value of the test is less than $\alpha = 0.001$. Either way, the null hypothesis is rejected, and it is reasonable to conclude that the RIDT has a true specificity greater than 90 percent.

6.3.3 Sequential Tests

A characteristic of classical hypothesis testing is that the sample size is fixed. It is determined prior to conducting the test and usually is set to achieve a desired power $(1 - \beta)$ for a specific alternative distribution and significance level (α). In contrast, as the name suggests, sequential tests are designed to sequentially collect data, only stopping when enough evidence is collected to conclude that one of two competing hypotheses is true.

The sequential probability ratio test (SPRT) of Wald (1947) is one well-known type of sequential test. A benefit of sequential tests is that they tend to require smaller sample sizes. In terms of health applications such as clinical trials, this often means the test can be concluded sooner. As Wald (1947, p. 1) says of the SPRT: "The sequential probability ratio test frequently results in a savings of about 50 per cent in the number of observations over the most efficient test procedure based on a fixed number of observations."

The SPRT works as follows. For two simple hypotheses, say $H_0 : \theta = \theta_0$ versus $H_a : \theta = \theta_1$, for $\theta_1 > \theta_0$, the SPRT calculates S_t, the sum of the *log-likelihood ratios* up to time t. The sum is usually iteratively calculated as

$$S_t = S_{t-1} + \ln\left(\frac{f(x_t; \theta_1)}{f(x_t; \theta_0)}\right), t = 1, 2, 3, \ldots,$$

starting with $S_0 = 0$. Which of the hypotheses is accepted and when follows from a *stopping rule* based on thresholds A and B:

- If $S_t \geq A$ accept H_a,
- else if $S_t \leq B$ accept H_0,
- else if $B < S_t < A$ take another sample at time $t + 1$, calculate S_{t+1}, and repeat.

The region (B, A) is referred to as the *indifference region* or *indifference zone*. The choices of A and B $(0 < B < A < \infty)$ depend on the desired probability of Type I and Type II errors, α and β (which have the same definitions as in classical hypothesis testing), where $A \approx \ln[(1 - \beta)/\alpha]$ and $B \approx \ln[\beta/(1 - \alpha)]$.

Given the parameters for a particular test, an ROC curve can be plotted just like in the case of a classical hypothesis test. However, unlike classical hypothesis testing, the ROC curve is not sufficient for choosing among sequential test alternatives. Rather, in addition to the ROC curve, the *average sample number* (ASN) is also needed. The ASN is the average number of observations (samples) required to reach a decision for a particular parameter value θ, and the ASN function is a plot over all possible values of θ. As Wald (1947, p. 27) says, "The OC [operating characteristic] function describes how well the [sequential] test procedure achieves its objective of making correct decisions, and the ASN function represents the price we have to pay, in terms of the number of observations required for the test."

Example 6.3. To conduct an SPRT for the hypotheses in Example 6.2, one must first define the indifference region. For this example, assume that the indifference region is 0.90 ± 0.03, which means that if the true specificity is within this region, one is indifferent as to whether the test concludes with the null or alternative hypothesis.

The SPRT test is then based on the simple hypotheses

$$H_0 : p = 0.87$$
$$H_a : p = 0.93$$

where, to fully define the test, one must also specify α and β. For the purposes of this example, set $\alpha = 0.01$ and $\beta = 0.10$. Then the thresholds are

$$A = \ln\left(\frac{1-\beta}{\alpha}\right) = \ln\left(\frac{1-0.1}{0.01}\right) = 4.50$$

$$B = \ln\left(\frac{\beta}{1-\alpha}\right) = \ln\left(\frac{0.1}{0.99}\right) = -2.29$$

Now, starting with $S_0 = 0$, sequentially take healthy individuals and determine whether the RIDT correctly classifies them as healthy, each time calculating

$$S_t = S_{t-1} + I_t, \quad t = 1, 2, 3, \ldots,$$

where if an individual is correctly classified as healthy, then

$$I_t = \ln\left(\frac{p_1}{p_0}\right) = \ln\left(\frac{0.93}{0.87}\right) = 0.0667$$

and if an individual is incorrectly classified as having H1N1, then

$$I_t = \ln\left(\frac{1-p_1}{1-p_0}\right) = \ln\left(\frac{0.07}{0.13}\right) = -0.619.$$

To illustrate how the test works, imagine that the RIDT has a true specificity of 0.95. Figure 6.6 is a plot of S_t versus t for one sequence of observations. The dips in the line occur each time the RIDT incorrectly classifies an individual as

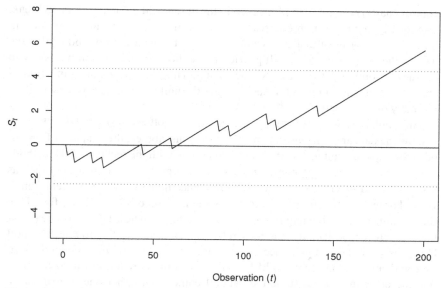

Figure 6.6. A plot S_t versus t for one sequence of observations where the SPRT concludes H_a at observation 182 when $S_{182} = 4.53 > A = 4.5$.

sick. The SPRT correctly concludes H_a, that the specificity of the test is greater than 0.93, at observation 182 when $S_{182} = 4.53 > A = 4.5$.

Of course, in Example 6.3, the stopping time of 182 is random and depends on the random times that the RIDT incorrectly classifies healthy individuals as sick. The ASN is the average time for the SPRT to signal. Using simulation to esti-mate the ASN for the example, ASN = $\mathbb{E}(t^*|p = 0.95) = 149.1$ (s.e. = 0.6), where t^* denotes the first time that either $S_t \geq A$ or $S_t \leq B$. Thus, the stopping time for the data in Figure 6.3 was actually longer than the expected stopping time.

6.3.4 How Early Event Detection Methods Differ

EED methods, to be described in more detail in the chapters to follow, are special types of sequential tests. Some methods, such as the Shewhart, are repeated classi-cal hypothesis tests; other methods such as the univariate CUSUM are equivalent to sequences of SPRTs, and the other methods take other forms. One common characteristic of all EED methods, like sequential tests and unlike binary clas-sification and classical hypothesis tests, is that they sequentially and repeatedly evaluate data over time. Usually the new data arrive at fixed time periods, such as daily, and the EED methods assess the data up to that point for evidence of an outbreak.

However, unlike the SPRT, EED methods never accept the null hypothesis that an outbreak is not occurring and thus stop sampling. Rather, EED methods (and control charts) continue sampling even in the absence of evidence of an outbreak. The idea is that even if an outbreak has not occurred up to a particular point in time, it does not mean that one cannot occur in the next time period or that the data in the next time period will provide the additional information necessary to identify an outbreak that has been occurring. Thus, EED methods (and control charts) continue to sample until such time as the null hypothesis is rejected, either correctly or incorrectly.

Although binary classification tests, classical hypothesis tests, and the SPRT all assume the data are independent and identically distributed, the data in EED methods are frequently autocorrelated. This, combined with the fact that EED methods never accept the null hypothesis, means that test performance measures such as sensitivity and specificity may not be well defined under the EED problem framework. For example, defining specificity as the fraction of observations for which the test fails to reject the null hypothesis does not work when the data or the statistics from the EED method are autocorrelated. In addition, failing to reject the null hypothesis is not the same as accepting it, at least in the sense of a sequential test.

Another difference between EED methods and the previous testing methods is that the other methods assume the data all come from either one of two states, and the point is to classify either the observations or parameters into one of those states. In contrast, in biosurveillance EED, the data may switch from the null state (no outbreak) to the alternate state (outbreak) and perhaps back again at unknown points in time. Thus, EED methods need to continuously assess whether a change has occurred from one state to the other, and the point is to determine if a change has occurred as quickly and reliably as possible.

Because of these differences, simply applying the previous testing methods to the EED problem can be inappropriate. As Sonesson and Bock (2003) say, "Many papers have addressed the problem of on-line surveillance, but the mistake of not noting the sequential type of decision situation is quite common." Rather, EED methods must correctly account for the sequential, nonstationary nature of the data, including the idea of transient outbreaks, and the methods must be evaluated using appropriate metrics.

6.4 Measuring Early Event Detection Performance

To evaluate the performance of an EED method or to implement one in practice and assess its performance, one must use the appropriate metrics. Metrics serve two purposes:

- For public health practitioners and biosurveillance system operators, metrics allow for effective implementation and assessment of biosurveillance operations, including managing the rate of false-positive signals.
- For researchers and academics, a common set of metrics allows for performance comparisons between methods, which facilitates improvements in the practice of EED.

For public health practitioners and biosurveillance system operators, the metrics should answer the following three questions:

- When there is an outbreak, how fast will the method detect the outbreak?
- When there is no outbreak, what is the time between false-positive signals?
- For a particular type of outbreak, what is the chance that the method will detect it at all?

As it turns out, metrics that are useful for answering these operational questions are also useful and quite appropriate for EED method design evaluation by researchers and academics.

The need for an answer to the first question is obvious and, resource constraints aside, faster is always preferred. However, for a given detection method, improving the speed of detection during an outbreak comes at the cost of increasing the number of false-positive signals. Thus, when setting a method's alerting threshold, it is absolutely critical to address the second question. Specifically, when choosing a threshold for an implementation, it should be set so that the rate of false signals is tolerably small, meaning the biosurveillance system operators have the necessary resources to investigate and adjudicate the signals (i.e., the determine whether the signals are true on false positives).

This approach will trouble some biosurveillance researchers and practitioners, because it makes the speed of detection secondary to daily operational considerations. They appropriately argue that one should set the threshold low enough so that a method signals a true outbreak very quickly. However, because threshold setting drives both true and false-positive signaling, if the threshold is set too aggressively, it will quickly result in an excessive number of (predomanantly false-positive) signals that the organization does not have the resources to investigate. And *an uninvestigated signal is as good as no signal at all.* As Shmueli and Burkom (2010) have said, "This frequent alerting leads users to ignore alarms and instead use the system to examine the data heuristically. As one user commented 'we hope that when there is a true alarm we will not ignore it.'" The only way to control this problem is to first set the threshold to operate with a tolerable false-positive rate and then allow that to drive the achievable detection speed for an actual outbreak.

The discussion thus far should make it clear that for EED, time is the critical measure of interest, in terms of both the time to detect an outbreak and the time between false-positive signals. Those familiar with the SPC literature will note that answering the first two questions leads to metrics that are similar to the *average run length* metrics used in industrial process control. However, unlike in industrial quality control, because outbreaks are transient, EED metrics based solely on time are not sufficient.

EED measures based solely on time are insufficient because it is possible to create detection methods that have a large time between false signals and a small time to detect outbreaks but that may also miss too many outbreaks. Of course, one would hope that a well-designed method that has a small time to detect an outbreak would also have a high probability of detecting transient outbreaks, but that may not always be the case. Thus, it is also important to ensure that EED methods have a high probability of detecting such transient outbreaks. This leads to a third measure that answers the third question, the probablity of successful detection of an outbreaks where the measure may be further tightened by requiring a high probability of detecting an outbreak within some small number of time periods.

6.4.1 Metrics for Temporal Methods

To be useful, a set of metrics must effectively address the two purposes previously discussed: (1) for practitioners, they must allow for effective implementation and assessment of biosurveillance operations, including managing the rate of false-positive signals, and (2) for researchers and academics, they must allow for clear and consistent performance comparisons between existing and proposed methods. In addition, they must also be practical in the sense that they can be easily calculated and understood.

Unfortunately, as yet there is no set of metrics that is commonly accepted throughout the biosurveillance community. Furthermore, many of those proposed and used in the literature fail to meet all of the criteria just listed. This text uses the following metrics, which do meet the criteria.

- *Average time between false signals* (ATFS) is the mean number of time periods it takes for the EED method to resignal after the method first signals, given that there are no outbreaks. Thus, the ATFS is the expected time between false signals.
- *Conditional expected delay* (CED) is the mean number of time periods it takes for the method to first signal, given that an outbreak is occurring *and* that the method signals during the outbreak. Thus, the CED is the expected number of time periods from the start of an outbreak until the first true signal during that outbreak.
- *Probability of successful detection* (PSD) is the probability the method signals during an outbreak, where the probability of detection is both a function of the EED method and the type of outbreak.

Thus, ATFS is a measure of the time between false-positive signals, CED is a measure of how fast a method will detect an outbreak, and PSD is a measure of how likely a method will detect a particular type of outbreak. Note that these metrics allow for effective implementation and assessment of biosurveillance system operations because they directly answer the three questions first posed on page 167:

- Question: *How fast will the method detect an actual outbreak?*
  Answer: CED is how fast a method will detect an outbreak on average.
- Question: *What is the time between false-positive signals?*
  Answer: ATFS is the average time between false-positive signals.

- Question: *What is the chance that the method will detect an outbreak?* Answer: PSD is the probability the method will detect an outbreak.

The metrics are mathematically defined as follows. Let T_t denote a generic EED method statistic T at time t, where T_0 is the value of the statistic when the method is first started. Let h denote the method's threshold, where if $T_t \geq h$ the method signals at time t. Also, let τ_s denote the first day of an outbreak, where the notation $\tau_s = \infty$ means that an outbreak never occurs, and let τ_l denote that last day of an outbreak, where if $\tau_s = \infty$ then by definition $\tau_l = \infty$. Finally, let t^* denote the first time the method signals, $t^* = \min(t : T_t \geq h)$, and let let t^{**} denote the next time the method signals, $t^{**} = \min(t : t > t^*$ and $T_t \geq h)$.
  Then

$$\text{ATFS} \triangleq \mathbb{E}(t^{**} - t^* | T_{t^*+1} = T_0 \text{ and } \tau_s = \infty), \tag{6.3}$$

$$\text{CED} \triangleq \mathbb{E}(t^* - \tau_s | \tau_s \leq t^* \leq \tau_l), \tag{6.4}$$

and

$$\text{PSD} \triangleq \mathbb{P}(\tau_s \leq t^* \leq \tau_l). \tag{6.5}$$

Mathematically, the ATFS metric as defined in Equation 6.3 is the same as the ARL_0 in SPC, where after each signal the method's statistic is reset to its starting value. However, some biosurveillance practitioners prefer not to reset after each signal, so in that case,

$$\text{ATFS} \triangleq \mathbb{E}(t^{**} - t^* | \tau_s = \infty). \tag{6.6}$$

Note the difference between Equation 6.3 and Equation 6.6: In the former, the statistic is reset to its starting value after each time the EED method signals, but in the latter, it is not. If the time series of EED statistics is autocorrelated, then the resulting ATFS performance can be very different since, with autocorrelation, after a signal has occurred in one time period more signals are likely to occur in subsequent periods. In this text, the ATFS as defined in Equation 6.3 (using resetting after each signal) will be used.

Under the condition that the statistic is not reset, Fraker *et al.* (2008) have proposed the *average time between signal events* (ATBSE) metric, where a *signal event* is defined as consecutive time periods during which an EED method signals. Under these conditions, the ATBSE may be a more informative measure because it quantifies the length of time between groups of signals, but it also may not provide sufficient information about the number of false-positive signals that will occur.

The CED is conceptually similar to the out-of-control average run length (ARL_1) in SPC, but in SPC, when a process goes out of control, it stays out of control. Thus, in SPC, $\text{ARL}_1 = \mathbb{E}(t^* - \tau_s | t^* \geq \tau_s)$. Because outbreaks are transient in biosurveillance, the definition differs because it must incorporate the idea that the signal occurs sometime during the duration of the outbreak.

Note that it will sometimes be useful to set $\tau_s = 1$ when estimating the CED. When doing so, the resulting estimate is referred to as the *zero state* or *initial state* CED because the EED method's statistic T_0 is in its initial state (which is zero for many EED methods) just before the outbreak occurs. Alternatively, if the estimates are based on a large τ_s where the method has been allowed to run for some time, so that T is not in its initial state, then it is referred to as the *steady state* CED.

PSD does not have an analogue in the SPC literature. As defined, it is the probability of detecting an outbreak at any time during the outbreak. For longer outbreaks, this definition may be too loose, meaning that detection later in the outbreak may not be medically useful. If that is the case, the definition by Sonesson and Bock (2003) may be more operationally relevant: $\text{PSD} = \mathbb{P}(t^* - \tau_s \le d | \tau_s \le t^* \le \tau_l)$, where d is the maximum delay required for a successful detection and where "successful detection" means early enough in the outbreak cycle that an intervention is medically effective.

6.4.2 Alternative Metrics

Fraker *et al.* (2008) note: "Substantially more metrics have been proposed in the public health surveillance literature than in the industrial monitoring literature." This plethora of metrics has made it difficult to advance the science and practice of biosurveillance because it is generally difficult and sometimes impossible to compare results across the literature, hence the focus of the previous section on a single set of preferred metrics. However, for completeness, this section summarizes the other metrics that have been proposed in the biosurveillance literature.

Run Length-Based Metrics

Run length-based metrics date back to Wald (1947, p. 34), who said, "Restricting ourselves to sequential tests of a given strength (α, β), a test may be regarded as more desirable the smaller the expected number of observations required by the test." In this vein, the *average run length* (ARL) is the standard metric for evaluating control charts. ARL_0 is referred to as the *in-control ARL* and ARL_1 is the *out-of-control ARL*. They are essentially equivalent to the ATFS and CED metrics for data that have the SPC data characteristics described in Table 6.1. A closely related metric is the *average time to signal* (ATS). When the ARL is based on the average number of observations until a signal, the ATS is the average number of time periods until a signal.

Although ARL and ATS have been used to evaluate the performance of EED methods, as discussed in the opening paragraph of this section, these metrics fail both to account for the transient nature of outbreaks and that the EED methods' statistics are often not reset after they signal. In comparison, when an SPC process goes out of control, it stays in that condition until the control chart signals and the cause is identified and corrected. Thus, in SPC, when a process goes out of control, any signal is a true signal, so the probability of signaling during an out-of-control condition is always 1. This is not the case in biosurveillance in which outbreaks are transient and after some period of time disappear. In this situation, it is possible for an EED method to fail to signal during an outbreak, after which a signal is a false signal.

To overcome the issues associated with applying the control chart ARL metrics to biosurveillance, various modifications have been proposed, including the ATBSE, in which a *signal event* is defined as consecutive time periods during which an EED method signals (Fraker *et al.*, 2008). They also define the *average signal event length* (ASEL) as how long, on average, an EED method signals over consecutive time periods.

The ATBSE and ASEL metrics are designed for how biosurveillance systems are often currently operated, where the EED methods are not reset after they signal. In this situation, biosurveillance system operators allow the EED methods to continue to run after they signal and interpret the resulting sequence of signals (or lack thereof) as additional information about a potential outbreak. Under these conditions, the ATBSE may be preferred to the ATFS metric.

Although these metrics are just as applicable to the EED problem, ATFS is recommended *under the assumption that EED methods are reset after each signal.* The reason for this preference is twofold:

- If the system is being used for bioterrorism, a bioterrorist attack cannot be detected during a natural disease outbreak with a system that is allowed to continuously signal.
- Even when used for natural disease surveillance, sequences of EED signals are at best crude indicators of the progression of an outbreak. Instead, given a correct EED signal, other measures of outbreak progression are likely to be more informative.

Most fundamentally, however, the preference for ATFS is based on the logic that biosurveillance systems should be structured so that every signal is taken as an alarm worthy of (and requiring) investigation. That is, biosurveillance systems should be designed and operated like any other alarm system. For example, it does not make much sense to design a fire alarm system so that the the firefighters wait for a second or third alarm before deciding to respond. The same is true with a burglar alarm, an aircraft collision early warning system, or any other type of alarm system. Biosurveillance EED signals should not be treated any differently.

Sensitivity, Specificity, and Timeliness Metrics

Sensitivity, specificity, and *timeliness* are probably the most commonly used biosurveillance metrics; their popularity likely stems from the medical community's familiarity with and widespread use of binary classification tests and classical hypothesis testing. Although these metrics are clearly defined and appropriate in standard medical and epidemiological settings, they are less so in the biosurveillance setting for a number of reasons.

First, in binary classification tests, one is generally classifying individual patients (sick or not), but in biosurveillance, one is classifying periods of time (an outbreak exists or not). In the former situation, with appropriate experimental design, one can reasonably assume the patients are independent, but independence is generally violated in biosurveillance. Specifically, biosurveillance data are usually autocorrelated and, even if such autocorrelation can be removed via modeling, the signaling statistics for EED methods that use historical data will still be autocorrelated.

Second, because the EED data and statistics are rarely independent and because EED methods never accept the null hypothesis, metrics such as sensitivity and specificity are not well defined. As Fraker *et al.* (2008, p. 454) say, "Specificity is not useful for the ongoing monitoring scenario because almost all surveillance schemes [i.e., EED methods] combine information over time and thus have autocorrelated surveillance statistics. In this situation it is difficult to interpret a false alarm probability because the decisions at each time period to signal or not are dependent and the 'false alarm probability' is not well-defined or directly related to the more meaningful time-to-signal performance."

To overcome this, researchers have struggled to redefine sensitivity and specificity for use in the biosurveillance context. Some definitions that have appeared in the literature include:

- "Sensitivity is defined as the number of days with true alarms divided by the number of days with outbreaks" (Reis *et al.*, 2003).
- "Sensitivity can be assessed by estimating the proportion of cases of a disease or health condition detected by the surveillance system. Sensitivity can also be considered as the ability of the system to detect unusual events" (Lawson & Kleinman, 2005, p. 14).
- "Sensitivity is the probability that a public health event of interest will be detected in the data given the event really occurred" (Lombardo & Buckeridge, 2007, p. 45).
- "Sensitivity is the probability of an alarm given an outbreak" (Lombardo & Buckeridge, 2007, p. 413).

However, none of these definitions overcomes the fundamental problem of the lack of independence. In addition, as Frisen and Sonesson (2005) say, "Evaluation [of EED methods] by the significance level, power, specificity, and sensitivity which is useful for a fixed sample is not appropriate in a surveillance situation without modification since they have no unique value unless the time period is fixed."

Third, "timeliness" is a concept, not a metric. It very appropriately suggests that EED methods should signal quickly, but there is no standard metric that precisely defines what it means to be timely. As previously discussed, the lack of a standard exacerbates the problem of synthesizing results across the biosurveillance literature.

These issues extend to other binary classification and classical hypothesis testing metrics, such as PVP and PVN, as well. In fact, suites of metrics that do not include any time-based metrics can give misleading results. Fraker *et al.* (2008) give an example in which two EED methods have exactly the same sensitivity, PVP, and PVN, yet one method has significantly better time to detection performance and is thus clearly to be preferred, a fact that is not evident without a time-based metric.

This is not to say that the conceptual approach to measuring EED performance in these three dimensions is undesirable, just that these terms are too imprecise to serve as *metrics* for biosurveillance. This lack of definitional precision has allowed each researcher to define his or her own set of metrics, some of which have been ill suited to the nature of EED as a sequential decision problem. On the other hand, the metrics discussed in Section 6.4.1 are both appropriate for the sequential nature of EED, and *they map directly onto the sensitivity, specificity, and timeliness performance dimensions*:

- CED is a timeliness metric. It measures the average time it takes an EED method to signal after the start of an outbreak, conditional on the method signaling sometime during the outbreak.
- PSD is a sensitivity-like metric. It measures the probability an EED method signals during an outbreak.
- ATFS is a specificity-like metric. It measures the frequency that an EED method does not signal when there is no outbreak.

Thus, one can think about PSD, ATFS, and CED as well-defined metrics that are appropriately measuring the "sensitivity," "specificity," and "timeliness" performance of EED methods.

Recurrence Interval Metrics

The *recurrence interval* (RI) is another biosurveillance metric that has been multiply defined. Intuitively, it is often thought of as the average number of time periods (or observations) between signals or signal events. However, this is the definition of the ATS, not the RI. Rather, the RI is "the fixed number of time periods for which the expected number of false alarms is one." See Fraker *et al.* (2008) and Woodall *et al.* (2008) for additional discussion on this point.

Kleinman (2005) defined the RI as

$$RI = \frac{1}{p\text{-value} \times S},$$

where S is the number of regions being simultaneously monitored and the p-value is the probability of observing a regional count as extreme or more extreme than the one observed in a particular time period.

When $S = 1$ and when the data and monitoring statistics are independent over time, then ATFS $= 1/p$, where p is the probability of a signal under a specific set of circumstances (e.g., that no outbreak is occurring). Under these conditions, the ATFS is the average time between false signals for a specific preset p, where p is the probability of a false signal and where a signal is generated when p-value $\leq p$.

However, this relationship between the RI and ATFS (or ARL_0) does not hold in general, either because of spatial correlation (when $S > 1$) or because the monitoring statistics are autocorrelated. In these situations, there is no relationship between the ATFS (or ARL_0) and the RI. As Fraker et al. (2008, p. 463) say, EED methods "with the same recurrence interval value can have widely different in-control [i.e., non-outbreak] time-to-signal properties." Furthermore, Fraker et al. (2008, p. 457) say, "If the marginal probabilities of signaling are not equal, then the number of time periods for which the expected number of signals is one is not constant and the recurrence interval is not well-defined."

Nonetheless, the recurrence interval is used in a number of biosurveillance EED applications and methods, including the small area regression and testing (SMART) method of Kleinman (2005) and the SatScan method of Kulldorff (2001).

Other Metrics

A number of metrics focused on generalizing the ROC curve have been proposed. Generalizations are necessary to incorporate some measure of timeliness. For example, Kleinman and Abrams (2006) proposed weighted ROC curves, where each point on the curve is weighted by a measure of timeliness. They also proposed a three-dimensional timeliness–receiver operating characteristic surface (TROS). Buckeridge et al. (2005) used an activity monitoring operating characteristic (AMOC) curve, which is a plot of a timeliness metric versus a false signal rate metric. For spatio-temporal methods, the free response operating characteristic (FROC) curve has been proposed, which is a plot of the fraction of outbreak locations detected versus the false-positive detection rate (Buckeridge et al., 2005).

These measures tend to have the same issues described in Section 6.4.2 because they are generally based (in whole or in part) on the same vague, inconsistently, or ill-defined "sensitivity," "specificity," and "timeliness" metrics. Furthermore, even if the metrics being plotted are well defined, it is important to note that ROC curves are plots over the entire possible range of thresholds ($-\infty \leq h \leq \infty$) when usually only a subset of all possible thresholds is of practical use. Thus, when judging performance, it is usually only necessary to compare curves over a smaller range of thresholds.

Sometimes these ROC-based metrics are motivated by a desire to distill the performance assessment of two EED methods down to a comparison between two univariate statistics. To do so, comparisons are made between the areas under the curves or surfaces. However, not only do these comparisons still suffer from the problems just described, but they also still fail to reduce the complexity of problem because multiple comparisons are still required for various types of outbreaks, background disease incidence patterns, and so on.

6.5 Discussion and Summary

This chapter describes and discusses some general principles for EED method design and metrics for evaluating EED method performance. In so doing, the focus has implicitly been on EED methods, which are described in detail in Chapters 7 and 8.

It is important to note that, as of this writing, the metrics described in Section 6.4 do *not* have general acceptance in either the biosurveillance research or operational communities. This lack of consensus is inhibiting the community's ability to synthesize research results and thus advance the state of biosurveillance EED science. The explicit focus on and exclusive use of ATFS, CED, and PSD in this text are intended to promote standardization, with the goal of bringing some order to the current babel of biosurveillance metrics.

Some may take umbrage at the ATFS, CED, and PSD metrics' departure from the classical sensitivity- and specificity-based methods so widely used in the medical and epidemiological communities, as well as their similarity to the SPC metrics. Hopefully Section 6.3 clearly explained the differences between EED methods and other statistical tests, and Section 6.4 made a convincing case for why the ATFS, CED, and PSD metrics are better suited to the biosurveillance problem. In the final accounting, what is important is that the metrics are effective in helping the research community develop the most effective EED methods and in helping public health practitioners operate biosurveillance systems to efficiently identify and effectively mitigate public health threats.

What Is "Effective" Early Event Detection?

In terms of EED, "effective" means detecting outbreaks as quickly and accurately as possible after the start of the outbreak. Quickness is what the CED metric measures, and accuracy is what the PSD metric measures. However, effectiveness can only be judged in the context of the ATFS.

As discussed in Section 6.4, at issue is that CED and PSD can always be improved by lowering the detection threshold. However, lowering the threshold also increases the number of false-positive signals, where the rate of false positives often increases dramatically with small decreases in the threshold.

Thus, the practical implementation of biosurveillance systems dictates that thresholds be set as low as possible, but they must be *constrained by an organization's resources for investigating signals.*

Isn't Explicitly Controlling the False-Positive Rate Backwards?

Explicitly controlling the false-positive rate in biosurveillance is equivalent to setting the Type II error rate in classical hypothesis testing and then accepting whatever Type I rate results, but hypothesis tests are usually set up to explicitly control the probability of a Type I error (α). This is based on the way hypothesis tests are designed, with the Type I error usually the more serious of the two possible errors.

For example, in criminal trials, the possible errors are either convicting an innocent person or letting a guilty person go free. US society generally believes that sending an innocent person to prison is the more serious error, and hence the null hypothesis is that a person is presumed innocent and must be proven guilty. By setting up the system this way, the chance of sending an innocent person to prison (the Type I error) is what is being explicitly controlled; the Type II error (a guilty person is let go free) is then a function of the observed alternative and test design (i.e., the trial process).

In biosurveillance, the possible errors are (1) failing to detect an outbreak or attack (a false negative) and (2) incorrectly signaling when there is no outbreak or attack (a false positive). Presumably, the first is the more significant error, which suggests biosurveillance systems should be structured to presume an outbreak exists unless proven otherwise. Returning to the trial example: What if the person incorrectly let free would release smallpox in the United States? Should the null hypothesis still be innocent until proven guilty or should it now be guilty until proven innocent?

However, always assuming an outbreak exists unless proven otherwise is completely impractical from an operational perspective for a number of reasons. First, structuring the problem this way would consume far too many resources, requiring organizations to continuously prove that everything is normal. Second, it is unclear how one would prove the lack of an outbreak, particularly given the natural variations in background disease incidence patterns. Third, such an approach negates the need for EED methods because one always assumes an outbreak exists until proven otherwise.

Instead, biosurveillance takes an equally appropriate approach to structuring the test, which is to make the alternative hypothesis the outcome that requires empirical proof. That is, prior to dedicating resources to investigating a possible outbreak, it is reasonable to require some evidence that an outbreak is (likely to be) occurring. A similar criterion is often used in classical hypothesis testing when deciding which hypothesis is the null and which is the alternative. However, a Type II error as serious as a missed bioterrorism attack implies that EED methods must have a high PSD and short CED should an attack occur.

This can be accomplished by both:

- Lowering detection thresholds to achieve a particular CED and PSD and allocating sufficient resources to investigate all of the resulting signals.
- Continuing to improve biosurveillance system design and operation so that better CED and PSD can be achieved for a given ATFS.

The latter should be the focus of a concerted and coordinated research effort aimed at things such as developing new EED methods, improving system design and operation to remove excess variation in the background data, and so on.

Additional Reading

Very little has been published in the literature about either effective EED method design principles or metrics. The citations within this chapter are the best place to begin for readers interested in delving deeper into these topics. Of these, in terms of metrics, the following are recommended:

- *Performance Metrics for Surveillance Schemes* (Fraker *et al.*, 2008) reviews various metrics that have been used in EED, with an emphasis on the recurrence interval. It also introduces and discusses the ATBSE and ASEL in more detail.
- *Optimal Surveillance* (Frisen & Sonesson, 2005), particularly Section 3.4.1, discusses metrics useful for EED performance assessment. Although the discussion retains a bit of an SPC flavor, it is also a more thorough development. The names of the CED and PSD metrics described in this chapter are taken from Sonesson and Bock (2003) and Frisen and Sonesson (2005).
- *Comparing Biosurveillance Detection Methods: EARS' Versus a CUSUM-based Methodology* (Fricker *et al.*, 2008a) and *Directionally Sensitive MCUSUM and MEWMA Procedures with Application to Biosurveillance* (Fricker *et al.*, 2008b) demonstrate how the ATFS, CED, and PSD metrics (although with alternate names) can be applied to compare the effectiveness of EED methods.

7

Univariate Temporal Methods

> At the present time, even a good surveillance system is perhaps best viewed as a "smoke detector." They may pick up important public health diagnoses or syndromes, but only labor-intensive follow-up investigations will distinguish genuine fires from backyard barbecues.
>
> Michael Grey and Kenneth Spaeth (2006, p. 76)

This chapter describes univariate temporal methods useful for early event detection (EED) and how to appropriately apply them to the biosurveillance problem. Biosurveillance systems often apply variants of standard univariate statistical process control (SPC) methods – the Shewhart, cumulative sum (CUSUM), and exponentially weighted moving average (EWMA) methods – for EED. A challenge in applying these methods to biosurveillance is that the data often violate classical SPC assumptions, particularly the assumptions of normality and independent and identically distributed observations.

When applied to biosurveillance, the Shewhart, CUSUM, and EWMA methods should be tailored to the biosurveillance problem and data. For example, biosurveillance is generally only focused on detecting increases in disease incidence, and thus the methods should be designed only to signal for increases. (In SPC parlance, these are "one-sided control chart" problems.) In addition, because biosurveillance data frequently contain various systematic effects, the methods should be applied to the residuals from a model designed to remove such effects, not the raw data itself. By making these and other adjustments, the classical SPC methods can often be appropriately applied to biosurveillance, and furthermore, in so doing, EED performance can often be improved.

This chapter begins by describing the historical limits method, a method commonly used in public health surveillance that is a particular variant of the Shewhart method. It then proceeds to describe and develop the Shewhart, CUSUM, and EWMA methods, both in an SPC context and then in a biosurveillance context. In the SPC context, these methods are referred to as *control charts*, but in the biosurveillance context, they are referred to as *EED methods*. For each, the control chart is first introduced followed by a discussion of how to modify and implement the method for biosurveillance. Following this, the chapter then discusses other methods that are commonly used in health surveillance, including the Early Aberration Reporting System (EARS) EED methods – which are actually variants of the Shewhart method, as well as scan statistics.

The discussions and examples in this chapter focus on the application of the EED methods to data that follow specific probability distributions. Although somewhat abstract, in so doing, the discussions make clear how to appropriately tailor the EED methods to particular types of data. Chapter 9 then demonstrates how to apply the methods to actual biosurveillance data.

Chapter Objectives

Upon completion of this chapter, the reader should be able to:

- Discuss the Shewhart, CUSUM, and EWMA univariate temporal methods, including
  - Specifying their traditional SPC formulations
  - Describing how they are modified for biosurveillance applications
  - Determining how to appropriately parameterize them for implementation
  - Applying them to achieve desired average time between false signals (ATFS), conditional expected delay (CED), and probability of successful detection (PSD) performance
- Describe the historical limits, temporal scan statistics, and EARS methods, including
  - Discussing how the methods are or can be used for surveillance and biosurveillance
  - Describing how the performance of these methods compare with Shewhart, CUSUM, and EWMA
  - Explaining why the EARS's C1 and C2 methods are not CUSUMs

Mathematical Notation

C	CUSUM statistic
D	Duration of outbreak
E	EWMA statistic
$\mathbb{E}(Y)$	Expected value of Y
f_0, f_1	Probability density functions (pdfs)
F_0, F_1	Cumulative distribution functions (cdfs)
F_t	Outbreak cdf at time t
F^{-1}	Inverse cdf
h	Threshold
k	Reference value parameter of CUSUM
L	Parameter for setting EWMA threshold
L_t	Log likelihood ratio at time t
M	Magnitude of outbreak
$\text{NBin}(r, l)$	Negative binomial distribution with parameters r and l
$N(0, 1)$	Normal distribution with mean 0 and variance 1
$\text{Pois}(\lambda)$	Poisson distribution with parameter λ
S	Shewhart statistic, scan statistic
$T_{i,j,k}$	Total number of reportable disease i, in week j and year k
Y	Observation
$\bar{Y}$	Sample mean of $Y_1, \ldots, Y_m$
$\hat{Y}_t$	Predicted value of Y for day t
Z	Standardized observation
λ	Smoothing parameter of EWMA
λ_0, λ_1	Poisson distribution parameters under F_0 and F_1, respectively
μ_i	Expected value of random variable with distribution F_i
$\hat{\mu}_i$	Estimated mean of random variable with distribution F_i
$\hat{\mu}_{i,j,k}$	Historical limits sample mean for reportable disease i in week j and year k
σ_0	Standard deviation of random variable with distribution F_0
$\hat{\sigma}_0$	Estimated standard deviation of random variable with distribution F_0
$\hat{\sigma}_{\bar{Y}}$	Estimated standard error of $\bar{Y}$
$\hat{\sigma}^2_{i,j,k}$	Historical limits sample variance for reportable disease i, in week j and year k
τ	(Unknown) time of change from F_0 to F_1
τ_l	Last time period of outbreak
τ_s	Start time period of outbreak

7.1 Historical Limits Detection Method

The *historical limits* method is commonly used by public health practitioners to compare data from a current time period with data from an equivalent historical period or periods. The idea is to assess whether the mean of the current data is significantly larger or smaller than the mean observed in the historical data after accounting for the natural variation inherent in the data.

An example of a system that uses historical limits is the Centers for Disease Control and Prevention (CDC) National Notifiable Diseases Surveillance System (NNDSS). NNDSS aggregates and summarizes data on specific diseases that health care providers are required by state law to report to public health departments. Reportable diseases include anthrax, botulism, plague, and tularemia.[1] Each week the states report counts of cases for each of the reportable diseases to the CDC.

A simple use of comparisons to historical data is Table I of the "Notifiable Diseases/Deaths in Selected Cities Weekly Information" report published online each week in the CDC's *Morbidity and Mortality Weekly Report* (*MMWR*). For each reportable disease, Table I provides the current week's national count total and a 5-year weekly average for an equivalent period. A significant deviation of the current count from the 5-year average is an indication of unusual activity in a particular week for any of the diseases. Table I also provides other useful statistics such as the cumulative number of cases reported for the year and the total number of cases reported for each of the past 5 years.

Figure I in the *MMWR's* "Notifiable Diseases/Deaths in Selected Cities Weekly Information" implements a more formal use of historical data by incorporating a measure of variation into limits. Specifically, the most recent 4-week totals for each of the notifiable diseases, $T_{i,j,k}$, for reportable disease i, in week j and year k, are compared with the mean number of cases reported for the same 4-week period, the preceding 4-week period, and the succeeding 4-week period for the previous 5 years as follows.

Calculating the mean of the 15 historical periods as

$$\hat{\mu}_{i,j,k} = \frac{1}{15} \sum_{s=1}^{5} \sum_{r=-1}^{1} T_{i,j-r,k-s},$$

and the variance as

$$\hat{\sigma}_{i,j,k}^2 = \frac{1}{14} \sum_{s=1}^{5} \sum_{r=-1}^{1} \left(T_{i,j-r,k-s} - \hat{\mu}_{i,j,k} \right)^2,$$

the historical limits for the ratio $T_{i,j,k}/\hat{\mu}_{i,j,k}$ are defined to be

$$1 \pm \frac{2\hat{\sigma}_{i,j,k}}{\hat{\mu}_{i,j,k}}. \tag{7.1}$$

---

[1] See www.cdc.gov/ncphi/disss/nndss/phs/infdis.htm for a complete list of reportable diseases.

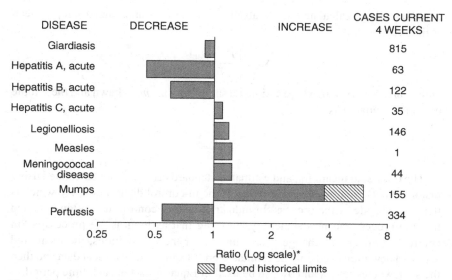

Figure 7.1. An example of Figure I from "Notifiable Diseases/Deaths in Selected Cities Weekly Information" for the week 47 of 2009 (CDC, 2009). For this week, the mumps count exceeded its historical limits.

Figure 7.1 is an example of Figure I from "Notifiable Diseases/Deaths in Selected Cities Weekly Information" for week 47 of 2009 (CDC, 2009), where for this week the mumps count exceeded its historical limits as shown by the crosshatched top of the bar. See Stroup *et al.* (1989) and Stroup *et al.* (1993) for additional discussion, including further discussion of the historical limits methodology used in the CDC's NNDSS and alternatives to that methodology.

Returning to Equation 7.1, multiplying through the equation by $\hat{\mu}_{i,j,k}$ shows that the idea of the historical method is to signal whenever the mean of the current data is larger then the mean of observed in the historical data plus two standard deviations, or it is smaller than the mean minus two standard deviations. That is, a signal is produced if

$$T_{i,j,k} \geq \hat{\mu}_{i,j,k} + 2\hat{\sigma}_{i,j,k} \tag{7.2}$$

or

$$T_{i,j,k} \leq \hat{\mu}_{i,j,k} - 2\hat{\sigma}_{i,j,k}. \tag{7.3}$$

As the next section will show, this is just a specific form of the Shewhart method with two standard deviation signal limits.

7.2 Shewhart Detection Method

The *Shewhart control chart* (Shewhart, 1931) is perhaps the best known of all univariate SPC methods and is widely applied in industry. One variant compares a test statistic S, calculated as the absolute value of a standardized sample mean at time t,

$$S_t = \left| \frac{\bar{Y}_t - \hat{\mu}_0}{\hat{\sigma}_{\bar{Y}}} \right|, \tag{7.4}$$

with a *threshold* $h > 0$, where at time t a sample of size m is drawn and the sample mean is calculated as

$$\bar{Y}_t = \frac{1}{m} \sum_{j=1}^{m} Y_{tj}.$$

The estimated mean, $\hat{\mu}_0$, and estimated standard error, $\hat{\sigma}_{\bar{Y}}$, are calculated using historical data from what is referred to as the in-control distribution, F_0, which is the desired state of the process. In industrial quality control, it is often assumed that the process mean is stationary, meaning that as long as the process is "in control," F_0 does not change over time. Under these conditions, the mean and standard deviation need only be estimated once from some historical data and then the same values for $\hat{\mu}_0$ and $\hat{\sigma}_{\bar{Y}}$ can be used in Equation 7.4 at each time period.

If S_t equals or exceeds the threshold, then a signal is generated. If it does not, then another sample is drawn, and the process is repeated.

The idea of the Shewhart control chart is that, if at some point in the future the observations have a new distribution F_1 with mean μ_1 (where $\mu_1 \neq \mu_0$), the resulting statistic S will be more likely to exceed h. The Shewhart chart is really just a repeated two-sided z- or t-test, where samples continue to be drawn and tested until the test statistic falls far enough out in one of the tails of the sampling distribution that a signal is generated.

For a reasonably large *iid* sample of size m, the sample mean has an approximately normal distribution via the Central Limit Theorem (CLT). This simplifies control chart implementation by eliminating the need to first determine F_0. Rather, for known $\sigma_{\bar{Y}}$ or for a reasonably large historical sample size, it follows that S is approximately distributed according to a standard normal distribution: $N(0, 1)$. This makes choosing thresholds relatively straightforward.

Note the correspondence between the Shewhart method in Equation 7.4 and the historical limits method. In particular, if $h = 2$, then the Shewhart method will signal if

$$\left| \frac{\bar{Y}_t - \hat{\mu}_0}{\hat{\sigma}_{\bar{Y}}} \right| \geq 2. \tag{7.5}$$

Rearranging Equation 7.5 results in equations equivalent to Equations 7.2 and 7.3, the main difference being that the historical limits method is monitoring totals but the Shewhart control chart usually monitors the process mean.

In industrial practice, two Shewhart control charts are often run simultaneously, one to monitor the process mean and the other the process variation. More complicated versions of the Shewhart chart also exist that are intended to be more sensitive to small shifts in the mean using what are called "runs rules."

Shewhart *individuals charts* can also be created for monitoring using individual observations, although the distribution of those individual observations must be either known or well estimated in order to appropriately set the thresholds. See Montgomery (2004) for additional details about the design and application of Shewhart control charts in the industrial SPC setting.

7.2.1 Modified for Biosurveillance

The fundamental idea of the Shewhart chart is to monitor data, comparing them with a distribution that reflects the "normal" state (F_0) until an observation is observed that is sufficiently rare under F_0 that it is rejected as truth. As with classical hypothesis testing, "rare" is defined by the alternative to be detected.

In biosurveillance, monitoring the data for unusual increases is of most interest. In addition, because the goal is often to detect an outbreak as quickly as possible, it is preferable to monitor the individual observations rather than waiting for enough data to accumulate to calculate sample averages. These conditions imply that the standard SPC implementation should be modified as follows.

Given only increases are relevant to detect, individual observations are used, and assuming F_0 is stationary, then the *Shewhart EED method* monitors

$$S_t = \frac{Y_t - \bar{Y}}{\hat{\sigma}_Y}$$

The sample mean and standard deviation are calculated from historical data distributed as F_0. That is, $\bar{Y}$ is an estimate of μ_0, and $\hat{\sigma}_Y$ is an estimate of the standard deviation of Y, σ_0.

If the distribution of the data is not stationary, which is the usual case in biosurveillance, apply the Shewhart method in two steps. First, model the systematic effects in the data, perhaps using one of the methods described in Chapter 5, and calculate the standardized residuals

$$Z_t = \frac{Y_t - \hat{Y}_t}{\hat{\sigma}_{Y-\hat{Y}}},$$

where $Y_t - \hat{Y}_t$ is the residual at time t and $\hat{\sigma}_{Y-\hat{Y}}$ is the estimated standard deviation of the residuals. Then monitor the residuals Z_t, where ideally, but not necessarily, $Z_t \sim N(0, 1)$. Regardless, the purpose of this first step is to remove the systematic effects from the data with the goal of achieving stationarity or near-stationarity of the residuals. If successful, then the Shewhart method is applied to the standardized residuals, where $Z_t \sim F_0$ for some distribution F_0.

The Shewhart method is applied to biosurveillance using the following "one-sided" scheme for monitoring the mean incidence: Choose a threshold h and observe a sequence of residuals over time. As long as $Z_t < h$, assume the F_0 is true and thus there is no evidence of an outbreak. However, if $Z_t \geq h$, signal that an outbreak may be occurring.

Example 7.1. To illustrate the Shewhart detection method, consider the following influenza-like illness (ILI) daily syndrome count data along with forecasts from a regression-based model (see Chapter 5) and the associated estimated standard deviations of the residuals, for days $t = 1, \ldots, 15$.

t	1	2	3	4	5	6	7	$\cdots$
y_t	20	18	21	24	17	22	23	$\cdots$
$\hat{y}_t$	20.222	17.274	21.143	25.715	16.932	20.718	23.212	$\cdots$
$\hat{\sigma}_{y-\hat{y}}$	0.959	0.984	0.976	0.991	1.016	0.983	1.038	$\cdots$

$\cdots$	8	9	10	11	12	13	14	15
$\cdots$	20	21	19	32	30	27	32	28
$\cdots$	21.016	20.465	20.100	30.543	26.848	25.371	29.466	26.443
$\cdots$	1.055	1.023	1.019	1.154	1.126	1.144	1.170	1.211

Calculate the standardized residuals, $z_1, \ldots, z_{15}$; plot them; and then for $h = 1.9$, determine whether an outbreak may have occurred.

Solution: The standardized residuals are:

t	1	2	3	4	5	6	7	$\cdots$
$z_t = \frac{y_t - \hat{y}_t}{\hat{\sigma}_{y-\hat{y}}}$	−0.231	0.738	−0.147	−1.731	0.067	1.304	−0.204	$\cdots$

$\cdots$	8	9	10	11	12	13	14	15
$\cdots$	−0.963	0.523	−1.079	1.263	2.799	1.424	2.166	1.286

Figure 7.2 is a time series plot of the residuals. It shows that for a threshold of $h = 1.9$, the Shewhart method signals at times 12 and 14, indicating a possible ILI outbreak. The signals are the result of large residuals, which occur because the observed values on days 12 and 14 significantly exceeded the forecast values.

For the (simulated) data in Example 7.1, the outbreak actually started on day 11. Thus, the Shewhart method with a threshold of $h = 1.9$ had a delay of one day between the start of the actual outbreak and when it first signaled. As is evident in Figure 7.2, the speed of detection can be improved by using a lower threshold. Indeed, if the threshold had been set below the residual value on day 11 (1.263), the Shewhart method would have signaled for days 11 to 15. However, note that this improved sensitivity comes at the cost of increased false-positive signals. For example, setting $h = 1.26$ would also have resulted in a false-positive signal on day 6.

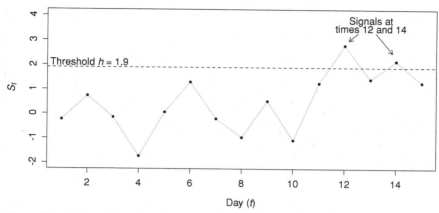

Figure 7.2. A plot of the residuals for the Shewhart EED method from Example 7.1. For a threshold of $h = 1.9$, the Shewhart method signals at times 12 and 14, indicating a possible ILI outbreak.

7.2.2 Implementation

To implement the Shewhart method, one must decide (1) which forecast model is most appropriate to use for a given set of data, (2) how to estimate the standard deviation of the residuals, and (3) how to set the threshold h. For forecast model alternatives, see Chapter 5. When estimating the standard deviation, the main question is how frequently it should be re-estimated and how much historical data should be used in the calculation. Setting these two issues aside, which must be decided in the context of the actual data in a specific situation, a critical issue is how to choose h.

The threshold h is chosen to achieve a desired level of performance as measured by the metrics described in Chapter 6. In particular, h is chosen to make the average time between false signals (ATFS) appropriately large, so that the rate of false-positive signals is low enough that the organization has the resources to investigate all resulting signals.

Assuming the residuals are independent and identically distributed according to F_0, then $\mathbb{P}(Z_t \geq h) = p$ for $t = 1, 2, 3, \ldots$. Under these conditions, the time until first signal has a geometric distribution with probability p, and thus the expected time to signal is $1/p$. Therefore, set $h = F_0^{-1}(1 - p)$ to achieve an ATFS $= 1/p$.

CED performance and PSD performance are functions of the outbreak distribution. In an industrial quality control context where $Z_t \sim F_1$ for $i = \tau, \tau + 1, \tau + 2, \ldots$, the average time until a true signal from the start of the outbreak is $1/p_1$, where $p_1 = 1 - F_1(h)$. In this situation, the PSD metric is unnecessary because, as long as $p_1 > 0$, the CED is finite, and thus the probability of eventual detection is 1. That is, when an outbreak continues indefinitely, the Shewhart method will eventually signal during the outbreak, so PSD $= 1$.

These results do not apply to an outbreak of finite duration, say of D periods. In this, the typical biosurveillance situation, assuming F_1 is stationary over the

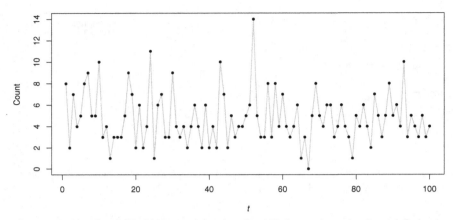

Figure 7.3. Simulated GI chief complaint data for 100 days, where the data were drawn randomly from a Poisson distribution with $\lambda_0 = 5$.

outbreak period, the CED is calculated as

$$\text{CED} = \sum_{i=1}^{D} i \left(1 - F_1(h)\right) F_1(h)^{i-1}. \tag{7.6}$$

The probability of detecting an outbreak of duration D, again assuming F_1 is constant over the outbreak period, is

$$\text{PSD} = \sum_{i=1}^{D} \left(1 - F_1(h)\right) F_1(h)^{i-1} = 1 - F_1(h)^{D}. \tag{7.7}$$

Now, if the outbreak distribution changes over time, $Z_{\tau_s} \sim F_{\tau_s}$, $Z_{\tau_s+1} \sim F_{\tau_s+1}, \ldots, Z_{\tau_s+D-1} \sim F_{\tau_s+D-1}$, then the CED is calculated as

$$\text{CED} = \left(1 - F_{\tau_s}(h)\right) + \sum_{i=2}^{D} \left[i \left(1 - F_{\tau_s+i-1}(h)\right) \prod_{j=1}^{i-1} F_{\tau_s+j-1}(h) \right] \tag{7.8}$$

and the probability of detecting an outbreak of duration D is

$$\text{PSD} = 1 - \prod_{i=1}^{D} F_{\tau_s+i-1}(h). \tag{7.9}$$

The following examples, starting with one using a discrete distribution, should make these definitions and ideas more concrete.

Example 7.2. Let the daily count for chief complaints corresponding to the gastrointestinal (GI) syndrome for a large metropolitan hospital follow a Poisson distribution with parameter $\lambda_0 = 5$. That is, $F_0 = \text{Pois}(5)$. Figure 7.3 shows what 100 observations drawn randomly according to F_0 look like.

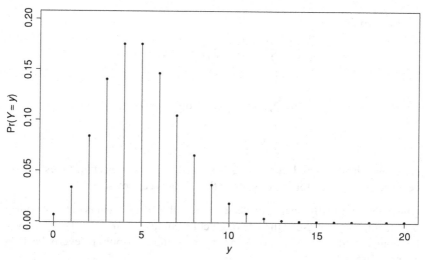

Figure 7.4. Probability mass function for a Poisson distribution with $\lambda_0 = 5$).

Question #1: What threshold h will achieve an ATFS of at least 100 days?

Solution: Figure 7.4 is the probability mass function for F_0. The goal is to determine the smallest h such that $\mathbb{P}(Y \geq h) \leq 0.01$. Looking up the probabilities in a table or software package gives $\mathbb{P}(Y \geq 11) = 0.0137$ and $\mathbb{P}(Y \geq 12) = 0.0055$. Thus, the appropriate choice of threshold is $h = 12$, which achieves an ATFS of about 182 days ($1/0.0055 = 181.8$), or roughly every 6 months.

Question #2: Given the threshold $h = 12$, what is the average time between signal events (ATBSE)?

Solution: Because Shewhart's detection method "resets" after every signal, ATBSE = ATFS = 182 days.

Question #3: Given the threshold $h = 12$, what is the expected time to detect an increase in the rate of GI chief complaints to $F_1 = \text{Pois}(10)$ *assuming the increase is constant and sustained*?

Solution: Again using a table or statistical software, calculate that for $Y \sim \text{Pois}(10)$, $\mathbb{P}(Y \geq 12) = 0.303$. Therefore, the expected time until a signal for a sustained outbreak is $1/0.303 = 3.3$ or a little over 3 days.

Question #4: Given the outbreak only lasts 5 days, what is the CED?

Solution: The CED is the average time it takes to detect an outbreak, starting from the first day of the outbreak, given an outbreak is occurring.

For this problem

$$\text{CED} = \sum_{i=1}^{D} i \, (1 - F_1(h)) \, F_1(h)^{i-1}$$

$$= \sum_{i=1}^{5} i \times (1 - 0.697) \times (0.697)^{i-1}$$

$$= 1.9 \text{ days.}$$

Note that the CED is less than the expected time to detect in Question #3 because (true) detection times greater than 5 days cannot occur.

Question #5: Finally, again given a threshold of $h = 12$, what is the probability of detecting an increase in the rate of GI chief complaints to $F_1 = \text{Pois}(10)$ over the course of the 5-day outbreak (after which the distribution reverts back to $F_0 = \text{Pois}(5)$)?

Solution: From Question #3, the probability of a signal on any one day with $F_1 = \text{Pois}(10)$ is 0.303. The probability of detecting the outbreak is one minus the probability that there are no signals on any of the outbreak days: $\text{PSD} = 1 - (1 - 0.303)^5 = 0.8355$, so there is an 83.6 percent chance of detecting the outbreak.

Alternate Solution: To directly calculate the probability of one or more signals over the course of the five days, let X be the number of signals over the five days, $X = 0, 1, \ldots, 5$. Then X follows a binomial distribution with $n = 5$ trials and probability of success $p = 0.303$. Using a table or statistical software, calculate that $\mathbb{P}(X \geq 1) = 0.8355$, which matches the previous solution.

Note that ATFS, the CED, and the PSD all trade-off depending on the choice of threshold. Whereas high thresholds result in large ATFS values, lower thresholds result in smaller ATFS values. As described in Chapter 6, the ATFS should be used to set the threshold, and it should be based on the resources available for adjudicating signals. The more resources available, the lower the threshold can be set and the more sensitive the system will be to detecting outbreaks.

The CED and PSD are then functions of the chosen threshold *and* the outbreak. They characterize the performance of the system in a particular situation where, obviously, smaller values for CED and larger values of the PSD are preferred. The lower the threshold, the smaller the CED and the higher the PSD. However, raising the threshold does not necessarily increase the CED. Rather, the CED is a concave function that initially increases with increasing thresholds but then decreases as thresholds get very large. Specifically,

$$\lim_{h \to -\infty} \text{CED} = 1,$$

because $F(h) \rightarrow 0$ as $h \rightarrow -\infty$, and

$$\lim_{h \rightarrow \infty} \text{CED} = 0,$$

because $F(h) \rightarrow 1$ as $h \rightarrow \infty$. Therefore, when judging performance, it is important to consider both the CED and PSD because as $h \rightarrow \infty$ the PSD $\rightarrow 0$.

Of course, these concepts apply equally to continuous distributions, as the next example illustrates.

Example 7.3. Let the standardized residuals from an adaptive regression model for the ILI syndrome counts in a county follow a standard normal distribution: $F_0 = N(0, 1)$. For $h = 2.7775$, assess the performance of Shewhart's method at detecting an 8-day outbreak that manifests as $F_{\tau_s + i} = N(\delta_i, 1)$, where $\delta_0 = 0.5, \delta_1 = 1.0, \delta_2 = 1.5, \delta_3 = 2.0, \delta_4 = 2.0, \delta_5 = 1.5, \delta_6 = 1.0, \delta_7 = 0.5$.

Question #1: Given $h = 2.7775$, what is the average time between false signals?

Solution: For $Y \sim N(0, 1)$, the $\mathbb{P}(Y \geq 2.7775) = 0.00274$. Therefore, the average time between false signals is $1/0.00274 = 365$ days, or about once a year.

Question #2: Given the outbreak described, what is the CED?

Solution: For this problem

$$\text{CED} = \left(1 - F_{\tau_s}(h)\right) + \sum_{i=2}^{D} \left[i \left(1 - F_{\tau_s + i - 1}(h)\right) \prod_{j=1}^{i-1} F_{\tau_s + j - 1}(h) \right]$$

$$= 1 \times 0.011 +$$
$$\quad 2 \times 0.038 \times 0.989 +$$
$$\quad 3 \times 0.101 \times 0.989 \times 0.962 +$$
$$\quad 4 \times 0.218 \times 0.989 \times 0.962 \times 0.899 +$$
$$\quad 5 \times 0.218 \times 0.989 \times 0.962 \times 0.899 \times 0.782 +$$
$$\quad 6 \times 0.101 \times 0.989 \times 0.962 \times 0.899 \times 0.782 \times 0.782 +$$
$$\quad 7 \times 0.038 \times 0.989 \times 0.962 \times 0.899 \times 0.782 \times 0.782 \times 0.899 +$$
$$\quad 8 \times 0.011 \times 0.989 \times 0.962 \times 0.899 \times 0.782 \times 0.782 \times 0.899 \times 0.962$$
$$= 2.3 \text{ days.}$$

Question #3: What is the probability of detecting the outbreak?

Solution: The probability of detecting the outbreak is

$$\text{PSD} = 1 - \prod_{i=1}^{D} F_{\tau_s + i - 1}(h)$$

$$= 1 - (0.989 \times 0.962 \times 0.899 \times 0.782 \times$$
$$0.782 \times 0.899 \times 0.962 \times 0.989) = 0.55.$$

Question #4: What do graphs of the ATFS, the CED, and the PSD for this outbreak as a function of the threshold, for $1.5 \leq h \leq 3$ show?

Solution: The plots are shown in Figure 7.5. The dotted lines show the values for each of the functions at $h = 2.7775$. Note how the ATFS is strictly increasing for increasing thresholds while the PSD is strictly decreasing. The CED, on the other hand, is concave. This occurs because when the threshold is smaller, increases make it more difficult to detect, and thus the CED increases. However, as the threshold continues to get larger, it reaches a point where most outbreaks are simply not detected and that then causes the CED to decrease. As previously discussed, in the limit as $h \to \infty$, CED $\to 0$.

Note how the plots show that increasing the PSD comes at the cost of decreasing the ATFS. Decreasing the ATFS is equivalent to increasing the rate of false-positive signals. For example, to achieve a PSD of 90 percent (up from 55 percent), the ATFS decreases to about 50 days (down from 365 days). Whether such a trade-off is desirable and achievable is a function of the resources available to adjudicate the signals. Also note how increasing the PSD also results in an increased CED – because more outbreaks are now being caught – and the increase is relatively modest.

7.3 Cumulative Sum Detection Method

The *CUSUM control chart* of Page (1954) and Lorden (1971) is a well-known SPC methodology that is also frequently applied in biosurveillance. Formally, the CUSUM is a sequential test for a change from a known distribution F_0 to a known alternative distribution F_1. The method monitors the statistic C_t, which satisfies the recursion

$$C_t = \max[0, C_{t-1} + L_t], \tag{7.10}$$

where the increment L_t is the log-likelihood ratio

$$L_t = \log \frac{f_1[Y_t]}{f_0[Y_t]}. \tag{7.11}$$

The method is usually started at $C_0 = 0$; it stops and concludes that $Y \sim F_1$ at the first time when $C_t \geq h$, for some threshold h that achieves a desired ATFS when $Y \sim F_0$ (i.e., when no outbreak is present).

If f_0 and f_1 are normal densities with common variance σ^2 and means μ_0 and $\mu_1 = \mu_0 + \delta\sigma$ ($\delta > 0$), respectively, then Equation 7.10 becomes

$$C_t = \max[0, C_{t-1} + (Y_t - \mu_0)/\sigma - k], \tag{7.12}$$

with $k = \frac{\mu_1 - \mu_0}{2\sigma} = \frac{\delta}{2}$, where k is commonly referred to as the *reference value*. If the Ys are independent and identically distributed according to f_0 before some

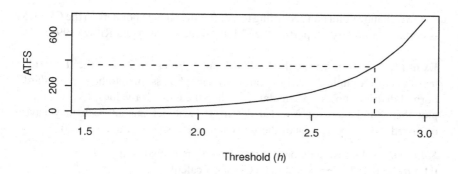

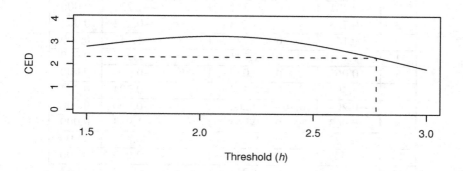

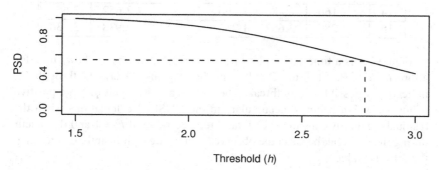

Figure 7.5. Graphs of ATFS, CED, and PSD as a function of the threshold, $1.5 \le h \le 3$, for the outbreak defined in Example 7.3.

unknown change point and according to f_1 after the change point, then the CUSUM has certain optimality properties. See Moustakides (1986) and Ritov (1990).

Example 7.4. To illustrate the CUSUM, apply Equation 7.12 to the ILI residuals data of Example 7.1 (which can reasonably be assumed to have a standard normal distribution). In particular, calculate the CUSUM values, $C_1, \ldots, C_{15}$, plot them, and then for $h = 1.0$ determine whether an outbreak may have occurred. For the purposes of these calculations, use $k = 1$ and $C_0 = 0$.

Solution: If the residuals have a standard normal distribution, $F_0 = N(0, 1)$, then $\mu_0 = 0$ and $\sigma = \sigma_0 = 1$. The CUSUM calculations are:

t	z_t	$C_{t-1} + z_t - k$			C_t
1	−0.231	$0 - 0.231 - 1$	=	−1.231	0.000
2	0.738	$0 + 0.738 - 1$	=	−0.262	0.000
3	−0.147	$0 - 0.147 - 1$	=	−1.147	0.000
4	−1.731	$0 - 1.731 - 1$	=	−2.731	0.000
5	0.067	$0 + 0.067 - 1$	=	−0.933	0.000
6	1.304	$0 + 1.304 - 1$	=	0.304	0.304
7	−0.204	$0.304 - 0.204 - 1$	=	−0.900	0.000
8	−0.963	$0 - 0.963 - 1$	=	−1.963	0.000
9	0.523	$0 + 0.523 - 1$	=	−0.477	0.000
10	−1.079	$0 - 1.079 - 1$	=	−2.079	0.000
11	1.263	$0 + 1.263 - 1$	=	0.263	0.263
12	2.799	$0.263 + 2.799 - 1$	=	2.062	2.062
13	1.424	$2.062 + 1.424 - 1$	=	2.486	2.486
14	2.166	$2.486 + 2.166 - 1$	=	3.652	3.652
15	1.286	$3.652 + 1.286 - 1$	=	3.938	3.938

Figure 7.6 is a time series plot of the CUSUM statistics. It shows that, for a threshold of $h = 1.0$, the CUSUM method signals on days 12 through 14, indicating a possible ILI outbreak. The signals are the result of large positive residuals, which begin to accumulate in the CUSUM calculations when the residuals regularly start to exceed the reference value of $k = 1$ and that occur during the outbreak because the observed counts are significantly greater than the forecast values.

To get some insight into how the CUSUM works, focus on the *increment* $(Y_t - \mu_0)/\sigma - k = (Y_t - \mu_0)/\sigma - \delta/2$, which is what gets added onto the cumulative sum at each iteration. In particular, note that when $Y \sim F_0$ that $\mathbb{E}\left[(Y_t - \mu_0)/\sigma - \delta/2\right] = (\mu_0 - \mu_0)/\sigma - \delta/2 = -\delta/2$. Hence, when the data are generated from F_0, the increment is negative (in an expected value sense), so the CUSUM statistic will have a downward drift. Because the CUSUM is bounded below by 0, under these conditions, the CUSUM will tend to be down around zero.

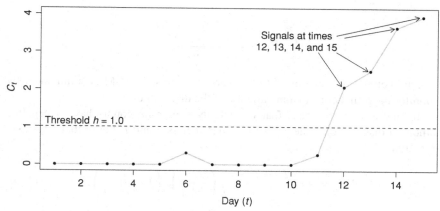

Figure 7.6. A plot of CUSUM statistics from Example 7.4. For a threshold of $h = 1.0$, the CUSUM method signals at for days 12 through 14 indicating a possible ILI outbreak.

On the other hand, when $Y \sim F_1$, then $\mathbb{E}\,[(Y_t - \mu_0)/\sigma - \delta/2] = (\mu_1 - \mu_0)/\sigma - \delta/2 = +\delta/2$. Thus, when the data are generated from F_1, the increment is positive, so the CUSUM statistic will have an upward drift. This positive drift will accumulate in the cumulative sum, which will then tend to exceed the threshold fairly quickly.

Equation 7.12 is a one-sided CUSUM, meaning that it will only detect increases in the mean. In industrial quality control, where it is often important to detect both increases and decreases in the mean, a second CUSUM control chart is used to detect decreases. The CUSUM can also be used to monitor process variability. For example, to monitor an increase in process variability, following Hawkins and Olwell (1998, p. 67), use the CUSUM recursion

$$V_t = \max[0,\, V_{t-1} + W_t - k],$$

where

$$W_t = \frac{\sqrt{|Y_t|} - 0.822}{0.394}.$$

As recommended by Hawkins and Olwell, the same value for k should be used in these CUSUMs for monitoring variability as in the CUSUMs for the mean.

Equation 7.12 is the CUSUM form routinely used even when the underlying assumptions are only approximately met. However, for other F_0 and F_1 distributions, the appropriate log-likelihood ratio (Equation 7.11) should be used and the CUSUM recursion adjusted.

For example, it may be reasonable to assume that the daily counts for some syndromes have a Poisson distribution. For $F_0 = \text{Pois}(\lambda_0)$ and $F_1 = \text{Pois}(\lambda_1)$ with $\lambda_1 > \lambda_0$, the CUSUM becomes

$$C_t = \max[0,\, C_{t-1} + Y_t - k], \tag{7.13}$$

where

$$k = \frac{\lambda_1 - \lambda_0}{\ln \lambda_1 - \ln \lambda_0}.$$

For the Poisson distribution, $\mathbb{E}(Y) = \mathrm{Var}(Y)$, so this CUSUM is simultaneously monitoring both the mean and variance of the distribution.

It may also be the case that other daily syndrome counts have a negative binomial distribution, where for given parameters r and l, the probability mass function is

$$\mathbb{P}(Y = y) = \binom{y + r - 1}{r - 1} \left(\frac{r}{r + l}\right)^r \left(1 - \frac{r}{r + l}\right)^y. \qquad (7.14)$$

Then for $F_0 = \mathrm{NBin}(r, l_0)$ and $F_1 = \mathrm{NBin}(r, l_1)$ (i.e., assuming r does not change) the CUSUM is

$$C_t = \max[0, C_{t-1} + Y_t - k], \qquad (7.15)$$

where

$$k = \frac{-r \ln\left[(r + l_0)/(r + l_1)\right]}{\ln\left[(l_1(r + l_0))/(l_0(r + l_1))\right]}.$$

For this parametrization of the negative binomial, $\mathbb{E}(Y) = l$ and $\mathrm{Var}(Y) = l + l^2/r$, so this CUSUM also simultaneously monitors both the mean and variance.

7.3.1 Modified for Biosurveillance

In industrial settings, the CUSUM is applied directly to the observations because some control is exhibited over the process such that it is reasonable to assume F_0 is stationary. If in fact biosurveillance data can reasonably be assumed *iid* according to a Poisson or negative binomial distribution, then the recursions using the increments from Equations 7.13 or 7.15, respectively, can be used to monitor disease incidence using the data themselves.

However, this is generally not the possible in biosurveillance because the data often have uncontrollable systematic trends, such as seasonal cycles and day-of-the-week effects. In this case, as with the Shewhart method, the CUSUM should be applied to the residuals of a model that accounts for and removes any systematic effects in the data. If the residuals are normally or nearly normally distributed, then the CUSUM in Equation 7.12 should be used. If the residuals are not normally distributed, then the correct log-likelihood ratio increment should be used in Equation 7.10 to derive the appropriate CUSUM. And, of course, because biosurveillance is focused on detecting increases in disease incidence, only a single CUSUM is necessary to monitor the mean.

7.3.2 *Implementation*

Implementing the CUSUM requires choosing a threshold h and setting the reference value k. The choice of threshold should be based on the smallest ATFS that can be accommodated. That is, to achieve the greatest sensitivity for detecting outbreaks, the threshold should be set as low as possible, subject to the constraint that sufficient resources are available to investigate the resulting signals.

In the CUSUM, the ATFS is also a function of the reference value, which itself is a function of the outbreak to be detected (e.g., μ_1 in Equation 7.12 or λ_1 in Equation 7.13 or l_1 in Equation 7.15). The choice of μ_1 or λ_1 or l_1 is a subjective judgment based on the smallest outbreak that is important to detect quickly.

For the CUSUM based on the normal distribution, given k, Table 7.1 can be used to determine the choice of h needed to achieve a desired ATFS. Alternatively, again for the CUSUM designed to detect a mean shift in a normal distribution, the following approximation for the expected time between false signals due to Siegmund (1985) can be used:

$$\text{ATFS} \approx \frac{\exp(2k(h + 1.166)) + 2k(h + 1.166) - 1}{2k^2}.$$

If the observations are not normally distributed, but the probability distribution of the observations or residuals can be specified, simulation can be used to determine the threshold to achieve a specific ATFS. For a given h and k, the following pseudo-code calculates the estimated ATFS and its standard error:

```
set h and k to desired values
   dimension tfs vector to size n
   loop from i = 1 to n
   {
   set CUSUM = 0
   set tfs[i] = 0
   while (CUSUM < h)
     {
     CUSUM = max(0, appropriate CUSUM recursion expression)
     tfs[i] = tfs[i] + 1
     }
   }
   print ATFS=average(tfs) and s.e.(ATFS) = s.d.(tfs)/√n
```

This simulation is iteratively run, starting with a relatively small n, to find the value of h that achieves a desired ATFS. As the approximate value of h is determined, n can be increased to obtain as precise an estimate as desired (and achievable within the computing resources available). The above pseudo-code can also be enclosed within additional code to automate the search for h.

Another alternative for calculating the expected time between false signals is the Markov chain approach of Brook & Evans (1972).

Table 7.1. ATFS for a CUSUM for the mean shift of a standard normal distribution as a function of k and h. Adapted from Hawkins & Olwell (1998, Table 3.1, p. 48)

k	0.00	0.25	0.50	0.75	1.00	1.25	1.50
h							
1.000	4.75	7.0	11.2	19.2	35.3	68.9	142.2
1.125	5.27	8.0	13.2	23.4	44.8	91.4	196.8
1.250	5.84	9.1	15.4	28.6	57.2	122.1	274.9
1.375	6.44	10.3	18.0	34.9	73.1	164.0	387.2
1.500	7.09	11.6	21.1	42.6	93.8	221.5	549.7
1.625	7.76	13.0	24.6	52.0	120.7	300.5	786.0
1.750	8.48	14.6	28.6	63.5	155.5	409.4	1,130.8
1.875	9.22	16.3	33.3	77.4	200.5	559.4	
2.000	10.00	18.2	38.5	94.3	258.7	766.2	
2.125	10.81	20.2	44.6	114.9	333.8	1,051.0	
2.250	11.66	22.4	51.5	139.7	430.7		
2.375	12.53	24.7	59.3	169.7	555.5		
2.500	13.43	27.3	68.2	206.0	716.0		
2.625	14.37	30.0	78.3	249.7	922.2		
2.750	15.33	32.9	89.8	302.5	1,187.0		
2.875	16.32	36.1	102.8	366.1			
3.000	17.35	39.5	117.6	442.8			
3.125	18.41	43.1	134.4	535.3			
3.250	19.50	47.0	153.4	646.9			
3.375	20.61	51.2	175.0	781.4			
3.500	21.76	55.7	199.6	943.7			
3.625	22.95	60.5	227.4	1,139.4			
3.750	24.16	65.7	259.0				
3.875	25.40	71.2	294.8				
4.000	26.68	77.1	335.4				
4.125	27.99	83.4	381.4				
4.250	29.32	90.2	433.6				
4.375	30.69	97.4	492.8				
4.500	32.09	105.1	559.9				
4.625	33.53	113.4	636.0				
4.750	34.99	122.2	722.3				
4.875	36.48	131.6	820.1				
5.000	38.01	141.7	930.9				
5.125	39.57	152.4	1,056.5				
5.250	41.15	163.9					
5.375	42.77	176.1					
5.500	44.42	189.2					
5.625	46.11	203.2					
5.750	47.82	218.0					
5.875	49.56	233.9					
6.000	51.34	250.8					

The following example illustrates how to apply and calculate the CUSUM in a specific biosurveillance scenario.

Example 7.5. The following data are the standardized residuals from an adaptive regression fit to daily ILI counts: $0.819, 0.557, 1.733, 0.415, 0.155, -3.173,$ $-0.549, -0.756, 1.060, 0.137, 0.744, 0.509, 1.206, 0.512, -1.347, 3.772,$ $1.142, 3.132, 2.846, 2.117.$

Under non-outbreak conditions, the standardized residuals are well characterized by the standard normal distribution.

Question #1: What reference value (k) should be used to detect a 2-standard deviation increase in the mean?

Solution: $k = \frac{\mu_1 - \mu_0}{2\sigma} = \frac{\mu_0 + 2\sigma - \mu_0}{2\sigma} = 1.$

Question #2: Given the k from the first question, what threshold should be used to achieve an average time between false signals of approximately 45 days?

Solution: Using Table 7.1, $k = 1$ and $h = 1.125$ gives an ATFS of 44.8 days.

Question #3: Given the threshold $h = 1.125$ and $k = 1$, what is the ATBSE?

Solution: Using simulation (based on the pseudo-code below), the average time between signal events is estimated as ATBSE $= 44.7$ (s.e. 0.14). In this case, the ATBSE is close to the ATFS, but that will not necessarily be case in general.

```
initialize h and k to desired values
    initialize counter1 to 0
    initialize counter2 to 1
    initialize CUSUM to 0
    dimension tbse vector to size n and set to a vector of
    1s loop from i = 1 to n
        {
        set lastCUSUM = CUSUM
        CUSUM = max(0, CUSUM +
            random standard normal deviate - k)
        counter1 = counter1 + 1
        if(CUSUM ≥ h & lastCUSUM < h)
            {
            TBSE[counter2] = counter1
            counter2 = counter2 + 1
            }
        if(CUSUM < h & lastCUSUM ≥ h)
            {
            counter1 = 1
            }
        }
    print ATBSE=average(tbse[2 to n])
    print s.e.(ATBSE) = s.d.(tbse[2 to n])/√n − 1
```

Table 7.2. CUSUM values for Example 7.5, where
$C_t = \max(0, C_{t-1} + Z_t - 1)$, both with and without resetting
after a signal. The bold C_t values are signal times, where
$$C_t \geq h = 1.125$$

		With re-setting		Without re-setting	
t	Z_t	C_{t-1}	C_t	C_{t-1}	C_t
1	0.819	0.000	0.000	0.000	0.000
2	0.557	0.000	0.000	0.000	0.000
3	1.733	0.000	0.733	0.000	0.733
4	0.415	0.733	0.148	0.733	0.148
5	0.155	0.148	0.000	0.148	0.000
6	−3.173	0.000	0.000	0.000	0.000
7	−0.549	0.000	0.000	0.000	0.000
8	−0.756	0.000	0.000	0.000	0.000
9	1.060	0.000	0.060	0.000	0.060
10	0.137	0.060	0.000	0.060	0.000
11	0.744	0.000	0.000	0.000	0.000
12	0.509	0.000	0.000	0.000	0.000
13	1.206	0.000	0.206	0.000	0.206
14	0.512	0.206	0.000	0.206	0.000
15	−1.347	0.000	0.000	0.000	0.000
16	3.772	0.000	**2.772**	0.000	**2.772**
17	1.142	0.000	0.142	2.772	**2.914**
18	3.132	0.142	**2.274**	2.914	**5.046**
19	2.846	0.000	**1.846**	5.046	**6.892**
20	2.117	0.000	1.117	6.892	**8.009**

Question #4: Calculate the CUSUM values over time, both when the CUSUM is reset after each signal and when it is not reset, and plot them on a chart showing the threshold. Is there any evidence of an outbreak?

Solution: Table 7.2 shows the CUSUM calculations and Figure 7.7 plots the CUSUM statistics over time. Both show that the first signal occurs at time $t = 16$ when the CUSUM statistic first exceeds h. After that time, the CUSUM that is reset signals intermittently, and the CUSUM that is not reset signals continuously. To understand whether and when it is appropriate to reset the CUSUM, see the discussion in Chapter 6 on pages 168 and 171.

This next example illustrates how to set up the CUSUM and then assess its performance for various types of outbreaks.

Example 7.6. Consider a biosurveillance system that, when there is no outbreak, the standardized residuals from a model of the daily counts have a standard normal distribution.

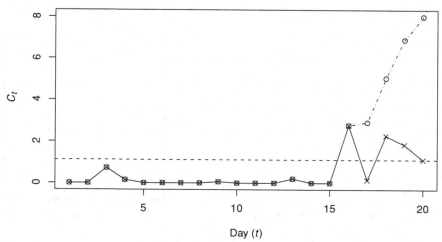

Day (t)

Figure 7.7. Plot of CUSUM statistics for Example 7.5. The solid line is the CUSUM with resetting, and the dotted line is the CUSUM without resetting. The horizontal dotted line is the threshold $h = 1.125$.

Question #1: What values of k and h should be used to detect a 1-standard deviation increase in the mean with an ATFS of roughly once every 40 days?

Solution: For standardized residuals $\mu_0 = 0$ and a 1-standard deviation increase means $\mu_1 = 1$, so that $k = 0.5$. Then, from Table 7.1, it follows that $h = 2.0$ results in an average of one false signal every 38.5 days.

Question #2: Using simulation, what are the zero-state CED and PSD of an outbreak characterized by a triangle-shaped mean shift with a duration (D) of 9 days and a maximum increase (M) of two standard deviations?[2]

Solution: Using a simulation based on the pseudo-code below, the zero-state CED is 4.34 days (s.e. = 0.01) with a PSD of 0.973. The pseudo-code:

```
set o = {0.0, 0.5, 1.0, 1.5, 2.0, 1.5, 1.0, 0.5, 0.0}
    dimension tfs vector to size n
    loop from i = 1 to n
    {
        set CUSUM = 0
        set tfs[i] = 0
        loop from j = 1 to 9
        {
            CUSUM = max(0, CUSUM + random normal variate + o[j] - 0.5)
            if(CUSUM ≥ 2 & tfs[i] = 0) then tfs[i] = j
        }
    }
    Assign to good.tfs vector only those tfs values greater than 0
    print CED=average(good.tfs), se(good.tfs), PSD=length(good.tfs)/n
```

---

[2] See Equation B.5 in Appendix B, with parameters $M = 2$ and $D = 9$.

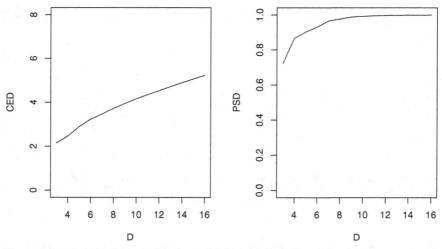

Figure 7.8. Plots of CED and PSD for Example 7.6 for $3 \leq D \leq 16$ and $M = 2$.

Question #3: Using simulation, plot the zero-state CED and PSD for $3 \leq D \leq 16$ and $M = 2$.

Solution: Figure 7.8 shows the plots. CED varies from 2.1 days for an outbreak of 3 days of duration to a CED of 5.2 days for an outbreak of 16 days of duration. The PSD varies from 0.72 for an outbreak of 3 days to 0.999 for an outbreak of duration of 16 days.

The following example illustrates the application of the CUSUM to data that follow a Poisson distribution. In such cases, the CUSUM based on Equation 7.12 would not be appropriate, particularly for Poisson distributions with very small means.

Example 7.7. In a biosurveillance system, in the absence of a flu outbreak, the daily counts of GI syndrome follow a Poisson distribution with $\lambda_0 = 5$. It is important to quickly detect a flu outbreak that increases the mean of the daily counts to $\lambda_1 = 10$.

Question #1: What is the value of k for a CUSUM monitoring this shift in the mean of a Poisson distribution?

Solution: For this CUSUM, $k = \frac{\lambda_1 - \lambda_0}{\ln \lambda_1 - \ln \lambda_0} = \frac{10-5}{\ln(10)-\ln(5)} = 7.213$.

Question #2: Using simulation, what is the threshold for this CUSUM that achieves an ATFS of approximately 30 days?

Solution: Via simulation, $h = 2.7$ gives an ATFS of 29.5 days (s.e. $= 0.1$).

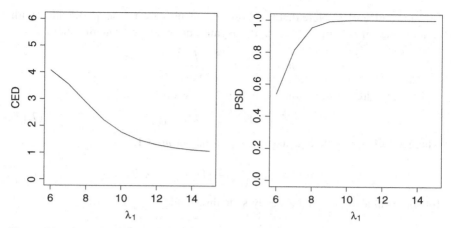

Figure 7.9. Plots of CED and PSD for Example 7.7 for $6 \leq \lambda_1 \leq 15$.

Question #3: Using simulation, what are the (estimated) CED and PSD for outbreaks with a duration of 8 days and with means from 6 to 15 (i.e., $6 \leq \lambda_1 \leq 15$)?

Solution: Figure 7.9 shows the simulation results in which CED varies from 4.1 days for an outbreak with $\lambda_1 = 6$ to a CED of 1.1 days for an outbreak with $\lambda_1 = 15$. The PSD varies from 0.54 to 1.0 over this range of λ_1 values.

7.4 Exponentially Weighted Moving Average Detection Method

The *EWMA control chart* of Roberts (1959) is another popular statistical process control method. It calculates

$$E_t = \lambda \bar{Y}_t + (1 - \lambda)E_{t-1}, \tag{7.16}$$

where $\bar{Y}_t$ is the sample mean of m observations taken at time t and $0 < \lambda \leq 1$ is the smoothing parameter.[3] Note the similarities to the EWMA models in section 5.2.2.1 of Chapter 5.

In Equation 7.16, E_t is a weighted average of past observations; smaller values of λ put more emphasis on past observations, and large values put more emphasis on recent observations. For $\lambda = 1$, the EWMA reduces to the Shewhart. The method starts at $E_0 = \mu_0$, where μ_0 is the expected value of the process under F_0, and a signal is generated at time t if $E_t \geq h$ or $E_t \leq -h$.

The threshold is set as

$$h = \mu_0 + L \frac{\hat{\sigma}}{\sqrt{m}} \sqrt{\frac{\lambda}{2 - \lambda}[1 - (1 - \lambda)^{2t}]}$$

---

[3] Potential notation confusion: λ_0 and λ_1 are parameters of the Poisson distribution, while λ is the EWMA smoothing parameter.

for some value of L. Note that the threshold changes over time, particularly with small values of t. Letting $t \to \infty$, the asymptotic or steady-state threshold is

$$h = \mu_0 + L \frac{\hat{\sigma}}{\sqrt{m}} \sqrt{\frac{\lambda}{2 - \lambda}}.$$

For individual observations, Equation 7.16 becomes

$$E_t = \lambda Y_t + (1 - \lambda) E_{t-1}, \tag{7.17}$$

where as before the method starts at $E_0 = \mu_0$. For $m = 1$,

$$h = \mu_0 + L\hat{\sigma} \sqrt{\frac{\lambda}{2 - \lambda}[1 - (1 - \lambda)^{2t}]}$$

for some value of L, and the steady-state threshold is

$$h = \mu_0 + L\hat{\sigma} \sqrt{\frac{\lambda}{2 - \lambda}}.$$

A nice property of the EWMA is that it can be robust to non-normality of the observations, a good property to have when working with individual observations. In particular, Borror *et al.* (1999) found the EWMA is robust for $0.05 \leq \lambda \leq 0.1$, and Borror *et al.* (1998) recommend using the EWMA form in Equation 7.17 for $Y \sim \text{Pois}(\lambda_0)$, setting $E_0 = \mu_0 = \lambda_0$.

7.4.1 Modified for Biosurveillance

The EWMA is a two-sided method, meaning that it is designed to detect both increases and decreases in the mean of a distribution. Because biosurveillance is only concerned with increases, the EWMA is "reflected" (in the spirit of the CUSUM) to improve its performance in detecting increases. In addition, in biosurveillance, the EWMA is either run on individual observations or residuals from a model of the systematic effects, so Equation 7.16 is modified to:

$$E_t = \max[\mu_0, \lambda Y_t + (1 - \lambda) E_{t-1}]. \tag{7.18}$$

The method starts at $E_0 = \mu_0$ and a signal is generated only when $E_t \geq h$, where for $\mu_0 = \mathbb{E}(Z)$ the threshold is

$$h = \mu_0 + L\hat{\sigma} \sqrt{\frac{\lambda}{2 - \lambda}[1 - (1 - \lambda)^{2t}]},$$

again for some value of L. When run on standardized residuals, so that $\mu_0 = 0$ and $\sigma = 1$, the threshold is

$$h = L \sqrt{\frac{\lambda}{2 - \lambda}[1 - (1 - \lambda)^{2t}]},$$

and asymptotically it is

$$h = L \sqrt{\frac{\lambda}{2 - \lambda}}.$$

Then Equation 7.18 becomes

$$E_t = \max[0, \lambda Z_t + (1 - \lambda)E_{t-1}]$$

with $E_0 = 0$.

Example 7.8. To illustrate the EWMA, apply Equation 7.18 to the ILI residuals data of Examples 7.1 and 7.4. Calculate the EWMA values, $E_1, \ldots, E_{15}$; plot them; and then for $h = 0.6$, determine whether an outbreak may have occurred. For the purposes of these calculations, use $\lambda = 0.2$ and $E_0 = 0$.

Solution: The EWMA calculations are:

t	z_t	$\lambda z_t + (1 - \lambda)E_{t-1}$			E_t
1	−0.231	$0.2 \times -0.231 + 0.8 \times 0$	=	−0.046	0.000
2	0.738	$0.2 \times 0.738 + 0.8 \times 0$	=	0.148	0.148
3	−0.147	$0.2 \times -0.147 + 0.8 \times 0.148$	=	0.089	0.089
4	−1.731	$0.2 \times -1.731 + 0.8 \times 0.089$	=	−0.346	0.000
5	0.067	$0.2 \times 0.067 + 0.8 \times 0$	=	0.013	0.013
6	1.304	$0.2 \times 1.304 + 0.8 \times 0.013$	=	0.271	0.271
7	−0.204	$0.2 \times -0.204 + 0.8 \times 0.271$	=	0.176	0.176
8	−0.963	$0.2 \times -0.963 + 0.8 \times 0.176$	=	−0.052	0.000
9	0.523	$0.2 \times 0.523 + 0.8 \times 0$	=	0.105	0.105
10	−1.079	$0.2 \times -1.079 + 0.8 \times 0.105$	=	−0.132	0.000
11	1.263	$0.2 \times 1.263 + 0.8 \times 0$	=	0.253	0.253
12	2.799	$0.2 \times 2.799 + 0.8 \times 0.253$	=	0.762	0.762
13	1.424	$0.2 \times 1.424 + 0.8 \times 0.762$	=	0.894	0.894
14	2.166	$0.2 \times 2.166 + 0.8 \times 0.894$	=	1.148	1.148
15	1.286	$0.2 \times 1.286 + 0.8 \times 1.148$	=	1.176	1.176

Figure 7.10 is a time series plot of the EWMA statistics. It shows that for a threshold of $h = 0.6$, the EWMA method signals on days 12 through 14, indicating a possible ILI outbreak.

7.4.2 Implementation

Implementing the EWMA requires choosing a threshold h and the smoothing parameter λ. As with the Shewhart and CUSUM methods, the choice of threshold should be based on smallest ATFS that can be accommodated.

For the EWMA, the ATFS is also a function of the smoothing parameter, the choice of which depends on the type of outbreak to be detected. Specifically, for larger and more immediate outbreaks, larger values of λ will result in an EWMA that more quickly detects the outbreak. As previously mentioned, with $\lambda = 1$, the EWMA reverts to the Shewhart, which is capable of detecting large outbreaks in

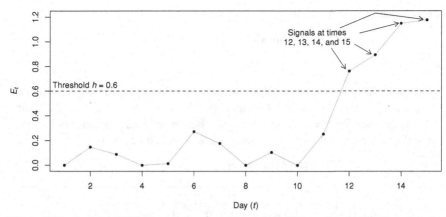

Figure 7.10. A plot of EWMA statistics from Example 7.8. For a threshold of $h = 0.6$, the EWMA method signals at for days 12 through 14, indicating a possible ILI outbreak.

one observation. Conversely, smaller outbreaks (of sufficient duration) are better detected with smaller values of λ.

For the EWMA based on standardized observations or residuals that are normally distributed, given a choice of λ, Table 7.3 can be used to determine the choice of h needed to achieve a desired ATFS.

Table 7.3. ATFS for an EWMA for the mean shift of a standard normal distribution as a function of λ and L determined via simulation. Standard errors of the estimates less than 0.1

λ	0.1	0.2	0.3	0.4	0.5	0.6	0.7	0.8	0.9
L									
1.000	10.4	8.2	7.2	6.8	6.5	6.2	6.1	6.2	6.2
1.125	13.5	10.3	9.0	8.2	7.8	7.5	7.4	7.4	7.4
1.250	17.5	12.9	11.1	10.0	9.5	9.2	9.0	9.1	9.2
1.375	22.6	16.4	13.8	12.5	11.7	11.4	11.2	11.2	11.4
1.500	29.3	20.7	17.4	15.7	14.6	14.1	13.9	14.0	14.3
1.625	37.7	26.4	22.0	19.7	18.5	17.8	17.6	17.8	18.2
1.750	49.2	34.0	28.2	25.3	23.7	22.8	22.5	22.8	23.6
1.875	63.9	43.4	36.3	32.6	30.6	29.6	29.3	29.8	30.9
2.000	83.6	57.0	47.5	42.6	40.1	38.8	38.6	39.4	41.1
2.125	100.0	75.0	62.5	56.5	53.3	51.8	51.7	52.9	55.2
2.250	145.8	99.5	83.6	75.9	71.9	70.1	70.2	71.8	75.5
2.375	195.4	133.8	113.0	103.2	98.3	96.3	96.6	99.2	104.9
2.500	264.6	182.4	155.0	142.7	136.5	134.2	135.1	139.2	147.4
2.625	362.3	252.0	215.9	200.1	192.8	190.2	192.0	198.2	210.5
2.750	503.3	353.3	305.2	285.1	276.2	274.0	276.9	286.4	304.5
2.875	708.5	502.8	438.3	412.3	402.5	400.4	405.9	420.1	447.5
3.000	1,014.9	727.2	639.6	606.4	595.1	594.7	604.0	625.6	667.3
3.125	1,470.7	1,068.7	948.6	905.9	894.4	897.7	912.8	946.1	1,009.6

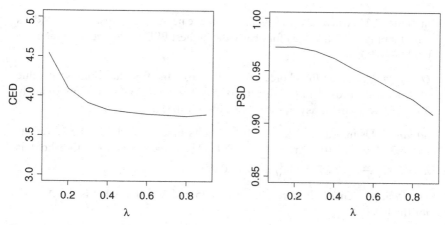

Figure 7.11. Plots of CED and PSD for Example 7.9 for $0.1 \leq \lambda \leq 0.9$ with $M = 1$ and $D = 10$.

If the observations are not normally distributed but the probability distribution of the observations or residuals can be specified, simulation can be used to determine the threshold to achieve a specific ATFS.

The following example illustrates how to apply and calculate the EWMA in the biosurveillance scenario first posed in Example 7.5.

Example 7.9. Using the data from an adaptive regression fit to daily ILI counts in Example 7.5 (0.819, 0.557, 1.733, 0.415, 0.155, −3.173, −0.549, −0.756, 1.060, 0.137, 0.744, 0.509, 1.206, 0.512, −1.347, 3.772, 1.142, 3.132, 2.846, 2.117), set up and repeat the analysis using the EWMA.

Question #1: What value of the smoothing parameter (λ) should be used to detect an outbreak 1 standard deviation in magnitude and 10 days in duration?

Solution: In the SPC literature, $0.1 \leq \lambda \leq 0.3$ is frequently recommended for detecting small changes in the mean. However, in biosurveillance terms, this recommendation is based on the assumption of an outbreak of infinite duration. When the duration is finite, as it will be in biosurveillance, the appropriate choice of λ likely depends on both the magnitude and duration of the outbreak.

Because there have not been any studies in the biosurveillance literature to guide the choice of λ, Figure 7.11 shows the results of a small simulation conducted to get some insight into the EWMA's behavior for various λ, in terms of CED and PSD, for this type of outbreak.

The simulation used the asymptotic form of the threshold equation with the parameter L set to achieve 30 days between false signals (by interpolating from Table 7.3). Then the zero-state CED and PSD were estimated using simulated random observations drawn from a $N(1, 1)$ distribution. The results are shown in Figure 7.11, where $\lambda = 0.3$ looks to achieve nearly the lowest CED (3.9 days out of a range of 3.8 to 4.5) for nearly the highest PSD (0.969 out of a range of 0.973 to 0.909).

Question #2: Given the choice of $\lambda = 0.3$ from the first question, what value of L should be used in the threshold to achieve an ATFS of approximately 30 days? What is the asymptotic threshold for that L?

Solution: Using Table 7.3, $L = 1.75$ results in 28.2, and $L = 1.875$ results in 36.3. Interpolating gives $L = 1.778$. Thus, the asymptotic threshold is $h = L\hat{\sigma}\sqrt{\frac{\lambda}{2-\lambda}} = (1.778)(1)\sqrt{\frac{0.3}{2-0.3}} = 0.75$.

Question #3: Given the threshold $h = 0.75$ and $\lambda = 0.3$, what is the ATBSE for the EWMA?

Solution: Using simulation (based on pseudo-code similar to that from Example 7.5, modified for the EWMA), the ATBSE is estimated to be 28.6 (s.e. = 0.09). In this case, the ATBSE is slightly shorter than the ATFS.

Question #4: Calculate the EWMA values over time, both when the EWMA is reset after each signal and when it is not reset, and plot them on a chart showing the threshold. Is there any evidence of an outbreak?

Solution: Table 7.4 shows the EWMA calculations, and Figure 7.12 plots the EWMA statistics over time. Both show that signals occur at times $t = 3$ and $t = 16$. The former is a false positive, and the latter is a true signal because day 16 was the first day of the outbreak. The false positive is a result of setting the threshold fairly aggressively to achieve an ATFS of 30 days: with 20 days of observations, the occurrence of a false positive is quite likely. This can be mitigated by choosing a larger ATFS, which will result in a higher threshold.

After time 16, both versions of the EWMA continue to signal, continuously for the EWMA that is not reset and intermittently for the EWMA that is reset. Again, see the discussion in Chapter 6 on pages 168 and 171.

Question #4: Using the results from this example and Example 7.5, how does the performance of the EWMA compare with the CUSUM?

Solution: Tables 7.2 and 7.4 (and the plots in Figures 7.7 and 7.12) show that both methods, whether reset or not, signal on day 16, the first day of the outbreak. As discussed in the solution to the previous question, the EWMA also has a false signal on day 3, and both methods give similar patterns of signals after day 16.

Returning to the scenario in Example 7.6, this next example illustrates how to set up the EWMA and then assess its performance for various types of outbreaks.

Table 7.4. EWMA values for Example 7.9, where
$E_t = \max(0, 0.3 \times Z_t + 0.7 \times E_{t-1})$, both with and without
resetting after a signal. The bold E_t values are signal times,
where $E_t \geq h = 0.75$

		With Resetting		Without Resetting	
t	Z_t	E_{t-1}	E_t	E_{t-1}	E_t
1	0.819	0.000	0.246	0.000	0.246
2	0.557	0.246	0.339	0.246	0.339
3	1.733	0.339	**0.757**	0.339	**0.757**
4	0.415	0.000	0.125	0.757	0.655
5	0.155	0.125	0.134	0.655	0.505
6	−3.173	0.134	0.000	0.505	0.000
7	−0.549	0.000	0.000	0.000	0.000
8	−0.756	0.000	0.000	0.000	0.000
9	1.060	0.000	0.318	0.000	0.318
10	0.137	0.318	0.264	0.318	0.264
11	0.744	0.264	0.408	0.264	0.408
12	0.509	0.408	0.438	0.408	0.438
13	1.206	0.438	0.669	0.438	0.669
14	0.512	0.669	0.622	0.669	0.622
15	−1.347	0.622	0.031	0.622	0.031
16	3.772	0.031	**1.153**	0.031	**1.153**
17	1.142	0.000	0.343	1.153	**1.150**
18	3.132	0.343	**1.180**	1.150	**1.745**
19	2.846	0.000	**0.854**	1.745	**2.075**
20	2.117	0.000	0.635	2.075	**2.088**

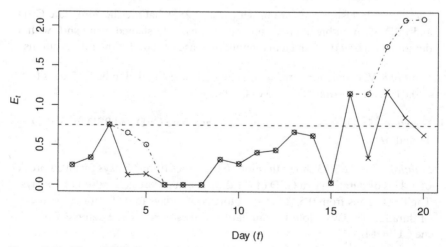

Figure 7.12. Plot of EWMA statistics for Example 7.9. The solid line is the EWMA with resetting, and the dotted line is the EWMA without resetting. The horizontal dotted line is the threshold $h = 0.75$.

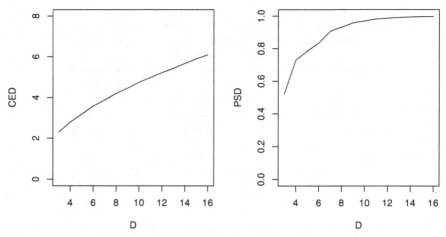

Figure 7.13. Plots of CED and PSD for Example 7.10 for $3 \leq D \leq 16$ and $M = 2$.

Example 7.10. Consider a biosurveillance system that, when there is no outbreak, the standardized residuals from a model of the daily counts has a standard normal distribution.

Question #1: Assuming $\lambda = 0.3$, what value of L should be used for an ATFS of once per quarter?

Solution: Defining a quarter as 91 days and interpolating from Table 7.3 with $L = 2.25$ for 83.6 days and $L = 2.375$ for 113 days gives $L = 2.28$.

Question #2: Using simulation, with $L = 2.28$, what are the zero-state CED and PSD of an outbreak characterized by a triangle-shaped mean shift with a duration (D) of 9 days and a maximum increase (M) of 2 standard deviations?

Solution: Via simulation, the zero-state CED is estimated to be 5.87 days (s.e. < 0.01) with an estimated PSD of 0.998.

Question #3: Using simulation, plot the zero-state CED and PSD for $3 \leq D \leq 16$ and $M = 2$.

Solution: Figure 7.13 shows the plots. CED varies from 2.3 days for an outbreak of 3 days of duration to a CED of 6.1 days for an outbreak duration of 16 days. The PSD varies from 0.522 for an outbreak of 3 days to 0.997 for an outbreak of duration 16 days. Note the similarity of these results to Example 7.6 with the CUSUM.

Question #4: Using the results from this example and Example 7.6, how does the performance of the EWMA compare with the CUSUM?

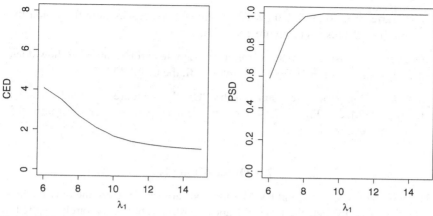

Figure 7.14. Plots of CED and PSD for Example 7.11 for $6 \leq \lambda_1 \leq 15$.

Solution: Comparing the results for the CUSUM in Figure 7.8 with the results for the EWMA in Figure 7.13, the EWMA seems to have a slightly lower PSD for similar CED values for the shorter duration outbreaks, and it has slightly higher CED values for similar PSD values for the longer duration outbreaks. This suggests the CUSUM is to be preferred for these types of outbreaks compared with the EWMA with smoothing parameter $\lambda = 0.3$. It is left as an exercise to see if another choice of λ would result in an EWMA with equivalent or better performance properties compared with the CUSUM.

The following example, based on the scenario of Example 7.7, illustrates the application of the EWMA to data that follow a Poisson distribution.

Example 7.11. In a biosurveillance system, in the absence of a flu outbreak, the daily counts of GI syndrome follow a Poisson distribution with $\lambda_0 = 5$. It is important to quickly detect a flu outbreak that increases the mean of the daily counts to $\lambda_1 = 10$.

Question #1: What value of L should be used to achieve an ATFS of 30 days for an EWMA with $\lambda = 0.3$ monitoring the shift in the mean of a Poisson distribution?

Solution: Using simulation on the standardized observations ($Z_t = (Y_t - 5)/\sqrt{5}$), $L = 1.88$ results in an ATFS of 30.1 days (s.e. = 0.1).

Question #2: Using simulation, what are the estimated CED and PSD for outbreaks with $2 \leq \lambda_1 \leq 15$ and a duration of 8 days?

Solution: Figure 7.14 shows the simulation results in which CED varies from 4.1 days with $\lambda_1 = 6$ to a CED of 1.1 days for an outbreak with $\lambda_1 = 15$. The

PSD varies from 0.59 to 1.0 over this range of λ_1s. Again, note the similarity to the CUSUM results in Figure 7.9 of Example 7.7.

Question #3: Using the results from this example and Example 7.7, how does the performance of the EWMA compare with the CUSUM?

Solution: Comparing the results for the CUSUM in Figure 7.9 with the results for the EWMA in Figure 7.14, the two methods perform very similarly for these outbreak scenarios.

7.5 Other Methods

The Shewhart, CUSUM, and EWMA methods are certainly not the only methods used for EED. In fact, the CUSUM and EWMA methods are rarely applied to biosurveillance even though they are popular in industrial quality control. Other methods that are used are scan statistics and methods first implemented in EARS where, interestingly, two of the original EARS methods are variants of the Shewhart method (but are often mistakenly called CUSUM methods).

7.5.1 *Temporal Scan Statistics*

The idea of the *temporal scan statistic* is to literally scan though a set of longitudinal data, looking at a fixed number of adjacent observations (a "window" of observations), typically with the goal of identifying the set of observations for which the total is largest.

Description
Mathematically, the temporal scan statistic for day t is defined as

$$S_t = \max_{1 \leq i \leq t} \sum_{j=\max(1, i-m+1)}^{i} Y_j$$

where m is the fixed window size. Literally, the sequence of data, $\{Y_1, Y_2, \ldots, Y_t\}$, is scanned, and S_t takes on the largest sum of m sequential observations. A signal is generated for time period t if $S_t \geq h$, for some threshold h.

For prospective monitoring, this approach is inefficient because at time t

$$S_t = \max\{S_{t-1}, T_t\}$$

where

$$T_t = \sum_{j=\max(1, t-m+1)}^{t} Y_j.$$

That is, at time t it is not necessary to re-scan through $\{Y_1, Y_2, \ldots, Y_{t-1}\}$ because it has already been scanned at time $t - 1$. This also means that, for prospective monitoring, it is only necessary to monitor T_t, reducing the temporal scan statistic to monitoring

$$T_t = \sum_{j=\max(1,t-m+1)}^{t} Y_j$$

and signaling at the first time $T_t \geq h$.

The temporal scan statistic is essentially SPC's moving average control chart, differing only in that the total of the window of observations are monitored rather than the average. It is also similar to the CUSUM and EWMA in the sense that it is monitoring the sum of the current observation and some historical data. However, it differs in the way the sum is calculated.

Performance Comparisons

Using standard SPC metrics, Han *et al.* (2009) found that the CUSUM and EWMA outperform the scan statistic for detecting increases in Poisson rates. Similarly, Joner *et al.* (2008a) found that the CUSUM performs better compared with the temporal scan statistic when monitoring for increases in incidence rates under the assumption of independent Bernoulli observations. However, they also concluded that the scan method may be preferred in some applications because of its simplicity at a cost of relatively little loss in performance efficiency. On the other hand, Woodall *et al.* (2008) showed that the temporal scan methods can be slightly more effective than the CUSUM when the duration of the outbreak is close to the width of the scan window.

7.5.2 Early Aberration Reporting System Methods and Associated Variants

EARS was designed to be a drop in biosurveillance system, meaning that it is intended to provide enhanced surveillance for a short duration around a discrete event (e.g., the Olympic Games or a national political convention), generally for which little or no prior data exists (Henning, 2004). Since September 11, 2001, the EARS system has also been increasingly used as a standard surveillance system (CDC, 2007) by state and local health departments. EARS uses three methods titled "C1-MILD," "C2-MEDIUM," and "C3-ULTRA." The C1, C3, and a modified form of the C2 methods were also implemented in BioSense 1.0. BioSense 2.0 currently only uses a modified form of the C2 method.

Description

The C1, C2, and C3 methods are often *incorrectly* described as CUSUM methods (Hutwagner *et al.*, 2003a; Zhu *et al.*, 2005). The EARS V4.5 User's Guide states that the EARS methods "were developed based on a one-sided positive CUSUM" (CDC, 2006e, p. 4). Even the latest BioSense 2.0 guidance incorrectly states that the EARS C2 method is "based on [a] cumulative sum control chart (CUSUM) methodology" (CDC, 2012b, p. 1).

However, as implemented in the EARS SAS code, the C1 and C2 are actually Shewhart variants that use a moving sample average and sample standard deviation to standardize daily counts. The C1 uses the seven days prior to the current observation to calculate the sample average and sample standard deviation. The C2 is similar to the C1 but uses the seven days prior to a two-day lag. The C3 is an *ad hoc* method that combines information from the current observation and previous two periods as described below.

Let Y_t be the observed count for period t representing, for example, the number of individuals arriving at a particular hospital emergency department with a specific syndrome on day t. The C1 calculates the statistic $C1_t$ as

$$C1_t = \frac{Y_t - \bar{Y}_t}{S_t} \qquad (7.19)$$

where $\bar{Y}_t$ and S_t are the moving sample mean and standard deviation, respectively, based on the previous seven day's observations:

$$\bar{Y}_t = \frac{1}{7} \sum_{i=t-1}^{t-7} Y_i \quad \text{and} \quad S_t = \sqrt{\frac{1}{6} \sum_{i=t-1}^{t-7} \left[Y_i - \bar{Y}_t \right]^2}.$$

If $S_t = 0$ then EARS sets it to a small positive number. As implemented in the EARS system, the C1 signals on day t when the C1 statistic exceeds a threshold h, which is fixed at three sample standard deviations above the sample mean: $C1_t > 3$.

The C2 is similar to the C1 but incorporates a two-day lag in the mean and standard deviation calculations. Specifically, it calculates

$$C2_t = \frac{Y_t - \bar{Y}_t^*}{S_t^*} \qquad (7.20)$$

where

$$\bar{Y}_t^* = \frac{1}{7} \sum_{i=t-3}^{t-9} Y_i \quad \text{and} \quad S_t^* = \sqrt{\frac{1}{6} \sum_{i=t-3}^{t-9} \left[Y_i - \bar{Y}_t^* \right]^2}.$$

As with the C1 method, if $S_t^* = 0$ then EARS sets it to a small positive number and the C2 method signals on day t when $C2_t > 3$.

The C3 combines current and historical data from day t and the previous two days, calculating the statistic $C3_t$ as

$$C3_t = \sum_{i=t}^{t-2} \max (0, C2_i - 1). \qquad (7.21)$$

The C3 method signals on day t when $C3_t > 2$.

BioSense Variants

BioSense 1.0 initially incorporated the original C1, C2, and C3 methods. It then replaced the C2 method with two modified forms it called the "W2 count" (W2c) and "W2 rate" (W2r) methods.

The W2c method calculated the mean and standard deviation separately for weekdays and weekends using the relevant prior seven days of data with a two-day lag. That is, the sample mean for weekdays was the average of seven weekdays occurring prior to a two-day lag, and the sample mean for weekends was the average of the seven weekend days prior to a two-day lag. The specific days included in the averages varied by day of the week.

The W2r method calculated a standardized statistic based on the proportion of visits for a particular syndrome out of the total number of visits to a health care facility on a given day. BioSense 1.0 allowed users to set the W2c and W2r method thresholds using a recurrence interval methodology. See Szarka *et al.* (2011) for additional details about both the W2c and W2r methods.

BioSense 2.0 introduced a new modified version of the EARS C2 method. This modification, which BioSense 2.0 calls the "C2 - Proportion Method," is similar to the W2r method in the sense that the observations (the Y_t in Equation 7.20) are the proportion of visits for a particular syndrome out of the total number of visits to a health care facility. Similar to the EARS C2 method, it uses a 2-day lag in the calculation of the average and standard deviation of the proportions, and it allows users to set the baseline period over which these statistics are calculated as either seven, fourteen, or twenty-eight days. The threshold default is 3.9 standard deviations, but the user can override the default with any value from 0.5 to 5.0. See CDC (2012b) for additional details.

Performance Comparisons

Fricker *et al.* (2008a) compared the CUSUM with the EARS C1, C2, and (original) C3 methods in the univariate and multivariate cases. They found that the CUSUM applied to residuals from an adaptive regression model with an eight-week sliding baseline outperformed the EARS methods. Szarka *et al.* (2011) compared the performance of the W2c and W2r methods with the Shewhart and EWMA methods using adaptive thresholds, concluding that EWMA performed better than the Shewhart and both the Shewhart and EWMA performed better than the W2r and W2c methods.

7.6 Discussion and Summary

The univariate temporal methods presented in this chapter are commonly used in biosurveillance, particularly the Shewhart variants in EARS and the CUSUM. The EWMA, although popular in industrial SPC, is less commonly used in biosurveillance.

The term "CUSUM" is sometimes used in the biosurveillance literature to incorrectly describe other methods such as the EARS C1, C2, and C3 methods.

Referring to section 7.3, it should be clear: *The EARS methods and their derivatives are not CUSUMs*. Indeed, the EARS C1 and C2 methods and associated variants are really just the Shewhart method applied to monitoring the standardized residuals of a moving average model (such as that described in section 5.2.1 of Chapter 5).

Industrial SPC research has demonstrated that the CUSUM and EWMA, with appropriate choices of k, λ, and thresholds, have very similar detection capabilities. It has also demonstrated that the CUSUM and EWMA can detect smaller sustained mean shifts quicker than the Shewhart, and the Shewhart can more quickly detect larger mean shifts. Presumably these broad results carry over to biosurveillance, although no research has been published that confirms this conjecture. In addition, more research is required to better understand how these methods behave in the biosurveillance context of transient outbreaks and, in particular, under what conditions each is to be preferred.

In biosurveillance, these industrial methods are sometimes incorrectly applied implicitly (and perhaps unknowingly), assuming the data are normally distributed. For example, the normal variant of the CUSUM (Equation 7.12) is often used with count data when, in fact, the Poisson or negative binomial variants (Equations 7.13 and 7.15) would likely be more appropriate. On the other hand, the normal CUSUM variant may be perfectly appropriate when monitoring the residuals of a model used to account for and remove systematic effects present in biosurveillance data.

A key point is that the choice of EED method should be based on the underlying probabilistic behavior of the data to which it will be applied and the type of shift to be detected. Current biosurveillance EED practice tends to focus only on a few of the most commonly known methods and applies them without much regard for the distribution of the data or that the methods are mainly designed to detect changes in distributional means. Similarly, the idea that the CUSUM or EWMA should be used if one is looking for smaller shifts or the Shewhart if one is looking for larger shifts does not seem to be well known.

Given that the industrial SPC literature is replete with many different types of control charts designed for many different situations and types of data, deeper mining of that literature would likely benefit biosurveillance. For example, the industrial literature has developed the notion of the *fast initial response* control chart, which is designed to more quickly detect changes that occur immediately after the chart is started. This idea is directly relevant to drop-in surveillance biosurveillance systems such as EARS.

Additional Reading

For those who would like to delve more deeply into univariate temporal methods, consider the following.

- "The Use of Control Charts in Health-Care and Public-Health Surveillance" (Woodall, 2006) is a comprehensive overview of medical and public health applications of control charts.

- Examples of the application of Shewhart, CUSUM, and EWMA detection methods in traditional medical settings and to public health surveillance include:
  - "Performance of Risk-adjusted Control Charts to Monitor In-hospital Mortality of Intensive Care Unit Patients: A Simulation Study" (Koetsier *et al.*, 2012)
  - "A Novel Experience in the Use of Control Charts for the Detection of Nosocomial Infection Outbreaks" (Gomes *et al.*, 2011)
  - "The Application of Statistical Process Control Charts to the Detection and Monitoring of Hospital-acquired Infections" (Morton *et al.*, 2001)
  - "Assessing the Early Aberration Reporting System's Ability to Locally Detect the 2009 Influenza Pandemic" (Hagen *et al.*, 2011)
  - "A One-Sided MEWMA Chart for Health Surveillance (Joner *et al.*, 2008b)
  - "Methods for Monitoring Influenze Surveillance Data" (Cowling *et al.*, 2006)
  - "Approaches to Syndromic Surveillance When Data Consist of Small Regional Counts" (Rogerson & Yamada, 2004a)
- *Introduction to Statistical Quality Control* (Montgomery, 2004) is an authoritative yet accessible introduction to statistical process control methods from an industrial quality control perspective.
- Useful control chart references:
  - CUSUM: *Cumulative Sum Charts and Charting for Quality Improvement* (Hawkins & Olwell, 1998) is a comprehensive treatment of the CUSUM, mainly from an industrial quality control perspective. See also Ewan (1963), Gan (1991), and Woodall and Adams (1993).
  - EWMA: Introduced by Roberts (1959). See also Crowder (1989), Lucas and Saccucci (1990), Crowder and Hamilton (1992), Borror *et al.* (1998), and Borror *et al.* (1999).

8

Multivariate Temporal and Spatio-temporal Methods

The real purpose of scientific method is to make sure Nature hasn't misled you into thinking you know something you don't actually know. There's not a mechanic or scientist or technician alive who hasn't suffered from that one so much that he's not instinctively on guard. That's the main reason why so much scientific and mechanical information sounds so dull and cautious. If you get careless or go romanticizing scientific information, giving it a flourish here and there, Nature will soon make a complete fool out of you.

Robert M. Pirsig (1999, pp. 108–109)

Current biosurveillance systems run multiple simultaneous univariate early event detection (EED) methods, each focused on detecting an increase in the time series of a single syndrome. Woodall and Ncube (1985) first proposed the application of simultaneous univariate cumulative sums (CUSUMs) in a multivariate application. Multiple simultaneous univariate methods have the advantages of ease of implementation and interpretation, but they can be less sensitive to some types of changes compared with multivariate methods. Also, unless the signal thresholds of the multiple simultaneous procedures are properly set, they can suffer from a higher than desired combined false alarm rate.

This chapter describes how to appropriately apply multivariate temporal methods to biosurveillance. Most existing multivariate statistical process control (SPC) charts are directionally invariant, meaning that they are designed to detect changes in a mean vector in all directions. Examples of such procedures include Hotelling's χ^2 (Hotelling, 1947), Crosier's multivariate CUSUM (Crosier, 1988), and the multivariate expotentially weighted moving average (MEWMA) control chart of Lowry et al. (1992). See Lowry and Montgomery (1995) for a more detailed discussion. The lack of directional sensitivity can be a limitation of these methods, particularly in biosurveillance in which practitioners are generally interested in detecting changes only in directions corresponding to increases in disease prevalence.

As with Chapter 7, the discussions and examples in this chapter focus on the application of the EED methods to data that follow specific probability distributions. Although somewhat abstract, in so doing, the discussions make clear how to appropriately tailor the EED methods to particular types of data.

Chapter Objectives

Upon completion of this chapter, the reader should be able to:

- Describe the advantages and disadvantages of using multivariate EED methods versus using multiple univariate EED methods.
- Define and apply multivariate temporal methods to biosurveillance:
  - Hotelling's χ^2
  - Multivariate CUSUM
  - MEWMA
- Describe other multivariate EED methods.
- Understand how to compare the performance of EED methods under various hypothetical scenarios and using simulated data.

Mathematical Notation

a_1, a_2	Parameters for spatio-temporal metrics
C	Multivariate cumulative sum (MCUSUM) statistic
D	Duration of outbreak
d_t	Statistical distance for day t in MCUSUM calculation
E	MEWMA statistic
$\mathbb{E}(Y)$	Expected value of Y
$\hat{f}$	Estimated (pdf)
f_0, f_1	probability density functions pdfs
F_0, F_1	Cumulative distribution functions (cdfs)
F_t	Outbreak cdf on day t
F^{-1}	Inverse cdf
$F_{m,n}$	F distribution with m and n degrees of freedom
h	Threshold
$\mathbf{I}$	Identity matrix
$\mathbf{k}, k$	MCUSUM parameters
L_t	Log likelihood ratio at time t
M	Magnitude of outbreak
$N_p(\boldsymbol{\mu}, \boldsymbol{\Sigma})$	Multivariate normal distribution of dimension p with mean $\boldsymbol{\mu}$ and covariance matrix $\boldsymbol{\Sigma}$
$\mathcal{O}_t$	Outbreak region at time t
o_t	Area of $\mathcal{O}_t$
p_1	Probability of a signal during an outbreak
$\mathbf{S}$	Intermediate sum vector in MCUSUM and MEWMA calculations
$\mathbf{S}'$	Transpose of $\mathbf{S}$ vector
$\mathcal{S}$	Subspace of $\mathbb{R}^p$
$\mathcal{S}_t$	Signal region at time t
s_t	Area of $\mathcal{S}_t$
t	Time index
t^*	Time of first signal from an EED method
t^{**}	Time of next signal from an EED method
$\mathcal{T}_t$	Generic EED statistic at time t
$\mathbf{Y}, \mathbf{y}$	Multivariate observation
$\bar{\mathbf{y}}$	Sample mean vector
$\mathbf{Z}, \mathbf{z}$	Standardized multivariate observation
χ^2, T^2	Statistic for Hotelling's method
λ	Smoothing parameter of MEWMA
$\boldsymbol{\mu}_i$	Mean vector for random variable with distribution F_i
ρ	Correlation
$\boldsymbol{\Sigma}_i$	Covariance matrix for random variable with distribution F_i
$\boldsymbol{\Sigma}^{-1}$	Inverse of covariance matrix $\boldsymbol{\Sigma}$
τ	(Unknown) time of change from F_0 to F_1
τ_l	Last time period of outbreak
τ_s	Start time period of outbreak

8.1 Multivariate Temporal Methods

8.1.1 Hotelling's χ^2

Hotelling's χ^2 *control chart* (Hotelling, 1947) is the multivariate generalization of the Shewhart control chart, testing whether the most recent observation falls in the "tail" of a multivariate normal distribution. For a p-dimensional observation at time t, $\mathbf{Y}_t = \{Y_1, \ldots, Y_p\}$ where $\mathbf{Y} \sim F_0 = N_p(\boldsymbol{\mu}_0, \Sigma_0)$, the χ^2 control chart computes

$$\chi_t^2 = (\mathbf{Y}_t - \boldsymbol{\mu}_0)' \Sigma_0^{-1} (\mathbf{Y}_t - \boldsymbol{\mu}_0), \tag{8.1}$$

where Σ_0^{-1} is the inverse of the variance–covariance matrix. Under these assumptions, as the notation implies, the statistic χ_t^2 has a chi-square distribution with p degrees of freedom.

The control chart stops at time t when $\chi_t^2 \geq h$ for some threshold h. The threshold h is a "statistical distance" that accounts for the correlation in the data. If an observation is far away from the mean of the distribution, as defined by h, then a signal is generated. Table 8.1 gives the probability α that the χ^2 statistic for a random observation from F_0 will be greater than or equal to a particular distance h from $\boldsymbol{\mu}_0$.

To illustrate, consider a bivariate normal distribution,

$$\mathbf{Y} \sim F_0 = N_2 \left(\begin{bmatrix} 0 \\ 0 \end{bmatrix}, \begin{bmatrix} 1 & \rho \\ \rho & 1 \end{bmatrix} \right),$$

with some correlation ρ, $-1 \leq \rho \leq 1$. Figure 8.1 shows the statistical distance contours (aka probability ellipses) for $h = 1, 2, 3$, and 4, and $\rho = 0.0, 0.3, 0.6$, and 0.9.

Note how the contours naturally account for the correlation in the data. Also note that because Equation 8.1 standardizes each observation, the probabilities in Table 8.1 apply to any bivariate normal distribution, although the probability ellipses in Figure 8.1 will change according to $\boldsymbol{\mu}_0$ and Σ_0.

Similar to the univariate Shewhart control chart, Hotelling's χ^2 control chart only uses the most recent observation to decide when to stop, and thus it can react quickly to large departures from F_0. On the other hand, the Hotelling's χ^2 control chart is also relatively insensitive to small mean shifts.

In industrial quality control settings, the χ^2 control chart is usually run on sample means. For moderate to large sample sizes, even if the underlying distribution of the individual observations is not normally distributed, the sample means are approximately normally distributed because of the Central Limit Theorem. Under these conditions, choosing h is simply a matter of calculating the appropriate quantile of a chi-square distribution with p degrees of freedom. That is, given $\chi_t^2 \sim G_0$, where G_0 is the cumulative distribution function for the chi-square distribution with p degrees of freedom, for a desired ATFS set $h = G_0^{-1}(1 - \alpha)$ with $\alpha = 1/\text{ATFS}$.

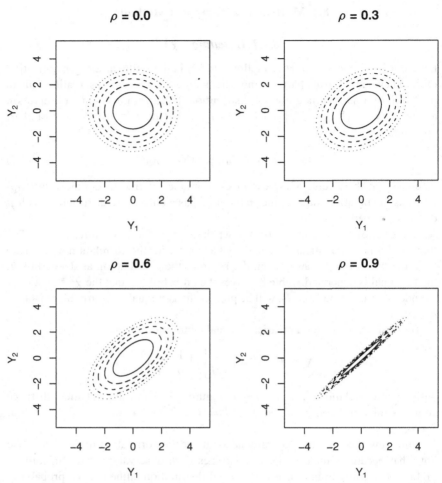

Figure 8.1. Statistical distance contours of $h = 1, 2, 3$, and 4 for bivariate normal distributions for $\rho = 0.0, 0.3, 0.6$, and 0.9.

Given that $\boldsymbol{\mu}_0$ and $\boldsymbol{\Sigma}_0$ are usually not known, they must be estimated from historical data distributed according to F_0. When the covariance matrix is estimated, Hotelling's method is called the T^2 control chart, and it is calculated as

$$T_t^2 = (\mathbf{Y}_t - \bar{\mathbf{y}})'\mathbf{S}^{-1}(\mathbf{Y}_t - \bar{\mathbf{y}}),$$

where $\bar{\mathbf{y}}$ is the mean of the historical data, $\bar{\mathbf{y}} = \{\bar{y}_1, \ldots, \bar{y}_p\}$ and $\bar{y}_i = \frac{1}{m}\sum_{j=1}^{m} y_{ij}$, and $\mathbf{S} = \frac{1}{m-1}\sum_{i=1}^{m}(\mathbf{y}_i - \bar{\mathbf{y}})(\mathbf{y}_i - \bar{\mathbf{y}})'$ is the sample covariance matrix estimating $\boldsymbol{\Sigma}_0$.

For a small number of dimensions, say $p < 5$, and a large historical sample size from which to estimate the covariance matrix, say $m > 100$, the chi-square distribution works reasonably well for setting approximate thresholds. When

Table 8.1. The probability α that a random
observation from F_0 will be at or more than a
distance h from μ_0 for $h = 1, \ldots, 10$

h	$\mathbb{P}(\chi^2 < h)$	$\alpha = \mathbb{P}(\chi^2 \geq h)$
1	0.393	0.607
2	0.632	0.368
3	0.777	0.223
4	0.865	0.135
5	0.918	0.082
6	0.950	0.050
7	0.970	0.030
8	0.982	0.018
9	0.989	0.011
10	0.993	0.007

$m \leq 100$ or when p is large (or both), the distribution of the T^2 test statistic deviates significantly from the chi-square distribution, so using it to calculate the threshold will result in performance that deviates from the desired ATFS. However,

$$T^2 \sim G_0 = \frac{p(m+1)(m-1)}{m(m-p)} F_{p,m-p},$$

so set $h = G_0^{-1}(1 - \alpha)$. See Montgomery (2004, chapters 11) for more information.

It is important to emphasize that the preceding results for calculating thresholds are all predicated on the data following a multivariate normal distribution. As with Shewhart's method, this does not mean that Hotelling's method cannot be applied to non-normal data, only that in such cases the distribution of test statistic (either χ^2 or T^2) will first need to be determined in order to correctly calculate the threshold h that achieves a desired control chart performance.

8.1.1.1 Modified for Biosurveillance

In biosurveillance, it is desirable to focus the χ^2 detection method on increases in incident rates. To accomplish this, Fricker (2007) modified the stopping rule so that it meets two conditions: (1) $\chi_t^2 \geq h$ and (2) $Z_t \in S$, where S is a particular subspace of $\mathbb{R}^p$ that corresponds to potential disease outbreaks. Under the assumption that a useful signal occurs only when at least one of the observed counts is greater than its mean, then define

$$S = \{z : z_i - \mu_i > 0 \text{ for at least one } i, i = 1, \ldots, p\}.$$

To illustrate S, consider

$$\mathbf{Z} \sim F_0 = N_2 \left(\begin{bmatrix} 0 \\ 0 \end{bmatrix}, \begin{bmatrix} 1 & \rho \\ \rho & 1 \end{bmatrix} \right),$$

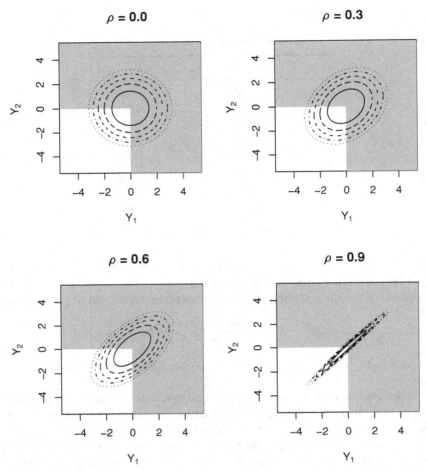

Figure 8.2. As in Figure 8.1, the curves are the statistical distance contours of $h = 1, 2, 3,$ and 4 for bivariate normal distributions with $\rho = 0.0, 0.3, 0.6,$ and 0.9. $\mathcal{S}$ is the shaded region, and a signal is generated for the χ^2 detection method only if an observation falls both outside the predefined probability ellipse and inside the shaded region.

for $\rho = 0.0, 0.3, 0.6,$ and 0.9. Then, as shown in the plots in Figure 8.2, $\mathcal{S}$ is the shaded region outside of the lower left quadrant, and a signal is generated only if an observation falls both outside the predefined probability ellipse *and* inside the shaded region.

The idea of using this region for $\mathcal{S}$ is that if F_1 represents a shift in the mean vector in any direction corresponding to an increase in one or more of the data streams, then the χ^2 detection method will have an increased probability of signaling, which should result in a decreased conditional expected delay. On the other hand, if F_1 represents a condition with a mean vector that corresponds to a

Table 8.2. χ^2 detection method ATFS values for a $N_2(\mathbf{0}, \mathbf{I})$ distribution as a function of the correlation ρ and the threshold h, determined via simulation. With high confidence, the estimated thresholds give ATFS values well within 1% of those listed in the table

ρ	0.0	0.1	0.2	0.3	0.4	0.5	0.6	0.7	0.8	0.9
ATFS										
30	6.22	6.18	6.14	6.09	6.05	5.99	5.93	5.87	5.79	5.68
60	7.61	7.57	7.53	7.48	7.43	7.38	7.32	7.26	7.18	7.08
91	8.44	8.41	8.35	8.31	8.27	8.21	8.15	8.08	8.01	7.90
182	9.84	9.79	9.75	9.70	9.65	9.60	9.54	9.47	9.38	9.29
273	10.65	10.61	10.56	10.50	10.47	10.40	10.33	10.27	10.21	10.10
365	11.23	11.17	11.12	11.10	11.04	11.00	10.94	10.86	10.79	10.69
547	12.05	11.99	11.94	11.87	11.84	11.78	11.74	11.66	11.56	11.51
730	12.61	12.57	12.52	12.45	12.43	12.37	12.32	12.25	12.17	12.08

decrease in all of the data streams, then the probability of signaling will decrease and the procedure will have less of a chance of producing a (false) signal.

8.1.1.2 Implementation

As with the univariate temporal methods, the threshold h is chosen to achieve a desired average time between false signals (ATFS). In particular, h is chosen to make the ATFS large enough that sufficient resources are available to investigate each and every signal generated.

Assuming that the observations (or the residuals from a model of the systematic effects) are independent and identically distributed according to F_0, the average time between false signals is $1/p_0$, where

$$p_0 = \int \int \cdots \int_{\{\mathbf{z}:\mathbf{z}\in S \text{ and } \chi^2 \geq h\}} f_0(\mathbf{z})d\mathbf{z}.$$

That is, under these conditions, the time until the first signal has a geometric distribution with probability p_0, and thus ATFS $= 1/p_0$.

Table 8.2 gives estimated thresholds to achieve various ATFS for the χ^2 detection method with data that are normally distributed for $p = 2$ and correlation ρ. Appendix C provides estimated thresholds for dimensions $p = 3, 4, \ldots, 10, 15,$ and 20.

The thresholds in Table 8.2 were estimated via simulation based on standard bivariate normal distributions (with a given positive correlation ρ). The simulations used the known variance–covariance matrix, and hence these thresholds apply to the χ^2 detection method. As with the χ^2 control chart, for large m where the variance–covariance matrix can be well estimated, these thresholds are still approximately correct.

However, for smaller m or larger p (or both), simulation should be used to estimate the appropriate threshold (because tabulating all possible combinations of m and p is not practical). Pseudo-code to estimate h is as follows:

```
initialize obs.dist vector of length nr.loops to all 0s
for (i in 1:nr.loops)
    generate y₁,...,yₘ random observations from F₀
    calculate the sample mean vector ȳ = {ȳ₁,...,ȳₚ}
    calculate the sample covariance matrix S₀ =
        1/(m-1) Σ_{j=1}^{m}(yⱼ - ȳ)(yⱼ - ȳ)'
    calculate S₀⁻¹
    generate a new observation from F₀, yᵢ = {yᵢ₁,...,yᵢₚ}
    if (yᵢⱼ - ȳᵢⱼ > 0 for at least one j, j = 1,...,p) then
        obs.dist[i] = (yᵢ - ȳ)'S₀⁻¹(yᵢ - ȳ)
    sort obs.dist vector from smallest to largest
    output est.threshold = obs.dist[ceiling(nr.loops*(1 - α))]
```

For the simulations used to generate the estimated thresholds in Table 8.2, where μ_0 and Σ_0 are assumed known, nr.loops was set to 10,000,000. However, the preceding pseudo-code is likely to require setting nr.loops higher to achieve the same precision because of the added variability introduced by the estimation of the mean vector and covariance matrix. In addition, the program will take longer to run because this estimation must be done for every loop of the program.

The average time until a true signal is a function of the outbreak distribution. Under the assumption that the outbreak continues indefinitely and that the outbreak distribution is stationary over the outbreak period, the average time until a true signal from the start of the outbreak is $1/p_1$, where

$$p_1 = \int \int \cdots \int_{\{z:z\in S \text{ and } \chi^2 \geq h\}} f_1(\mathbf{z})d\mathbf{z}.$$

Assuming F_1 is known, the probability p_1 can be estimated via simulation as follows:

```
initialize h
initialize ind.vector of length nr.loops to all 0s
for (i in 1:nr.loops)
    generate a new observation from F₁, yᵢ = {yᵢ₁,...,yᵢₚ}
    if (yᵢⱼ - μ₀ⱼ > 0 for at least one j, j = 1,...,p) and
       ((yᵢ - μ₀)'Σ₀⁻¹(yᵢ - μ₀) ≥ h) then
        set ind.vector[i] = 1
output hat.p1 = sum(ind.vector)/nr.loops
output se.p1 = sqrt((hat.p1*(1-hat.p1))/nr.loops)
```

Of course, the assumption that an outbreak continues indefinitely is generally not appropriate for a real biosurveillance application in which outbreaks are of finite duration, say D periods. In this, the typical biosurveillance situation, assuming F_1 is stationary over the outbreak period, the contitional expected delay (CED) can be estimated as

$$\text{CED} = \sum_{i=1}^{D} i\,(\hat{p}_1)\,(1 - \hat{p}_1)^{i-1},\tag{8.2}$$

where $\hat{p}_1$ is first estimated via simulation. Then, the probability of successfully detecting an outbreak of duration D, again assuming F_1 is constant over the outbreak period, is

$$\text{PSD} = 1 - (1 - \hat{p}_1)^{D},\tag{8.3}$$

where PSD is probability of successful detection.

Now, if the outbreak distribution changes over time, $Z_{\tau_s} \sim F_{\tau_s}$, $Z_{\tau_s+1} \sim F_{\tau_s+1}, \ldots, Z_{\tau_s+D-1} \sim F_{\tau_s+D-1}$, then the PSD and CED are more easily estimated directly via simulation as follows, where the pseudo-code below assumes F_0 is known.

```
initialize h
initialize start.outbreak and end.outbreak
initialize tfs.vector of length nr.loops to all 0s
initialize good.signal.vector of length nr.loops to all 0s
for (i in 1:nr.loops)
    initialize test.statistic to starting value
    initialize counter to 1
    initialize S.ind to 0
    while (test.statistic < h) or (S.ind = 0)
        if (i < start.outbreak or i > end outbreak) generate
            a new observation yi from F0
        else generate the new observation yi from the
            appropriate F1 distribution
        test.statistic = ((yi - μ0)'Σ0⁻¹(yi - μ0))
        if (yij - μ0j > 0 for at least one j, j = 1,...,p)
            then set S.ind = 1
        set counter = counter + 1
    set tfs.vector[i] = counter
    if (start.outbreak ≤ tfs.vector[i] ≤ end.outbreak) then
        set good.signal.vector[i] = 1
assign to good.tfs vector only those tfs.vector[i] values
    for which good.signal.vector[i]=1
print CED=average(good.tfs),
    se(good.tfs)=sd(good.tfs)/sqrt(length(good.signal.vector)),
    PSD=length(good.tfs)/nr.loops
```

The following example illustrates how to apply Hotelling's method to a hypothetical syndromic surveillance problem.

Example 8.1. A hospital simultaneously monitors influenza-like illness (ILI) and gastrointestinal (GI) syndromes using the residuals from a predictive model. When there is no outbreak, the residuals can reasonably be assumed to follow a bivariate normal distribution with correlation $\rho = 0.4$. Compared with multiple simultaneous univariate methods, because of the positive correlation between ILI and GI, the use of a multivariate method can be expected to have more power to detect outbreaks.

Question #1: What threshold h will achieve an ATFS of approximately once every 6 months?

Solution: Via Table 8.2, for $\rho = 0.4$, use a threshold of $h = 9.65$. That is, for $h = 9.65$, and for F_0, a bivariate normal distribution with $\rho = 0.4$, the χ^2 detection method will have an average time between false signals of 182 days.

Question #2: Given the threshold $h = 9.65$, what is the average time between signal events (ATBSE)?

Solution: Because the χ^2 detection method "resets" after every signal, ATBSE = ATFS = 182 days.

Question #3: Given $h = 9.65$, what is the expected time to detect an outbreak with

$$F_1 = N_2 \left(\begin{bmatrix} 1 \\ 1 \end{bmatrix}, \begin{bmatrix} 1 & 0.4 \\ 0.4 & 1 \end{bmatrix} \right)$$

and *assuming the outbreak is constant and sustained?*

Solution: Estimated via simulation, $\hat{p}_1 = 0.0494$, so the CED $= 1/\hat{p}_1 = 20.24$ days. That is, if the F_1 distribution is characterized by a mean shift to $\mu_1 = (1, 1)'$, then the χ^2 detection method will take on average slightly more than 20 days to detect the shift.

Question #4: Given an outbreak of duration 5 days, what is the CED?
Solution:

$$CED = \sum_{i=1}^{5} i(\hat{p}_i)(1 - \hat{p}_i)^{i-1}$$
$$= 1 \times 0.0494 + 2 \times 0.0494 \times 0.9506 + 3 \times 0.0494 \times 0.9506^2$$
$$+ 4 \times 0.0494 \times 0.9506^3 + 5 \times 0.0494 \times 0.9506^4$$
$$= 0.65 \text{ days.}$$

Question #5: What is the PSD over the course of the 5-day outbreak?

Solution:

$$PSD = 1 - (1 - \hat{p}_1)^D$$
$$= 1 - (1 - 0.0494)^5$$
$$= 0.224.$$

So, the solutions to Questions 4 and 5 show that the χ^2 detection method will only detect this type of outbreak 22.4 percent of the time. When it detects, it does so on average in just 0.65 days, but this means that the χ^2 detection method either detects this type of outbreak immediately or misses it completely.

Question #6: How do the CED and PSD change for a 5-day outbreak if $\mu_1 = (2, 2)'$?

Solution: Now, $\hat{p}_1 = 0.298$, so

$$CED = \sum_{i=1}^{5} i(0.298)(1 - 0.298)^{i-1}$$
$$= 1 \times 0.298 + 2 \times 0.298 \times 0.702 + 3 \times 0.298 \times 0.702^2$$
$$+ 4 \times 0.298 \times 0.702^3 + 5 \times 0.298 \times 0.702^4$$
$$= 1.93 \text{ days.}$$

and $PSD = 1 - (1 - 0.298)^5 = 0.83$. Thus, for this type of outbreak, the χ^2 detection method will detect it 83 percent of the time and on average in just under 2 days.

Question #7: Now, consider a 5-day outbreak where $\mu_{1,1} = (1, 1)'$, $\mu_{1,2} = (2, 2)'$, $\mu_{1,3} = (3, 3)'$, $\mu_{1,4} = (2, 2)'$, and $\mu_{1,5} = (1, 1)'$. What is the CED and PSD?

Solution: Via simulation, for $\mu_{1,3} = (3, 3)'$, $\hat{p}_1 = 0.736$, so

$$PSD = 1 - \prod_{i=1}^{5}(1 - \hat{p}_{1,i})$$
$$= 1 - (1 - 0.0494)(1 - 0.298)(1 - 0.736)(1 - 0.298)(1 - 0.0494)$$
$$= 0.882$$

and

$$CED = \hat{p}_{1,1} + \sum_{i=2}^{5} i(\hat{p}_{1,i}) \prod_{j=1}^{i-1} (1 - \hat{p}_{1,j})$$

$$= 0.0494 +$$

$$+ 2 \times 0.298 \times 0.9506$$

$$+ 3 \times 0.736 \times 0.9506 \times 0.702$$

$$+ 4 \times 0.298 \times 0.9506 \times 0.702 \times 0.264$$

$$+ 5 \times 0.0494 \times 0.9506 \times 0.702 \times 0.264 \times 0.702$$

$$= 2.34 \text{ days.}$$

So, for this type of outbreak, the χ^2 detection method will detect it more than 88 percent of the time and, when it does, it does so on average in 2.34 days.

The next example illustrates the application of Hotelling's method to a more complicated monitoring problem in five dimensions ($p = 5$).

Example 8.2. A public health department is simultaneously monitoring the ILI syndrome at five hospitals using the residuals from a predictive model. When there is no outbreak, the residuals can reasonably assumed to follow a multivariate normal distribution with the following variance–covariance matrix:

$$\Sigma_0 = \begin{pmatrix} 1 & 0.2 & 0.3 & 0.4 & 0.5 \\ 0.2 & 1 & 0.2 & 0.3 & 0.4 \\ 0.3 & 0.2 & 1 & 0.2 & 0.3 \\ 0.4 & 0.3 & 0.2 & 1 & 0.2 \\ 0.5 & 0.4 & 0.3 & 0.2 & 1 \end{pmatrix}$$

Question #1: What threshold h will achieve an ATFS of 60 days?

Solution: From Appendix C, the thresholds range from 13.4 to 13.7. Setting to the middle of the range gives $h = 13.55$. Checking the threshold via simulation shows gives an estimated ATFS $= 59.9$ ($s.e. = 0.46$).

Question #2: Given $h = 13.55$, what is the expected time to detect an increase in the rate of ILI complaints if $\mu_1 = (2, 2, 0, 0, 0)'$ and *assuming the increase is constant and sustained*?

Solution: Via simulation, $\hat{p}_1 = 0.666$, so the CED $= 1/\hat{p}_1 = 1.5$ days.

Question #3: Given an outbreak of duration 5 days, what is the CED?

Solution:

$$CED = \sum_{i=1}^{5} i(0.666)(1 - 0.666)^{i-1}$$

$$= 1 \times 0.666 + 2 \times 0.666 \times 0.334 + 3 \times 0.666 \times 0.334^2$$
$$+ 4 \times 0.666 \times 0.334^3 + 5 \times 0.666 \times 0.334^4$$

$$= 1.47 \text{ days.}$$

Question #4: What is the PSD over the course of the 5-day outbreak?

Solution: PSD $= 1 - (1 - 0.666)^5 = 0.996$. Thus, for this type of outbreak, the χ^2 detection method will detect it 99.6 percent of the time and on average in just less than 1.5 days.

Question #5: Now consider a 5-day outbreak where $\mu_{1,1} = (0, 1, 0, 0, 0)'$, $\mu_{1,2} = (1, 2, 1, 1, 0)'$, $\mu_{1,3} = (2, 3, 2, 1, 0)'$, $\mu_{1,4} = (1, 2, 1, 1, 0)'$, and $\mu_{1,5} = (0, 1, 0, 0, 0)'$. What are the CED and PSD?

Solution: Via simulation, for $\hat{p}_{1,1} = \hat{p}_{1,5} = 0.052$, $\hat{p}_{1,2} = \hat{p}_{1,4} = 0.319$, and $\hat{p}_{1,3} = 0.873$, so

$$PSD = 1 - \prod_{i=1}^{5}(1 - \hat{p}_{1,i})$$

$$= 1 - (1 - 0.052)(1 - 0.319)(1 - 0.873)(1 - 0.319)(1 - 0.052)$$

$$= 0.947$$

and

$$CED = \hat{p}_{1,1} + \sum_{i=2}^{5} i(\hat{p}_{1,i}) \prod_{j=1}^{i-1}(1 - \hat{p}_{1,j})$$

$$= 0.052$$
$$+ 2 \times 0.319 \times 0.948$$
$$+ 3 \times 0.873 \times 0.948 \times 0.681$$
$$+ 4 \times 0.319 \times 0.948 \times 0.681 \times 0.127$$
$$+ 5 \times 0.052 \times 0.948 \times 0.681 \times 0.127 \times 0.681$$

$$= 2.47 \text{ days.}$$

So, for this type of outbreak, the χ^2 detection method will detect it almost 95 percent of the time and, when it does, on average in 2.47 days.

8.1.2 Crosier's Multivariate Cumulative Sum

Crosier (1988) proposed an *MCUSUM control chart* that at each time t calculates the CUSUM

$$\mathbf{S}_t^* = \mathbf{S}_{t-1} + \mathbf{Y}_t - \boldsymbol{\mu}_0$$

and the statistical distance

$$d_t = \sqrt{\mathbf{S}_t^{*\prime} \Sigma_0^{-1} \mathbf{S}_t^*},$$

where $\boldsymbol{\mu}_0$ is the mean and Σ_0 is the variance–covariance matrix of $\mathbf{Y} \sim F_0$. It then "shrinks" the CUSUM by

$$\mathbf{S}_t = \begin{cases} \mathbf{S}_t^*(1 - k/d_t), & d_t > k \\ \mathbf{0}, & d_t \le k \end{cases}, \tag{8.4}$$

where k is a predetermined statistical distance and calculates the statistic

$$C_t = \sqrt{\mathbf{S}_t' \Sigma_0^{-1} \mathbf{S}_t}.$$

The procedure starts with $\mathbf{S}_0 = \mathbf{0}$ and it concludes that a change has occurred at the first time when $C_t \ge h$, for some threshold h that achieves a desired ATFS. In terms of choosing k, Crosier (1988) states, "In the univariate [CUSUM] case, the quantity $S_{t-1} + (Y_t - \mu)$ is shrunk towards 0 by k standard deviations. If this is to hold for the multivariate case, $\mathbf{k}$ must satisfy $\mathbf{k}'\Sigma^{-1}\mathbf{k} = k^2$ – that is, $\mathbf{k}$ must be of length k, where the length is defined by using the covariance matrix Σ."

The literature contains a number of MCUSUM control charts. In fact, Crosier's MCUSUM control chart described above is one of a number of other multivariate CUSUM-like algorithms he proposed, but Crosier generally preferred the above procedure after extensive simulation comparisons. Pignatiello and Runger (1990) proposed other multivariate CUSUM-like algorithms but found that they performed similar to Crosier's. Healy (1987) derived a sequential likelihood ratio test to detect a shift in a mean vector of a multivariate normal distribution. However, although Healy's procedure is more effective when the change is to the precise mean vector to be detected, it is less effective than Crosier's for detecting other types of shifts, including mean shifts that were close to but not precisely the specified mean vector.

8.1.2.1 Modified for Biosurveillance

For the biosurveillance problem, an advantage of Crosier's MCUSUM formulation is that it is easy to modify to only look for positive increases. As described in Fricker (2007), the motivation for this modification is the univariate CUSUM where directionality is achieved because the CUSUM statistic is bounded below by zero. In the MCUSUM detection method, directionality is similarly achieved by bounding each component of the cumulative sum vector by zero. In particular,

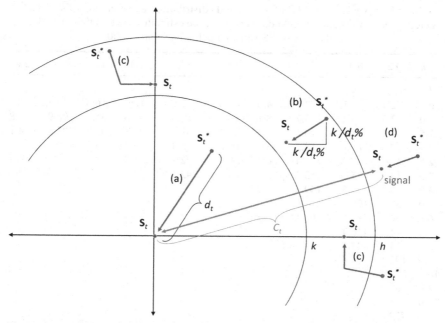

Figure 8.3. Graphical illustration of the MCUSUM detection method based on Equation 8.5 for $p = 2$.

for detecting the positive increases relevant in the biosurveillance problem, limit S_t to be non-negative in each dimension by modifying Equation 8.4 to

$$S_t = \begin{cases} \max[0, S_t^*(1 - k/d_t)], & d_t > k \\ 0, & d_t \le k \end{cases}, \tag{8.5}$$

where the maximum function is applied componentwise.

Figure 8.3 illustrates how the MCUSUM detection method works in two dimensions. In (a), the distance from S_t^* to $\mathbf{0}$ is less than k (i.e., $d_t \le k$), so S_t is set to $\mathbf{0}$. This is the result of the second line in Equation 8.5. In (b), S_t^* falls in between k and h (i.e., $k < C_t < h$), so S_t is calculated by shrinking S_t^* in each dimension by k/d_t. In (c), two examples are shown of S_t^*, for which one of the components is negative. In these cases, the S_t^* is shrunk, as in (b) and then any negative components of the resulting vector are set to zero. Finally, in (d), after S_t^* is shrunk the distance from S_t to $\mathbf{0}$ is greater than h (i.e., $C_t \ge h$), and a signal is produced.

8.1.2.2 Implementation

Implementing the MCUSUM requires choosing the parameter k and the threshold h. Unlike with the univariate CUSUM, however, because of the MCUSUM's ad hoc derivation, there is no theory or other guidance upon which to base the choice of k. Furthermore, k and h interact in the performance of the MCUSUM.

Table 8.3. MCUSUM ATFS for a $N_2(\mathbf{0}, \mathbf{I})$ distribution as a function of k and h determined via simulation. Standard errors of the estimates are less than 0.1. Blank cells have ATFS values much larger than 1,000

k	0.2	0.4	0.6	0.8	1.0	1.2	1.4	1.6	1.8	2.0
h										
0.5	2.1	2.5	3.1	4.0	5.3	7.5	10.9	16.6	26.3	43.4
1.0	3.3	4.2	5.7	8.1	12.2	19.1	31.6	55.0	98.9	184.8
1.5	5.1	7.0	10.3	16.4	28.1	51.5	98.8	202.2	423.8	914.1
2.0	7.5	11.1	18.2	33.2	66.8	145.3	338.3	823.7		
2.5	10.5	17.0	31.4	66.4	159.4	422.1	1,201.2			
3.0	14.2	25.2	53.5	133.0	384.2	1,242.4				
4.0	24.8	53.5	149.9	535.2						
5.0	39.6	108.1	421.6							
6.0	60.9	215.1	1,200.1							
7.0	91.1	426.4								
8.0	133.0	847.5								
9.0	192.1									
10.0	274.1									
11.0	388.5									
12.0	549.0									
13.0	773.0									

Table 8.3 gives the MCUSUM ATFS for the $F_0 = N_2(\mathbf{0}, \mathbf{I})$ distribution as a function of k and h determined via simulation. Standard errors of the estimates are less than 0.1, and blank cells have ATFS values much larger than 1,000. Appendix C contains tables of the ATFS for various values of k and h for standard multivariate normal distributions with $p = 3, 4, \ldots, 10, 15$, and 20.

The standard multivariate normal is a special case, perhaps only arising in practice when monitoring the residuals from a model of systematic effects. If the F_0 distribution is not the standard bivariate normal, the ATFS performance of the MCUSUM can be determined using simulation, where the pseudo-code below assumes μ_0 and Σ_0 are known. If they are not known, as is the likely case in practice, then they will need to be appropriately estimated within the simulation.

```
initialize h
initialize k
initialize run.vector of length nr.runs to all 0s
for (i in 1:nr.runs)
    initialize counter to 0
    initialize C to 0
    initialize S to 0
    while (C < h)
        generate a new observation y from F0
        calculate d = [(S + y − μ0)′Σ0⁻¹(S + y − μ0)]^(1/2)
```

```
if d > k then for j = 1, 2, ..., p calculate
    S_j = max[0, (S_j + Y_j − μ_j)(1 − k/d)]
    else S = 0
calculate C = (S'Σ_0^{-1}S)^{1/2}
set counter=counter+1
set run.vector[i] = counter
output est.ATFS = average(run.vector)
output est.se.ATFS = std.dev(run.vector)/sqrt(nr.runs)
```

Example 8.3. As in Example 8.1, a hospital simultaneously monitors ILI and GI syndromes using the residuals from a predictive model, and when there is no outbreak, the residuals can reasonably be assumed to follow a bivariate normal distribution with correlation $\rho = 0.4$. Assess the performance of the MCUSUM and compare it with the χ^2 method.

Question #1: For $k = 0.6$, what threshold h will achieve an ATFS of approximately once every 6 months?

Solution: Via Table 8.3, for $k = 0.6$ a threshold of $h = 4.0$ gives an ATFS = 149.9 days (for $\rho = 0.0$).

Question #2: Via simulation, assess whether $\rho = 0.4$ affects the ATFS and adjust h as necessary to achieve ATFS = 182 days.

Solution: Via simulation, with $\rho = 0.4$, $h = 4.0$ gives ATFS = 182.9 days (s.e. = 1.8). So, $h = 4.0$ is the appropriate threshold for this F_0.

Question #3: Given the threshold $h = 4.0$, if the MCUSUM is not reset, what is the ATBSE?

Solution: Via simulation, the ATBSE = 138.6 days (s.e. = 1.7). This means that if the MCUSUM is not reset, the time between signal events will be just under 140 days. And compared with ATFS, the ATBSE is about 44 days shorter.

Question #4: Given $h = 4.0$, what is the expected time to detect an outbreak with

$$F_1 = N_2 \left(\begin{bmatrix} 1 \\ 1 \end{bmatrix}, \begin{bmatrix} 1 & 0.4 \\ 0.4 & 1 \end{bmatrix} \right)$$

and *assuming the outbreak is constant and sustained?*

Solution: Estimated via simulation, the CED = 6.2 days (s.e. = 0.03). This is significantly faster than the χ^2 detection method that will take on average slightly more than 20 days to detect this type of outbreak.

Question #5: Given an outbreak of duration 5 days, what are the zero-state CED and PSD, estimated via simulation?

Solution: Estimated via simulation, the CED = 3.9 days (s.e. = 0.01), and the PSD = 0.492 (s.e. = 0.005). Compared with a CED of 0.65 days and a PSD of 0.224 for the χ^2 method, the MCUSUM more than doubles the probability of detecting this type of outbreak. The CED is longer for the MCUSUM, but this is the result of the increased probability of detection.

Question #6: How do the CED and PSD change for a 5-day outbreak if $\mu_1 = (2, 2)'$?

Solution: Estimated via simulation, the CED = 2.71 days (s.e. = 0.008), and the PSD = 0.995 (s.e. = 0.0007). Comparing this with the χ^2 detection method with CED = 1.93 days and PSD = 0.83, the MCUSUM again has a higher probability of detection. Although this results in a higher CED, the MCUSUM is preferred for this type of outbreak because it is virtually certain to detect it.

Example 8.4. As in Example 8.2, a public health department is simultaneously monitoring the ILI syndrome at five hospitals using the residuals from a predictive model. When there is no outbreak, the residuals follow a multivariate normal distribution with the following variance–covariance matrix:

$$\Sigma_0 = \begin{pmatrix} 1 & 0.2 & 0.3 & 0.4 & 0.5 \\ 0.2 & 1 & 0.2 & 0.3 & 0.4 \\ 0.3 & 0.2 & 1 & 0.2 & 0.3 \\ 0.4 & 0.3 & 0.2 & 1 & 0.2 \\ 0.5 & 0.4 & 0.3 & 0.2 & 1 \end{pmatrix}$$

Question #1: For $k = 0.6$, find the threshold h for F_0 with Σ_0 that achieves an ATFS of 60 days.

Solution: From Appendix C, $h = 5.0$ gives ATFS = 39.3 for $\rho = 0.0$. Simulation shows that for Σ_0 this results in an ATFS of 63.9 days (s.e. = 0.6). Through further simulations, $h = 4.92$ gives ATFS = 59.8 (s.e. = 0.55).

Question #2: Given $h = 4.92$, what is the expected time to detect an increase in the rate of ILI complaints if $\mu_1 = (2, 2, 0, 0, 0)'$ and *assuming the increase is constant and sustained*?

Solution: Via simulation, the CED = 2.35 days (s.e. = 0.006), which is almost 1 day slower (on average) than the χ^2 detection method CED of 1.5 days.

Question #3: Given an outbreak of duration 5 days, what are the CED and PSD?

Solution: Via simulation, the CED = 2.35 days (s.e. = 0.006) and PSD = 0.9997 (s.e. = 0.0002) compared with the χ^2 detection method CED of 1.47 days and PSD of 0.996.

8.1.3 Multivariate Exponentially Weighted Moving Average

Lowry *et al.* (1992) introduced the MEWMA control chart as a generalization of the univariate EWMA of Roberts (1959). When the process is in control, denote the mean of Y_t as μ_0 and let Σ_0 be the covariance matrix. Then at time t, the MEWMA calculates

$$S_t = \lambda(Y_t - \mu_0) + (1 - \lambda)S_{t-1}. \qquad (8.6)$$

S_t is a weighted average of the current observation standardized around μ_0 and the previous S statistic. As in the univariate EWMA, the smoothing parameter $0 < \lambda \leq 1$ controls how much emphasis is placed on the new observation vector.

The covariance matrix for S_t is

$$\Sigma_{S_t} = \Sigma_0 \left(\frac{\lambda \left[1 - (1 - \lambda)^{2t} \right]}{2 - \lambda} \right).$$

Taking the limit as $t \to \infty$,

$$\Sigma_{S_\infty} = \frac{\lambda}{2 - \lambda} \Sigma_0.$$

Σ_{S_∞} is then used to calculate the MEWMA test statistic E_t, where

$$E_t = S_t' \Sigma_{S_\infty}^{-1} S_t.$$

The MEWMA signals whenever E_t equals or exceeds a predetermined threshold h, which is set to achieve a desired ATFS. If $E_t < h$, then the MEWMA iterates through the next time step with a new observation vector, recalculating the test statistic and continuing until such time as the $E_t \geq h$.

8.1.3.1 Modified for Biosurveillance

In the spirit of the reflected EWMA of Crowder and Hamilton (1992), the MEWMA detection method proposed by Joner *et al.* (2008b) calculates

$$S_t = \begin{cases} \max[0, \lambda(Y_t - \mu_0) + (1 - \lambda)S_{t-1}], & \text{for } t > 0 \\ 0, & \text{for } t = 0 \end{cases},$$

where the maximum function is applied componentwise.

As with the MEWMA control chart, Σ_{S_∞} is used to calculate E_t where

$$E_t = S_t' \Sigma_{S_\infty}^{-1} S_t.$$

As before, the MEWMA detection method signals whenever E_t equals or exceeds the threshold h, which is set to achieve a desired ATFS.

8.1.3.2 Implementation

Implementation of the MEWMA requires choosing the smoothing parameter λ and the threshold h. As with the EWMA, the choice of λ can cause the MEWMA to be more like χ^2 detection method or the MCUSUM detection method. In particular,

Table 8.4. MEWMA ATFS for a $N_2(\mathbf{0}, \mathbf{I})$ distribution as a function of λ and h determined via simulation. Standard errors of the estimates are less than 0.1

λ	0.1	0.2	0.3	0.4	0.5	0.6	0.7	0.8	0.9
h									
1.0	7.5	5.1	4.2	3.7	3.5	3.3	3.2	3.2	3.2
2.0	14.6	9.5	7.6	6.7	6.1	5.8	5.7	5.6	5.7
3.0	24.2	15.7	12.6	11.1	10.2	9.8	9.5	9.6	9.8
4.0	37.8	24.7	20.1	17.8	16.4	15.9	15.7	15.9	16.6
5.0	58.1	38.2	31.5	28.3	26.6	25.8	25.9	26.4	27.8
6.0	88.0	59.0	49.3	44.8	42.7	42.0	42.3	43.9	46.6
7.0	133.2	91.1	77.6	71.5	68.9	68.3	69.5	72.3	77.6
8.0	202.3	141.3	122.2	114.3	111.5	111.5	114.2	119.9	129.4
9.0	309.3	202.5	193.7	183.6	181.1	182.9	188.2	198.4	215.1
10.0	475.9	346.4	308.8	296.7	295.4	300.2	310.7	328.4	357.3
11.0	737.4	547.3	494.8	480.6	483.1	494.1	513.1	543.5	593.3
12.0	1,149.3	869.3	796.7	781.7	791.5	814.0	848.0	899.7	984.5

note that for $\lambda = 1$, $\Sigma_{\mathbf{Z}_\infty} = \Sigma_0$, and thus for the "unreflected" version (Equation 8.6), it follows that

$$E_t = \mathbf{S}_t' \Sigma_{\mathbf{S}_\infty}^{-1} \mathbf{S}_t$$
$$= (\mathbf{Y}_t - \boldsymbol{\mu}_0)' \Sigma_0^{-1} (\mathbf{Y}_t - \boldsymbol{\mu}_0) = \chi_t^2.$$

For smaller λ, as illustrated in Chapter 10, the MEWMA EED method can perform very similarly to the MCUSUM EED method, although not enough research has been conducted to draw any general conclusions.

Table 8.4 gives the MEWMA ATFS for $F_0 = N_2(\mathbf{0}, \mathbf{I})$ distribution as a function of λ and h determined via simulation. Standard errors of the estimates are less than 0.1.

As with Tables 8.2 and 8.3, the ATFS values in Table 8.4 are applicable only in the case of a standard bivariate normal F_0 distribution. Appendix C contains tables of the ATFS for various values of λ and h for standard multivariate normal distributions with $p = 3, 4, \ldots, 10, 15$, and 20.

If the F_0 distribution is not the standard bivariate normal, the ATFS performance of the MEWMA can be determined using simulation, where the pseudo-code below assumes $\boldsymbol{\mu}_0$ and Σ_0 are known. If they are not known, as is the likely case in practice, then they will need to be appropriately estimated within the simulation.

```
initialize h
initialize λ
initialize run.vector of length nr.runs to all 0s
for (i in 1:nr.runs)
    initialize counter to 0
    initialize E to 0
    initialize S to 0
```

```
while (E < h)
    generate a new observation y from F₀
    calculate S = max[0, λ(y − μ₀) + (1 − λ)S]
    calculate E = S'Σ⁻¹_{S∞}S
    set counter=counter+1
set run.vector[i] = counter
output est.ATFS = average(run.vector)
output est.se.ATFS = std.dev(run.vector)/sqrt(nr.runs)
```

Example 8.5. As in Examples 8.1 and 8.3, a hospital simultaneously monitors ILI and GI syndromes using the residuals from a predictive model, and when there is no outbreak, the residuals can reasonably, assumed to follow a bivariate normal distribution with correlation $\rho = 0.4$. Assess the performance of the MEWMA and compare it with the χ^2 and MCUSUM methods.

Question #1: For $\lambda = 0.3$, what threshold h will achieve an ATFS of approximately once every 6 months?

Solution: Via Table 8.4, for $\lambda = 0.3$ a threshold of $h = 8.0$ gives an ATFS = 122.2 days and $h = 9.0$ gives an ATFS = 193.7 days (for $\rho = 0.0$). Simply interpolating gives $h = 8.8$.

Question #2: Via simulation, assess whether $\rho = 0.4$ affects the ATFS and adjust h as necessary to achieve ATFS = 182 days.

Solution: Via simulation, with $\rho = 0.4$, $h = 8.5$ gives ATFS = 179.5 days (s.e. = 1.8). So, $h = 8.5$ is the appropriate threshold for this F_0.

Question #3: Given the threshold $h = 8.5$, if the MEWMA is not reset, what is the ATBSE?

Solution: Via simulation the ATBSE = 170.9 days (s.e. = 1.8). Compared with the MCUSUM with an ATBSE of 138.6 days and an ATFS of 182.9 days, the MEWMA ATBSE is much closer to its ATFS.

Question #4: Given $h = 8.5$, what is the expected time to detect an outbreak with

$$F_1 = N_2 \left(\begin{bmatrix} 1 \\ 1 \end{bmatrix}, \begin{bmatrix} 1 & 0.4 \\ 0.4 & 1 \end{bmatrix} \right)$$

and *assuming the outbreak is constant and sustained?*

Solution: Estimated via simulation, the CED = 6.6 days (s.e. = 0.04). This is significantly faster than the the χ^2 detection method, which will take on average slightly more than 20 days to detect this type of outbreak, and slightly slower than the MCUSUM, which will take 6.2 days on average to detect this outbreak.

Question #5: Given an outbreak of duration 5 days, what are the zero-state CED and PSD, estimated via simulation?

Solution: Estimated via simulation, the CED = 3.7 days (s.e. = 0.01), and the PSD = 0.494 (s.e. = 0.005). Compared with a CED of 0.65 days and a PSD of 0.224 for the χ^2 method, the MEWMA more than doubles the probability of detecting this type of outbreak. The MEWMA CED and PSD are also just slightly better than the MCUSUM's (CED = 3.9, PSD = 0.492).

Question #6: How do the CED and PSD change for a 5-day outbreak if $\mu_1 = (2, 2)'$?

Solution: Estimated via simulation, the CED = 2.49 days (s.e. = 0.008) and the PSD = 0.992 (s.e. = 0.0009). Comparing the EWMA with the χ^2 detection method with CED = 1.93 days and PSD = 0.83, the MEWMA again has a higher probability of detection, and it is very similar to the MCUSUM (CED = 2.71 days; PSD = 0.995). Although both the MEWMA and MCUSUM have higher CEDs, they are preferred for this type of outbreak because they are virtually certain to detect it.

Example 8.6. As in Examples 8.2 and 8.4, a public health department is simultaneously monitoring the ILI syndrome at five hospitals using the residuals from a predictive model. When there is no outbreak, the residuals follow a multivariate normal distribution with the following variance–covariance matrix:

$$\Sigma_0 = \begin{pmatrix} 1 & 0.2 & 0.3 & 0.4 & 0.5 \\ 0.2 & 1 & 0.2 & 0.3 & 0.4 \\ 0.3 & 0.2 & 1 & 0.2 & 0.3 \\ 0.4 & 0.3 & 0.2 & 1 & 0.2 \\ 0.5 & 0.4 & 0.3 & 0.2 & 1 \end{pmatrix}$$

Question #1: For $\lambda = 0.3$, find the threshold h for F_0 with Σ_0 that achieves an ATFS of 60 days.

Solution: From Appendix C, $h = 10.0$ gives ATFS = 43.0 for $\rho = 0.0$. Simulation shows that for Σ_0, this results in an ATFS of 64.6 days (s.e. = 0.6). Through further simulations, $h = 9.79$ gives ATFS = 60.0 (s.e. = 0.57).

Question #2: Given $h = 9.79$, what is the expected time to detect an increase in the rate of ILI complaints if $\mu_1 = (2, 2, 0, 0, 0)'$ and *assuming the increase is constant and sustained*?

Solution: Via simulation, the CED = 2.00 days (s.e. = 0.006), which is a half-day slower (on average) than the χ^2 detection method CED of 1.5 days and a third of a day faster than the MCUSUM (CED = 2.35 days).

Question #3: Given an outbreak of duration 5 days, what are the CED and PSD?

Solution: Via simulation, the CED = 2.00 days (s.e. = 0.007), and PSD = 0.9998 (s.e. = 0.0001) compared with the χ^2 detection method CED of 1.47 days and PSD of 0.996 and the MCUSUM with CED = 2.35 days and PSD = 0.9997.

8.1.4 Other Multivariate Temporal Methods

Recent work on directional multivariate procedures includes Follmann (1996), Testik and Runger (2006), and Mei (2010). Follmann (1996) introduced a variant to Hotelling's χ^2 procedure, where the χ^2 statistic is calculated as usual,

$$\chi_t^2 = (\mathbf{Y}_t - \boldsymbol{\mu}_0)' \Sigma_0^{-1} (\mathbf{Y}_t - \boldsymbol{\mu}_0), \qquad (8.7)$$

but the stopping rule is modified so that $\chi_t^2 \geq h$ and $\sum_{i=1}^{p}(y_{t,i} - \mu_i) > 0$. That is, the test signals when the test statistic exceeds a predefined threshold h and the sum of the elements of the observed vector exceeds the sum of the mean vector. In a sense, this stopping rule is requiring the directionality of the shift to be more positive than negative.

In terms of biosurveillance, this means that one component could show a positive increase in disease incidence, but because it is offset by another component that is slightly more negative, no signal would be generated. However, one could reasonably want an increase in any component to generate a signal, which is the logic behind the χ^2 detection method described in Section 8.1.1, where the signal conditions can be expressed as $\chi_t^2 \geq h$ and $\max_i (y_{t,i} - \mu_i) > 0$.

On the other hand, the χ^2 detection method can allow a signal resulting from a large negative shift as long as one of the components is ever so slightly more positive than its mean. These types of shifts would produce signals that likely turn out to be false positives. Therefore, the χ^2 detection method is potentially erring on the side of sensitivity, perhaps at the expense of specificity.

In any case, no comparisons have been made between these two possible stopping rules in the context of biosurveillance. Thus, the conditions under which each is to be preferred are an open question.

Testik and Runger (2006), building on the work of Follmann (1996), Perlman (1969), and Kudô (1963), developed a number of other directional multivariate procedures. In particular, Testik and Runger developed and compared multivariate procedures that look for (1) a positive shift in one or more components of the mean vector without any negative shifts, (2) a positive shift in a prespecified subset of the components of a mean vector while allowing the remaining components to either increase or decrease, and (3) a shift of the mean vector in the direction of a specific vector.

Unfortunately, no comparisons among these methods based on Hotelling's χ^2 statistic have appeared in the literature, so which one performs better than the others and under what conditions is still an open question.

Mei (2010) has derived a method for monitoring p time series, using p univariate CUSUM statistics. As described in Chapter 7, the univariate CUSUM for the ith time series is defined as

$$C_{t,i} = \max[0, C_{t-1,i} + L_{t,i}],$$

where the increment $L_{t,i}$ is the log likelihood ratio

$$L_{t,i} = \log \frac{f_1[Y_{t,i}]}{f_0[Y_{t,i}]}.$$

Rather than monitoring each CUSUM separately, each against its own threshold, in Mei's scheme, the sum of the CUSUM statistics is monitored, where for some predefined threshold h, a signal is generated at the first time t when $\sum_{i=1}^{p} C_{t,i} \geq h$.

Again, no comparisons have been made between Mei's procedure and the MCUSUM detection method. However, Mei (2010) does prove that his procedure is optimal in the sense that it asymptotically minimizes the detection delays for each and every possible combination of affected time series, subject to a global false alarm constraint.

Other temporal methods that have been proposed or are in use for biosurveillance include wavelets (see Goldenberg et al., 2002; Zhang et al., 2003; Shmueli, 2005; and the discussion in Shmueli and Burkom, 2010) Bayesian networks (see Wong et al., 2005; Rolka et al., 2007); hidden Markov models (see LeStrat & Carrat, 1999); Bayesian dynamic models (see, e.g., Sebastiani et al., 2006) and rule-based methods (see, e.g., Wong et al., 2003).

8.2 Spatio-temporal Methods

Spatio-temporal methods are designed to monitor disease incidence both over time and space. Ideally, signals from these methods have the potential to be very useful in biosurveillance because they would indicate not only *when* an outbreak is occurring but also *where* it is occurring. However, this additional information comes at the cost of more complicated methods whose applied performance in prospective biosurveillance is still largely unknown.

8.2.1 SaTScan

The most commonly used spatial method in public health is the scan statistic, particularly as implemented in the SaTScan software (http://www.satscan.org). Originally developed to retrospectively identify disease clusters (see Kulldorff, 1997), the method has been applied prospectively in biosurveillance systems (see Kulldorff, 2001). For example, it was used as part of a drop-in syndromic surveillance system in New York City after the September 11, 2001, attack (Ackelsberg et al., 2002). Although it has been studied by the the BioSense program, it has not yet been implemented in the BioSense system.

The basic idea in SaTScan is to count the number of cases that occur in a cylinder of "space," where the circle is the geographic base and the height of the cylinder corresponds to time. The cylinder is moved around the geographic area of interest, varying the radius of the circle (up to a maximum radius that includes 50 percent of the monitored population), and the height of the cylinder, and counts of cases for the geographic regions whose centroids fall within the circle for the period of time specified by the height of the cylinder are summed. When used for prospective biosurveillance, the start date of the height of the cylinder is varied, but the end date is fixed at the most current time period. Conditioning on the expected spatial distribution of observations, SaTScan reports the most likely cluster (in both space and time) and its p-value.

Some aspects of the prospective application of the SaTScan methodology have been questioned, particularly the use of recurrence intervals and performance comparisons between SaTScan and other methods. See Woodall *et al.* (2008) for further details. Also see Kulldorff (2001) for other methods for disease mapping and for testing whether an observed pattern of disease is due to chance.

8.2.2 Repeated Two-Sample Rank

Fricker and Chang (2008) proposed the repeated two-sample rank (RTR) method as prospective spatio-temporal biosurveillance method. The general idea is that it looks for changes in the spatial distribution of disease incidence over time. It works as follows.

Consider a sequence of bivariate observations $\mathbf{Y}_i = \{Y_{1,i}, Y_{2,i}\}$, where each $\mathbf{Y}_i$ is the latitude and longitude of, for example, the home address of each individual with a particular syndrome who presents to a hospital emergency room. Assume $\mathbf{Y}_1, \ldots, \mathbf{Y}_{\tau-1}$ are independent and identically distributed (*iid*) according to some density f_0, that corresponds to the normal state of disease incidence and $\mathbf{Y}_\tau, \mathbf{Y}_{\tau+1}, \ldots$ are *iid* according to anther density f_1, which corresponds to an increase in disease incidence in at least some portion of the region being monitored. The densities f_0 and f_1 are unknown. The change point τ is the time when the normal background disease incidence state changes to an elevated disease incidence state.

Assume that a historical sample of data $\mathbf{Y}_{1-N}, \ldots, \mathbf{Y}_0$ is available. The disease incidence is assumed to have been in a non-outbreak state throughout the historical sample, so that the historical observations are distributed according to f_0. The historical sample is followed by new data $\mathbf{Y}_1, \mathbf{Y}_2, \ldots$, whose density may change from f_0 to another density at some unknown time. Also consider a set of the $w + 1$ most recent data points $\mathbf{Y}_{n-w}, \ldots, \mathbf{Y}_n$, which will be used to decide whether or not the process is in an outbreak state at the time when observation n arrives.

The RTR procedure uses a kernel estimate $\hat{f}_n$ formed from the historical sample data and the new data, defined as follows. Given a kernel function k (which is usually a density on $\mathbb{R}^2$) and a bandwidth $b > 0$,

$$
\hat{f}_n(\mathbf{y}) =
\begin{cases}
\dfrac{1}{N+n} \displaystyle\sum_{i=1-N}^{n} k_b(\mathbf{y}, \mathbf{Y}_i), & n < w + 1 \\[3ex]
\dfrac{1}{N+w+1} \displaystyle\sum_{i=n-w-N-1}^{n} k_b(\mathbf{y}, \mathbf{Y}_i), & n \geq w + 1
\end{cases}
\tag{8.8}
$$

where $k_b(\mathbf{y}, \mathbf{Y}_i) = b^{-2} k\left[(y_1 - Y_{1,i}, y_2 - Y_{2,i})/b \right]$, and where $\mathbf{y} = \{y_1, y_2\}$ is the point in the plane at which the function is evaluated. The density estimate $\hat{f}_n$ is evaluated at each historical point and each data point in the new data, obtaining the values

$$
\underbrace{\hat{f}_n(\mathbf{Y}_{1-N}), \ldots, \hat{f}_n(\mathbf{Y}_0)}_{\text{historical observations}}, \underbrace{\hat{f}_n(\mathbf{Y}_1), \ldots, \hat{f}_n(\mathbf{Y}_n)}_{\text{new observations}}
\tag{8.9}
$$

when $n < w + 1$ or

$$
\underbrace{\hat{f}_n(\mathbf{Y}_{n-w-N-1}), \ldots, \hat{f}_n(\mathbf{Y}_{n-w-1})}_{\text{historical observations}}, \underbrace{\hat{f}_n(\mathbf{Y}_{n-w}), \ldots, \hat{f}_n(\mathbf{Y}_n)}_{\text{new observations}}
\tag{8.10}
$$

when $n \geq w + 1$.

Then the RTR method performs a Kolmogorov-Smirnov hypothesis test on the ranks at each time when a new observation arrives and signals the first time the test rejects the hypothesis that the ranks of the estimated density heights of the new sample of data are uniformly distributed among the ranks of the density heights of the historical sample. For notational convenience, assume $n \geq w + 1$ and let $\hat{J}_n$ denote the empirical distribution function of the density heights $\hat{f}_n(\mathbf{Y}_{n-w}), \ldots, \hat{f}_n(\mathbf{Y}_n)$ for the new data, defined by

$$
\hat{J}_n(z) = \frac{1}{w+1} \sum_{i=n-w}^{n} I\left\{ \hat{f}_n(\mathbf{Y}_i) \leq z \right\},
\tag{8.11}
$$

where I denotes the indicator function. Similarly, for the historical sample, define

$$
\hat{H}_N(z) = \frac{1}{N} \sum_{i=n-w-N-1}^{n-w-1} I\left\{ \hat{f}_n(\mathbf{Y}_i) \leq z \right\}.
\tag{8.12}
$$

The Kolmogorov-Smirnov statistic at the time when observation n arrives is

$$
S_n = \max_z \left| \hat{J}_n(z) - \hat{H}_N(z) \right|.
\tag{8.13}
$$

In summary, the RTR method proceeds as follows.

1. Choose a historical sample size N, a new sample size $w + 1$ (where $N \gg w + 1$), and set a threshold h to achieve a desired ATFS.

2. Collect an historical sample of data points during which the background disease incidence is in a non-outbreak state and set $n = 1$.
3. Using $w + 1$ of the most recent data points, calculate the estimated density heights for the historical sample and the new data using Equation 8.8.
4. Calculate the Kolmogorov-Smirnov statistic S_n according to Equation 8.13:
   - If $S_n \geq h$, stop and signal that an outbreak may be occurring.
   - If $S_n < h$, when a new observation arrives, increment n, update the historical and new data sets, and go to step 3 and repeat.

See Fricker and Chang (2008) for additional details about how to implement the RTR, including how to set the threshold.

8.2.3 Generalized Linear Mixed Models

Kleinman *et al.* (2004) and Lazarus *et al.* (2002) proposed a generalized linear mixed model (GLMM) to simultaneously monitor disease counts over time in a region divided into smaller sub-areas (zip codes). This is statistically attractive because it uses information across the entire region while appropriately adjusting for the smaller areas.

As described in Kleinman *et al.* (2004), there are two forms of the model depending on whether individual data and covariates are available versus aggregated counts and covariates by zip code. In the former case, the model is

$$\mathbb{E}(Y_{ijt}|b_i) = p_{ijt} \text{ and } \text{logit}(p_{ijt}) = \mathbf{x}_{ijt}\boldsymbol{\beta} + b_i, \tag{8.14}$$

where y_{ijt} is an indicator for whether or not person j in area i is a case on day t, p_{ijt} is the probability he or she is a case, $\mathbf{x}_{ijt}$ is a vector of observed covariates on person j and/or area i over time up to and including day t, $\boldsymbol{\beta}$ is a vector of fixed effects, and b_i is a random effect for area i. When no individual-level covariate information is available, the most likely situation, the model is

$$\mathbb{E}(Y_{it}|b_i) = p_{it} \text{ and } \text{logit}(p_{it}) = \mathbf{x}_{it}\boldsymbol{\beta} + b_i, \tag{8.15}$$

where $y_{it} = \sum_{j=1}^{n_{it}} y_{ijt}$. In this model, p_{it} can be thought of as the probability that an individual in area i will be a case on day t.

Having fit the model, z cases are observed on day $t + 1$. The rarity of the observed count is assessed by calculating

$$\Pr(Z \geq z \text{ cases}) = 1 - \sum_{k=1}^{z-1} \binom{n_{it}}{k} \hat{p}_{it}(1 - \hat{p}_{it})^{n_{it}-k}, \tag{8.16}$$

where $\hat{p}_{it}$ is calculated from the estimated coefficients in the usual way for logistic regression and $1/(\hat{p}_{it} \times \text{number of tests conducted})$ is proposed as the recurrence interval: the number of time periods for which the expected number of counts of z or more cases is 1 (Woodall *et al.*, 2008). Waller (2004b) recommends an alternate calculation for the recurrence interval, and Woodall *et al.* (2008) take issue with both the use of and recommended calculations for the recurrence interval.

The small area regression and testing (SMART) method implemented in BioSense 1.0 (see the BioSense User Guide, CDC, 2006d) was based on the Kleinman *et al.* (2004) and Lazarus *et al.* (2002) GLMM approach. However, as implemented in BioSense 1.0, it only used spatial information to bin data into separate time series, the output of which is subsequently combined using a Bonferroni correction. Hence, the BioSense 1.0 SMART method was, strictly speaking, only a temporal method.

It is worth noting that the GLMM in the SMART method is just a model of the disease incidence. As such, the residuals from this model could be monitored using the recurrence interval approach, as was done in BioSense 1.0, but they could also just as well be monitored using the χ^2, MCUSUM, or MEWMA detection methods. In fact, the use of the recurrence interval is simply a conservative Shewhart-like method because (1) only the most recent observation (in a given region) is used and (2) the multiplication term (of the number of tests conducted) in the denominator is a Bonferroni correction applied typically in classical hypothesis testing situations to account for multiple testing. As such, it is quite likely that the implementation of the SMART method in BioSense 1.0 was less sensitive to detecting outbreaks than if the methods described in this chapter had been used to monitor the GLMM residuals, particularly for modest outbreaks with spatial correlation.

8.2.4 Other Methods

Other spatio-temporal approaches include Sonesson (2007), who applies a CUSUM methodology to scan statistics, and Rogerson and Yamada (2004b), who apply CUSUM methods to the spatial distribution of cases. Diggle *et al.* (2004b) use a spatio-temporal Cox point process methodology based on the counts in subregions. Also see Diggle *et al.* (2004a). Olson *et al.* (2005) and Forsberg *et al.* (2006) assess possible disease clusters, using M-statistics based on the distribution of pairwise distances between cases.

See Lawson and Kleinman (2005) and Waller (2004a) for additional exposition and methods and Lawson (2004) and Mandl *et al.* (2004) for further discussion on spatial and spatio-temporal modeling issues. For spatial methods with application to more traditional public health data and problems, see Waller and Gotway (2004).

8.2.5 Metrics for Spatio-temporal Methods

The performance metrics for spatio-temporal methods are more challenging than those for purely temporal EED methods. The issue is that in the temporal problem, a successful detection simply requires a method signal during an outbreak (or perhaps within d days of the start of the outbreak). However, in the spatio-temporal problem, this is insufficient because a successful detection requires a method to both signal during an outbreak and to accurately identify the location of the outbreak.

Whether an EED method is purely temporal or spatio-temporal, as first discussed in Chapter 6 (see pages 167 through 168), the necessary performance metrics still must be able to answer the following questions:

- When there is an outbreak, how fast will the method detect the outbreak?
- When there is no outbreak, what is the time between false-positive signals?
- For a particular type of outbreak, what is the chance that the method will detect it at all?

Thus, although the questions do not change, what does change is how the metrics must be defined in order to answer the second and third questions. That is, they must be modified to account for the fact that any definition of a successful detection must have both a temporal and spatial component.

To begin, let $\mathcal{O}_t$ denote the outbreak region at time t and $\mathcal{S}_t$ denote the signal region at time t. That is, $\mathcal{O}_t$ is the location or locations in (two-dimensional) space of the outbreak at time t, where the area of $\mathcal{O}_t$ is 0 when there is no outbreak. Similarly, $\mathcal{S}_t$ is the location (or locations) where a spatio-temporal method indicates that an outbreak is occurring at time t, where the area of $\mathcal{S}_t$ is 0 when there is no signal. Finally, denote the area of $\mathcal{O}_t$ as o_t, the area of $\mathcal{S}_t$ as s_t, the area of $\mathcal{O}_t \cap \mathcal{S}_t$ as os_t, and the area of $\overline{\mathcal{O}}_t \cap \mathcal{S}_t$ as $\overline{os}_t$.

Sensitivity- and specificity-like measures can then be used to quantify the performance of the method for time period t^* when the spatio-temporal method signals. That is, given a signal, the fraction of the outbreak region contained in the signal region is os_{t^*}/o_{t^*}. This is a measure of sensitivity. Similarly, the ratio of the signal region outside the outbreak region to the non-outbreak region is $\overline{os}_{t^*}/\overline{o}_{t^*}$. One minus this is a measure of specificity. For an ideal signal from a spatio-temporal method, $os_{t^*}/o_{t^*} = 1$ and $1 - \overline{os}_{t^*}/\overline{o}_{t^*} = 1$. In practice, though, $0 \leq os_{t^*}/o_{t^*} \leq 1$ and $0 \leq \overline{os}_{t^*}/o_{t^*} \leq 1$.

As with the temporal metrics, let t^* denote the first time the method signals, $t^* = \min(t : \mathcal{T}_t \geq h)$, and let let t^{**} denote the next time the method signals, $t^{**} = \min(t : t > t^* \text{ and } \mathcal{T}_t \geq h)$. Given this, the spatio-temporal metrics are defined as:

$$\text{ATFS} \triangleq \mathbb{E}(t^{**} - t^* | \mathcal{T}_{t^*+1} = \mathcal{T}_0 \text{ and } \tau_s = \infty),$$

$$\text{CED} \triangleq \mathbb{E}\left(t^* - \tau_s \mid \tau_s \leq t^* \leq \tau_l, os_{t^*}/o_{t^*} \geq a_1, \text{ and } 1 - \overline{os}_{t^*}/\overline{o}_{t^*} \geq a_2\right),$$

and

$$\text{PSD} \triangleq \mathbb{P}\left(\tau_s \leq t^* \leq \tau_l, os_{t^*}/o_{t^*} \geq a_1, \text{ and } 1 - \overline{os}_{t^*}/\overline{o}_{t^*} \geq a_2\right).$$

What remains is to determine a_1 and a_2, which are parameters that specify how well a spatio-temporal method must identify an outbreak region to be useful and, like d in the PSD metric, they must be specified by the public health community based on medical and operational considerations. Furthermore, the CED and PSD performance of a spatio-temporal EED methods can and should be assessed over a range of a_1 and a_2 values, where it is likely that trade-offs will occur between the detection speed of a true signal and the spatial accuracy of the estimated outbreak location.

Note that the spatial conditions for CED and PSD are specifically formulated in terms of area and *not* in terms of the affected or non-affected individuals in those regions. There are three reasons for this. First, the goal of a spatio-temporal method is to accurately identify the outbreak region, not the affected individuals. Obviously, it would be ideal if a spatio-temporal method could actually identify the specific affected individuals, but this will generally not be possible, particularly if the data are aggregated by subregions. Second, it is likely that the outbreak region will contain both affected and non-affected individuals simply because not everyone in the outbreak region will be exposed or get sick (or both). Thus, even a method that perfectly identifies the outbreak region will not achieve a sensitivity of 1 if sensitivity is defined at the individual level. Furthermore, and third, if sensitivity were calculated at the individual level, then two methods that both perfectly identified the same outbreak region could have different specificities if either the disease prevalence or the population size in the outbreak region is changed. Because the spatio-temporal detection method cannot control either disease prevalence or the population distribution, the performance metrics should not be dependent on these factors.

8.3 Discussion and Summary

To date, the multivariate Hotelling, CUSUM, and EWMA methods discussed in this chapter have not been incorporated into operational biosurveillance systems. Generally speaking, current biosurveillance systems tend to use multiple univariate methods, sometimes combined with spatio-temporal methods. As discussed in the introduction to this chapter, multiple simultaneous univariate methods have the advantages of ease of implementation and interpretation, but they can be less sensitive to some types of changes compared with multivariate methods. Also, unless the signal thresholds of the multiple simultaneous procedures are properly set, they can suffer from a higher than desired combined false alarm rate. On the other hand, signals from multivariate methods require additional evaluation to determine the source of the signal.

Comparisons

As with the univariate methods in Chapter 7, in the SPC literature, it is well established that the Hotelling χ^2 control chart is better for detecting large shifts and the MCUSUM control chart is better for small to moderate shifts. And, again similar to the univariate methods, through the appropriate choice of λ, the MEWMA can be made to perform similar to either the Hotelling χ^2 control chart or the MCUSUM control chart.

In addition, it is also well established in the SPC literature, in comparisons between multiple univariate control charts and multivariate charts, that multiple univariate charts perform better when the shift is in only one or a small number of dimensions. In contrast, multivariate methods generally perform better when the shift is in more than a few dimensions, particularly in directions not along one or more axes, and when there is correlation among the time series being monitored. In one comparison of multiple univariate CUSUMs versus various directionally invariant multivariate CUSUMs for monitoring spatial patterns in disease incidence, Rogerson and Yamada (2004b) find: "When the degree of spatial autocorrelation is low, the univariate method is generally better at detecting changes in rates that occur in a small number of regions; the multivariate is better when change occurs in a large number of regions."

Temporal scan methods are compared with other methods in Han *et al.* (2009) and Woodall *et al.* (2008). In particular, under the typical SPC scenario of a sustained increase in Poisson rates, Han *et al.* (2009) compare the temporal scan method with the CUSUM and EWMA. They conclude that the CUSUM and EWMA generally outperformed the temporal scan method. They also conclude that whereas the CUSUM performed better than the EWMA for larger shifts with later time changes, the EWMA performed better for smaller shifts and early change times. In contrast, in a comparison between the CUSUM and temporal scan statistics, Woodall *et al.* (2008) found that for shifts of limited duration the better method depended on the duration of the shift.

Comparisons in the biosurveillance literature under conditions appropriate for that data are much more limited. Fricker *et al.* (2008b) compared the performance of the MCUSUM and MEWMA detection methods and found that, as in the SPC literature, they can be made to perform very similarly in biosurveillance applications. They conclude,

> Because there is seemingly no performance advantage in using one method over the other, this result leads us to prefer the MEWMA for procedural reasons. Specifically, it is relatively easy to develop an intuitive appreciation for how to choose λ and much more difficult to understand how to appropriately choose **k**. That is, unlike the *k* in the univariate CUSUM which has a clear interpretation, namely it is one-half of the smallest mean shift that is to be detected quickly, the *k* in Crosier's MCUSUM is a parameter in a multiplicative "shrinkage factor" for which there is no literature or research to guide one in the trade-offs that must result from various choices of *k*.

Joner *et al.* (2008b, p. 514) compare the MEWMA detection method described in this chapter to the "MC1" MCUSUM method of Pignatiello and Runger (1990) and multiple univariate CUSUMs. They conclude that

> the proposed one-sided MEWMA chart is superior to the other monitoring techniques that we considered, namely the MC1 chart and the system of multiple univariate CUSUM charts. The one-sided MEWMA chart is, on average, the fastest to signal even when the increase is different from the increase the chart was designed to detect optimally. The MC1 chart, on the other hand, has inferior performance. We feel that the MC1 chart should not be used in surveillance because of the credit that can build up when this chart is used.

Additional Reading

For those who would like to delve more deeply into multivariate methods, consider:

- *Introduction to Statistical Quality Control* Montgomery (2004) is a good introduction to multivariate SPC methods from an industrial quality control perspective.
- In terms of the specific methods described in this chapter:
  - *Hotelling's* χ^2: Hotelling (1947) developed the original directionally invariant method. Fricker (2007) introduced the directional form described in this chapter. Testik and Runger (2006), building on the work of Follmann (1996), Perlman (1969), and Kudô (1963), developed a number of alternative directional variants.
  - *MCUSUM*: There are a number of multivariate CUSUMs and CUSUM-like variants. These include Crosier (1988), Pignatiello and Runger (1990), and Healy (1987). The directional variant in this chapter, based on Crosier (1988), was introduced by Fricker (2007). For a review of MCUSUMs from a statistical process control perspective, see chapter 8 of Hawkins & Olwell (1998).
  - *MEWMA*: Lowry *et al.* (1992) introduced the MEWMA. Joner *et al.* (2008b) modified it to create the directional MEWMA described in this chapter.
- Other useful references include chapter 9 of Lawson and Kleinman (2005), which summarizes some general approaches to multivariate surveillance.

Part IV

Putting It All Together

9

Applying the Temporal Methods to Real Data

> ...the fact that the criterion we happen to use has a fine ancestry of highbrow statistical theorems does not justify its use. Such justification must come from empirical evidence that it works.
>
> Walter A. Shewhart (1891–1967)

This chapter brings together everything from the past eight chapters, demonstrating the application of early event detection (EED) methods for both natural disease detection and bioterrorism detection. In so doing, it highlights that effective detection depends on specifically defining the surveillance purpose. Current biosurveillance system design and practice typically do not do so. However, it does not follow that a system operated for detecting natural diseases will be most effective at detecting bioterrorism and vice versa.

In particular, determining whether an abnormality is present requires defining the normal background disease incidence. For seasonal outbreak detection, normal disease incidence should be characterized using historical data from periods without seasonal outbreaks. In contrast, for short-term outbreaks such as bioterrorism, seasonal outbreaks are part of the normal disease incidence and thus must be incorporated into the background disease incidence. For example, during flu season, EED methods looking for bioterrorism must account for the elevated flu incidence before assessing whether a bioterrorism attack may or may not have occurred.

Specifying the surveillance purpose should also drive whether the detection methods are "reset" after a signal (meaning the EED method's statistic is reset to its starting value) or whether it is not reset and thus likely continues to signal in subsequent time periods. Typically, current biosurveillance practice is not to reset after a signal because the continuing signals are often interpreted as additional information about the existence and extent of the outbreak. However, when the surveillance purpose is bioterrorism detection (and it has been determined that no attack has taken place), resetting after a signal has occurred may be critical for detecting an attack.

This chapter begins with examples of the application of EED methods for natural disease surveillance followed by applications for bioterrorism surveillance. In both cases, it illustrates EED performance with and without resetting. In addition to the policies of never resetting and always resetting after every signal, it describes an intermediate method for automatically resetting after an outbreak has subsided. The chapter then illustrates how the performance of EED methods can be compared using information about known outbreaks, in this case the H1N1 outbreaks of 2009.

Chapter Objective

The goal of this chapter is to illustrate the application of EED methods for detecting both natural disease outbreaks and bioterrorism attacks. Upon completion of the chapter, the reader should:

- Understand how to effectively apply EED methods to actual data, including how to accommodate the underlying probabilistic behavior of the data, and how to appropriately set the threshold to achieve a desired ATFS.
- Have gained some appreciation of the limitations of estimating EED performance using one set of real data, which include the issues that (1) it is almost impossible to authoritatively and accurately identify actual outbreaks in the data and (2) it is very difficult to quantify EED performance precisely.
- Understand the effects of resetting and not resetting EED statistics after signaling, including discussing the effect that not resetting can have on the ability of a biosurveillance system to detect a bioterrorism attack.

Note that the results presented herein are meant to be illustrative. While the results are informative with respect to the performance of the particular EED methods compared herein, definitive conclusions should follow only after these results have been replicated and additional comparisons under other conditions have been made.

Mathematical Notation

$\widehat{\text{ATFS}}$	Estimated average time between false signals (ATFS)
C_t	Cumulative sum (CUSUM) statistic for day t
$\widehat{\text{CED}}$	Estimated conditional expected delay (CED)
D	Outbreak duration
$\hat{F}_t$	Estimated distribution function at time t
$\hat{F}_t^{-1}$	Inverse estimated distribution function at time t
h	EED method threshold
k	CUSUM parameter
L	Parameter for calculating exponentially weighted moving average (EWMA) threshold
M	Outbreak magnitude
$\widehat{\text{PSD}}$	Estimated probability of successful detection (PSD)
r, p	Negative binomial distribution parameters
$\hat{r}, \hat{p}$	Estimated parameters of negative binomial distribution
s	Parameter of Montes de Oca *et al.* (2010) methodology for automatically resetting EED methods
S_t, S_t^*	Sample standard deviations in Early Aberration Reporting System (EARS) method calculations
y_t	Observation y for day t
z_t	Standardized observation z for day t
$\hat{\beta}_0$	Estimated intercept of fitted regression line
$\hat{\beta}_1$	Estimated slope of fitted regression line
λ	EWMA parameter
λ_0, λ_1	Poisson distribution parameters
$\hat{\lambda}_t$	Adaptively estimated Poisson distribution parameter
$\hat{\mu}_0$	Estimated mean daily disease incidence during non-outbreak period
$\hat{\sigma}_0$	Estimated standard deviation of disease incidence during non-outbreak period

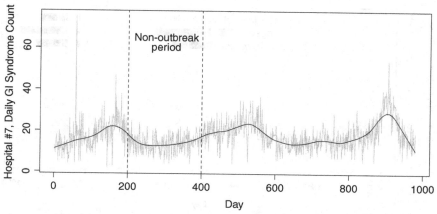

Figure 9.1. Plot of Hospital #7 GI syndrome data. The dotted lines indicate a period of "normal" (i.e., nonseasonal outbreak) disease incidence from days 220 to 400.

9.1 Using Early Event Detection Methods to Detect Outbreaks and Attacks

9.1.1 Detecting Seasonal Outbreaks

Consider the problem of detecting seasonal flu outbreaks in hospital data. Figure 9.1 is a plot of $2\frac{1}{2}$ years of gastrointestinal (GI) syndrome data for Hospital #7, where, in retrospect, three episodes of seasonal increases in GI are visually obvious. One way to illustrate prospectively detecting seasonal increases is to hypothetically turn the clock back to day 400 to define the parameters of the EED methods and then run the methods forward from day 401 to day 980.

So, given the historical data from days 1 to 400, one might decide that days 200 to 400, delineated by the dotted lines in Figure 9.1, best characterize normal (i.e., nonseasonal outbreak) disease incidence. For this period, the mean incidence is estimated as $\hat{\mu}_0 = \frac{1}{201} \sum_{t=200}^{400} y_t = 13.6$ per day with an estimated standard deviation of $\hat{\sigma}_0 = \left[\frac{1}{200} \sum_{t=200}^{400} (y_t - \hat{\mu}_0)^2 \right]^{1/2} = 4.5$.

Ignoring day and other effects, one approach is to simply standardize future observations with

$$z_t = \frac{y_t - \hat{\mu}_0}{\hat{\sigma}_0} = \frac{y_t - 13.6}{4.5}, t = 401, 402, \ldots$$

and apply the Shewhart, CUSUM, and EWMA detection methods to the z_t (without resetting after signals). For an average time between false signals (ATFS) of 365 days, assuming the standardized values are approximately normally distributed (which a Q-Q plot shows is reasonable) set $h = 2.7775$ for the Shewhart, $h = 1.35$ and $k = 1.5$ for the CUSUM, and $L = 2.815$ and $\lambda = 0.3$ for the EWMA.

The results are shown at the top of Figure 9.2, where the signaling times for each detection method are indicated by the short vertical lines. The figure shows

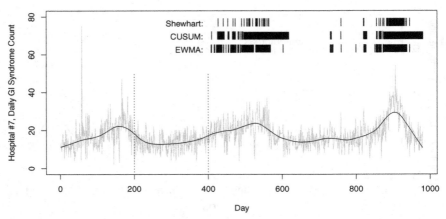

Figure 9.2. Plot of Hospital #7 GI syndrome data with signal times, where the Shewhart, CUSUM, and EWMA detection method signaling times are indicated with the vertical lines. Thresholds were set with an ATFS of 365 days and the methods are not reset after signals.

that all three detection methods clearly indicate the two large seasonal increases (after day 400) in GI. However, there are some differences in how they indicate the duration of the outbreaks and because the methods are not reset, the CUSUM's and EWMA's signals are more persistent.

In particular, note how the CUSUM continues to signal well after the two seasonal increases have subsided. In addition, the EWMA and CUSUM detection methods tend to signal earlier because of the gradual increase in GI counts at the start of the outbreaks. Finally, note that there are a couple of smaller potential outbreaks in between the two larger outbreaks that are now more obvious given the signals.

To Reset or Not to Reset?

This example raises the issue of whether simply allowing the CUSUM and EWMA methods to run after they signal without resetting is a good policy. Not resetting them provides useful information early in an outbreak that the outbreak is continuing. However, as an outbreak is ending, not resetting can result in inertia from the prior outbreak data, causing the methods to continue to signal even after the outbreak is over.

Figure 9.3 zooms in on days 201 to 700, showing the GI incidence with the CUSUM statistics $C_{201}, \ldots, C_{700}$ (heavy solid line) and the CUSUM threshold $h = 1.35$ (light dotted line) overlaid. As before, the CUSUM signals are indicated by the short vertical lines. The figure shows how the persistent CUSUM signals result from the inertia build up in the CUSUM statistic, where it takes 55 days from the peak of the signal on day 565 to return to below the threshold on day 620.

Resetting after every signal, on the other hand, results in fewer signals early in an outbreak, but then each subsequent signal can be interpreted as confirmation

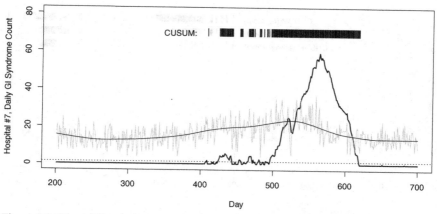

Figure 9.3. Plot of Hospital #7 GI syndrome data for days 201 to 700) with the CUSUM statistics $C_{201}, \ldots, C_{700}$ (heavy solid line) and the CUSUM threshold $h = 1.35$ (light dotted line) overlaid. As before, the CUSUM signals are indicated by the short vertical lines.

that the outbreak is continuing. Compare Figure 9.4, in which each of the methods was reset to its initial value each time after a signal, with Figure 9.2.

In Figure 9.4, the signals now better show the end of the outbreak periods but less consistently indicate when they start. This suggests a strategy of not resetting until an outbreak is either obvious or confirmed, after which the detection method is reset after each signal so that the end of the outbreak is more readily detected.

However, in biosurveillance systems monitoring a large number of data streams, it may be impractical to manually observe each data stream and make a decision about resetting for every signal. In such situations, the methodology proposed by Montes de Oca *et al.* (2010) can be used to automatically reset the CUSUM and

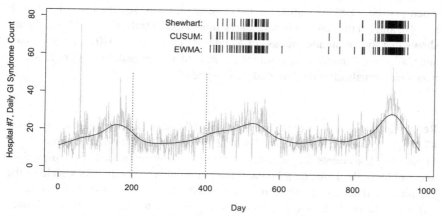

Figure 9.4. Plot of Hospital #7 GI syndrome data with signal times where the Shewhart, CUSUM, and EWMA detection method signaling times are indicated with the vertical lines. Thresholds set with an ATFS of 365 days and the methods are reset after each signal.

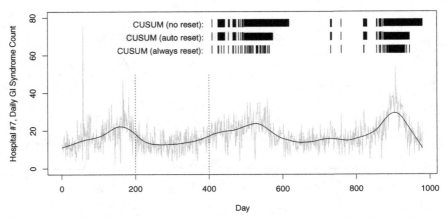

Figure 9.5. Comparison of the signals for the CUSUM run on the Hospital #7 GI syndrome data when (1) the CUSUM statistic is never reset, (2) it is automatically reset with $s = 16$, and (3) the CUSUM statistic is reset every time it exceeds the threshold.

EWMA statistics. It works as follows. Whenever a signal is generated, say $C_t \geq h$ for the CUSUM, regress $C_t, C_{t-1}, \ldots, C_{t-s}$ on $t, t - 1, \ldots, t - s$. If the estimated slope of the line is statistically negative (i.e., $\hat{\beta}_1 < 0$ with a p value < 0.05) then set $C_t = 0$. Otherwise, leave C_t unchanged and repeat the next time a signal is generated.

The idea is to assess the trend in the CUSUM and EWMA statistics, automatically resetting them when there is sufficient evidence after a signal of a downward trend in those statistics. The choice of s can be based on one-half the duration of the expected outbreak, where if the statistic peaks in the middle of the outbreak, then it will automatically reset roughly at the end of the outbreak.

Figure 9.5 compares the signals for the CUSUM run on the Hospital #7 data when (1) the CUSUM statistic is never reset, (2) it is automatically reset with $s = 16$, and (3) the statistic is reset every time it exceeds the threshold. The figure shows that the automatic method of Montes de Oca *et al.* (2010) provides a balance, allowing consistent signaling at the start of an outbreak without excessively persistent signals after the outbreak has subsided.

Additional Examples

Returning to the problem of detecting seasonal flu outbreaks, compare the Hospital #7 GI syndrome data in Figure 9.1 with $2\frac{1}{2}$ years of GI data from Hospital #2 in Figure 9.6. The counts for Hospital #2 are much lower than those for Hospital #7 and, unlike in the Hospital #7 data, there are no obvious outbreaks visible in the Hospital #2 data. More importantly, the standardized counts for Hospital #2 *do not* have a normal distribution, so it is inappropriate to apply the approach used on the Hospital #7 data to the Hospital #2 GI syndrome data.

However, again using days 200 to 400 as the "historical data," the mean incidence is $\hat{\mu}_0 = 3.6$ per day with a standard deviation of $\hat{\sigma}_0 = 3.5$. Thus, it is

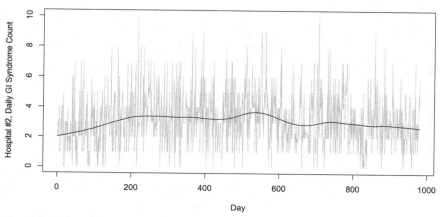

Figure 9.6. Plot of Hospital #2 data.

reasonable to assume the data come from a Poisson distribution with $\lambda_0 = 3.6$ and apply the Poisson versions of the Shewhart, CUSUM, and EWMA methods.

For the Shewhart detection method, $h = 10$ results in an ATFS of 244 days where, because of the discreteness of the Poisson, this gets as close to the desired ATFS of 365 days as possible (e.g., $h = 11$ gives an ATFS of 770 days). For the CUSUM, assuming the detection of a 2–standard deviation increase in the mean is desired, set

$$k = \frac{\lambda_1 - \lambda_0}{\ln \lambda_1 - \ln \lambda_0} = \frac{7.34 - 3.6}{\ln(7.34) - \ln(3.6)} = 5.25.$$

Via simulation, $h = 5.8$ results in an ATFS of 376.1 days ($s.e. = 1.2$). Similarly, for the EWMA, assuming smoothing parameter $\lambda = 0.3$, via simulation $L = 14.2$ results in an ATFS of 370.5 days ($s.e. = 1.1$).

Figure 9.7 shows the results, where the CUSUM and EWMA statistics were designed to automatically reset with $s = 16$: the CUSUM signals on days 552 to 555 and the EWMA on days 552, 553, and 563. The Shewhart fails to signal, but given the subtlety of this possible outbreak, its failure to signal should not be surprising.

Note that the CUSUM and EWMA signals occur during the first large outbreak in Figure 9.2 for Hospital #7. This, combined with the slight bump in the smoothed line in Figure 9.7, suggests that Hospital #2 also experienced a small GI outbreak even though it is not obviously visible in the data.

As another example, consider the clinic influenza like illness (ILI) data that, when standardized, is not normally distributed, nor does a Poisson distribution fit because of overdispersion. However, using days 1 to 50 as the "historical data" (delineated by the dotted line in Figure 9.8), it is reasonable to assume that the data come from a negative binomial distribution with a mean ILI incidence of 20.6 per day and a variance of 27.1.

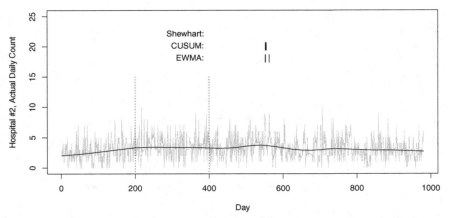

Figure 9.7. Plot of Hospital #2 data with signal times where the Shewhart, CUSUM, and EWMA signaling times are indicated with the vertical lines. Thresholds were set with an expected time between false signals of approximately 365 days.

For the first 50 days of the data, the method of moments (see page 339) fits the negative binomial distribution $Y \sim \text{NBin}(\hat{r}, \hat{p})$, where

$$\hat{r} = \frac{\bar{y}^2}{s^2 - \bar{y}} = \frac{20.6^2}{27.1 - 20.6} = 65.2$$

and

$$\hat{p} = \frac{\bar{y}}{s^2} = \frac{20.6}{27.1} = 0.76.$$

Applying the negative binomial versions of the Shewhart, CUSUM, and EWMA methods, for the Shewhart, $h = 38$ results in an ATFS of 492 days where, again

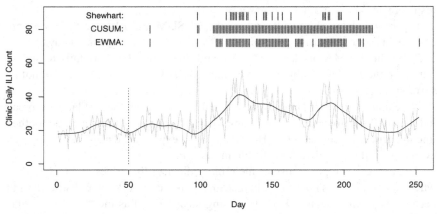

Figure 9.8. Plot of clinic ILI syndrome data with signal times, where the Shewhart, CUSUM, and EWMA detection method signaling times are indicated with the vertical lines. Thresholds set with an ATFS of 365 days or greater.

because of distributional discreteness, this is as close to but still greater than the desired 365 days between false signals that can be achieved (e.g., $h = 37$ gives an ATFS of 310 days). For the CUSUM, assuming the detection of a 2–standard deviation increase in the mean is desired, set

$$k = \frac{-r \ln\left[(r + \lambda_0)/(r + \lambda_1)\right]}{\ln\left[(\lambda_1(r + \lambda_0))/(\lambda_0(r + \lambda_1))\right]}$$

$$= \frac{-65.2 \ln\left[(65.2 + 20.6)/(65.2 + 31)\right]}{\ln\left[(31(65.2 + 20.6))/(20.6(65.2 + 31))\right]}$$

$$= 25.4.$$

Via simulation, $h = 14.5$ results in an ATFS of 362.7 days ($s.e. = 1.1$). And for the EWMA, assuming $\lambda = 0.3$, via simulation $L = 63.9$ results in an ATFS of 360.4 days ($s.e. = 1.1$).

As in the previous examples, Figure 9.8 shows that the three methods all indicate the increase in ILI over days 100 to 200+. The CUSUM and EWMA signals were automatically reset with $s = 16$. The CUSUM and EWMA again generally signal before the Shewhart because of the moderate increase early in the outbreak. Prior to the large outbreak, all three methods also signal on day 98 because of the large outlier on that day. And the CUSUM and EWMA both also signal on day 65, when it appears there was a small increase in ILI incidence for a few days.

9.1.2 Detecting a Bioterrorism Attack

When monitoring for bioterrorism attacks, natural outbreaks are simply part of the "normal" background disease incidence. Thus, using the approach from the previous section, where observations are standardized using non-outbreak period data is not sufficient because bioterrorism attacks will not be detectable during outbreak periods. To be able to detect a bioterrorism attack at any time of the year, it is necessary to characterize the typical behavior at each time in the year and then monitor for departures (increases) from that typical behavior.

To do this, some research has focused on building and fitting complex models that attempt to predict the seasonal variation in the data. These models require years of data and generally do a poor job of predicting seasonal variation because natural outbreaks such as the flu vary from year to year, both in terms of when they occur and in their severity (duration and magnitude). In addition, years of data are often not available, and even when they are, they may not be reliable because of changes in population demographics or behavior.

Now, even if years of accurate data are available, long-term prediction models are not what is most relevant to the bioterrorism problem. Rather, when monitoring for bioterrorism, what is most relevant is identifying departures (unusual increases) from recent past behavior. Given this, the questions are (1) how to best model the recent past behavior and (2) how to best detect departures.

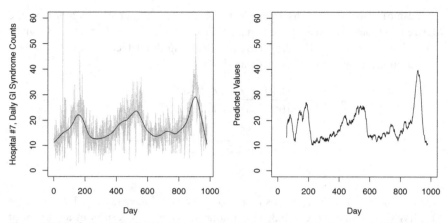

Figure 9.9. Left plot: Hospital #7 GI syndrome data (without injected outbreaks). Right plot: Fitted values from the adaptive regressions using linear regression and a 56-day baseline.

To illustrate one approach for implementing the univariate temporal methods for detecting a bioterrorism attack (or any outbreak of short duration), consider the Hospital #7 data with outbreaks artificially "injected" into the real data. Using this approach ensures the methods must contend with all the complexity of real data while allowing the simulated attacks to be completely known. See Appendix B for more discussion on simulating biosurveillance data, including injecting outbreaks into actual data.

Because the daily counts in these data are relatively large, recent past behavior is modeled using adaptive regression with a sliding baseline to model and remove the systematic effects in the data. See Chapter 5 for a detailed description of adaptive regression. Each day's prediction is based on the past 8 weeks of data, which are subtracted from the observed value, and the resulting residuals are monitored over time. Large residuals are evidence of a possible bioterrorism attack.

The left plot in Figure 9.9 shows the Hospital #7 GI syndrome data, and the plot on the right is the adaptive regression predicted values; comparing the two shows that the predicted values capture the overall trends in the data well. Furthermore, the residuals in the left plot of Figure 9.10 demonstrate that adaptive regression seems to have removed the major systematic effects, and the quantile-quantile plot on the right shows that the residuals are normally distributed.

Given the actual data, three outbreaks are then injected. They followed Equation B.5 with $M = 12$ and $D = 11$, the first starting on day 450, the second starting on day 700, and the third on day 940. Then each of the detection methods was run on the data, the Shewhart with $h = 2.7775$, the CUSUM with $k = 1$ and $h = 1.35$, and the EWMA with $\lambda = 0.3$ and $L = 2.815$. Thus, all three methods were designed for ATFS of 365 days when run on standardized residuals that are normally distributed.

The outbreak periods are shown in Figure 9.11 by the dotted lines, where the first outbreak occurs during a natural outbreak when the GI incidence is increasing,

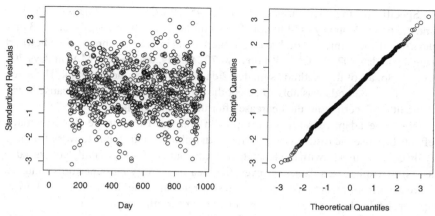

Figure 9.10. Left plot: Residuals from the adaptive regression fitted to Hospital #7 GI syndrome data. Right plot: Quantile-quantile plot of the residuals.

the second outbreak occurs in the middle of a non-outbreak period, and the third was after the peak of the second large outbreak. Comparing Figure 9.11 with Figure 9.4, it is clear that the injected outbreaks would not be observable in a biosurveillance system designed to detect seasonal outbreaks when the methods are not reset.

The short vertical lines in Figure 9.11 indicate the methods' signals, where there are many fewer signals (compared with Fig. 9.4) because the methods were run to automatically reset with $s = 5$. Nonetheless, Figure 9.11 shows that all three methods signal during the first two injected outbreaks, sometimes more than once, and they also signal during the naturally occurring outbreaks.

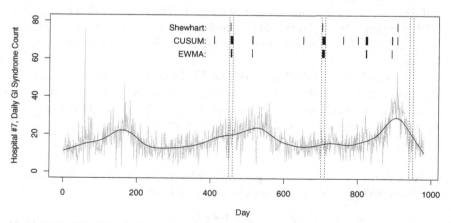

Figure 9.11. Plot of Hospital #7 data with bioterrorism signal times where the Shewhart, CUSUM, and EWMA signaling times are indicated with the short vertical lines. The injected outbreak periods are indicated by the vertical dotted lines. Procedure thresholds set with an expected time between false signals of approximately 365 days.

Specifically, the Shewhart signals on day 453, the CUSUM on days 453 to 459, and the EWMA on days 454 to 456. So, all of the methods first signal either 3 or 4 days into the first injected outbreak. For the second injected outbreak, the Shewhart signals on day 702, the CUSUM on days 702 to 709, and the EWMA on days 702 to 707. So, all of the methods signaled 2 days into the second outbreak. However, none of the methods was able to detect the third injected outbreak because it was difficult to discern amid the decrease after the larger outbreak.

Now, the adaptive regression approach was used to remove the systematic effects because the residuals are normally distributed. This tends to work for large daily counts, such as with the Hospital #7 data, but not for small daily counts, such as with Hospital #2's data. However, the idea of identifying departures (unusual increases) from recent past behavior is still relevant. The difference is in how to appropriately characterize recent past behavior for other types of data.

Additional Examples

Consider the Hospital #2 GI syndrome data as an example of daily counts too small for using the adaptive regression approach. However, as Section 9.1.1 demonstrates, the Poisson distribution is a good fit to the data. So, characterize recent past behavior by letting λ adaptively change over time. The idea is to re-estimate λ each day as

$$\hat{\lambda}_t = \frac{1}{n} \sum_{i=t-n-1}^{t} y_i, t = n+1, \ldots, 980,$$

where n controls how much of the past data is used in the estimate. For the purposes of comparison, set $n = 56$ for consistency with the previous example. In other applications, choosing n is a matter of how much the data changes over time and whether there are periodic systematic effects. The more the data change, the smaller n should be, and it should be a multiple of the smallest periodic trend in the data. Figure 9.12 is a plot of the $\hat{\lambda}_t$ values, $t = 57, \ldots, 980$, for the Hospital #2 data.

Now to apply the Shewhart, CUSUM, and EWMA detections methods, adaptive thresholds must be employed so that on any given day with an estimated $\hat{\lambda}$, the threshold is set to achieve an ATFS of approximately 365 days. For example, for $\hat{F}_t = \mathrm{Pois}(\hat{\lambda}_t)$, the (daily) threshold for the Shewhart is

$$h_t = \hat{F}_t^{-1}(364/365).$$

For a CUSUM to detect a 2-sigma standard deviation increase in the mean of a Poisson random variable, the adaptive reference interval is

$$\hat{k}_t = \frac{(\hat{\mu}_t + 2\hat{\sigma}_t) - \hat{\mu}_t}{\ln(\hat{\mu}_t + 2\hat{\sigma}_t) - \ln(\hat{\mu}_t)} \tag{9.1}$$

$$= \frac{2\sqrt{\hat{\lambda}_t}}{\ln(1 + 2/\sqrt{\hat{\lambda}_t})} \tag{9.2}$$

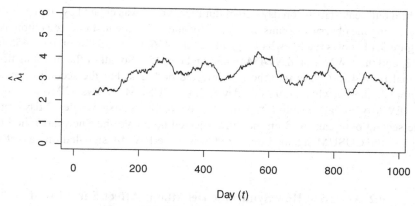

Figure 9.12. Plot of the estimated λ values.

because $\hat{\mu}_t = \hat{\lambda}_t$ and $\hat{\sigma}_t = \sqrt{\hat{\lambda}_t}$. Then, using simulation the CUSUM thresholds were found that achieve ATFS ≈ 365 for various λ. In particular, for $2.3 \leq \lambda_t \leq 4.3$, the associated thresholds are $5.0 \leq h_t \leq 6.3$. Similarly, for the EWMA with smoothing parameter $\lambda = 0.3$, simulation was used to find L_t so that ATFS ≈ 365, where, for $2.3 \leq \lambda_t \leq 4.3$, the associated thresholds are $10.5 \leq L_t \leq 16.4$.

Figure 9.13 shows the results for three injected outbreaks. The injected outbreaks were created by adding additional observations to those in the actual data as follows. Starting on day 450, an outbreak of duration 11 days was created by sequentially increasing the observed counts by 1, 1, 1, 2, 2, 3, 2, 2, 1, 1, and 1. A similar second outbreak starting on day 900 of duration 11 days was created by sequentially increasing the observed counts by 1, 1, 1, 2, 2, 3, 2, 2, 1, 1, and 1. And

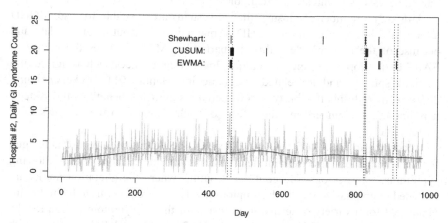

Figure 9.13. Plot of Hospital #2 data where the Shewhart, CUSUM, and EWMA signaling times are indicated with the short vertical lines. The injected outbreak periods are indicated by the vertical dotted lines. Thresholds were set with an expected time between false signals of approximately 365 days.

a third outbreak starting on day 820 of duration 5 days was created by sequentially increasing the observed counts by 1, 6, 12, 6, and 1. For the first injected outbreak, Figure 9.13 shows the Shewhart signals on day 456, the CUSUM on days 455 to 463, and the EWMA on days 454 to 457 and day 459. So, all of the methods first signal from 4 to 6 days into the first injected outbreak. For the second injected outbreak, the Shewhart signals on day 822, the CUSUM on days 822 to 828, and the EWMA on days 822 to 825. So, all of the methods first signaled 2 days into the second outbreak. And on the third injected outbreak, the Shewhart failed to signal, the CUSUM signaled on day 908, and the EWMA signaled on days 906 and 907.

9.2 Assessing How Syndrome Definitions Affect Early Event Detection Performance

The previous section illustrated how to apply EED methods to biosurveillance data either for natural disease outbreak detection or for bioterrorism detection. This section illustrates how to use real biosurveillance data to compare and contrast the performance of various EED methods. In particular, this section compares the EARS and CUSUM EED methods for various ILI syndrome definitions. The results in this section are drawn from joint research with Katie Hagen, Krista Hanni, Suzie Barnes, and Kristy Michie. See Hagen *et al.* (2011) for complete details.

The Monterey County Health Department (MCHD) uses EARS V4.5 to monitor chief complaint data from four hospital emergency rooms (ERs) and six public health clinics, particularly as an alert system for various types of disease outbreaks, which may include those naturally occurring (e.g., influenza), accidental (e.g., fire-related illnesses), or intentional (e.g., bioterrorism).

Although a number of biosurveillance systems are available for use, MCHD uses EARS because it allows MCHD to maintain local control of the data and because of the system's flexibility. In particular, MCHD values the ability in EARS to develop syndromes for unique, local circumstances such as agriculture pesticide spraying and fire-related illness tracking (Hanni, 2011; Fricker & Hanni, 2010). Although this flexibility is considered a significant benefit of the system, it is important to understand the effects of such changes on the system's EED performance.

According to the EARS baseline ILI syndrome definition, a record is flagged for ILI when the chief complaint field contains any one or more of the following symptoms: "sore throat" or "cold" or "cough," where the quotation marks are intended to emphasize that each symptom involves searching through chief complaint text for a variety of terms, from just 1 for the flu symptom to 236 for the sore throat symptom. Table 9.1 shows the EARS baseline definition along with two alternative definitions.

The impact of changing the syndrome definitions is quite dramatic, at least in terms of the total number of individuals classified with the ILI syndrome.

Table 9.1. The EARS baseline ILI definition is what is used by EARS V4.5. The MCHD-expanded and restricted definitions are variants created by MCHD

ILI Definitions	Symptom Combination Logic
EARS Baseline:	"cold" *or* "cough" *or* "sore throat"
MCHD Expanded:	"cold" *or* "cough" *or* "fever" *or* "chills" *or* "muscle pain" *or* "headache" *or* ("flu" *and not* "shot")
MCHD Restricted:	("fever" *and* "cough") *or* ("fever" *and* "sore throat") *or* ("flu" *and not* "shot")

For example, for 1 year of Monterey County data, the EARS baseline definition resulted in just under 6 percent of the record being classified with the ILI syndrome (9,093 of 153,696 records). In contrast, the MCHD expanded definition resulted in a 53 percent increase in the number of records classified as the ILI syndrome (13,956 records or 9 percent of the total), and the MCHD restricted ILI resulted in a 92 percent reduction of the number of records (734 or just 0.5 percent of the total).

9.2.1 Determining the Outbreak Periods

To judge how the definitional changes affect EED performance, it is first necessary to establish when the seasonal ILI and 2009 H1N1 pandemic outbreaks actually occurred within Monterey County. As anyone who has attempted to do this will recognize, establishing some sort of universal "ground truth" about precisely when an outbreak started is often elusive. Not only can the timing of the outbreak vary by geography and subpopulation, but the data can also be quite imprecise. Furthermore, the determination can at times be circular in the sense that knowledge of the start of an outbreak is required to judge EED method performance, but the EED methods are sometimes the most effective way to determine the outbreak start.

In this case, as shown in Figure 9.14, four sources of information were used to assess the outbreak periods. The figure shows the reported weekly percentage of patients classified with ILI from September 28, 2008, to January 2, 2010, along with locally weighted smoothing lines to better show the underlying trends, using data from (1) the California Sentinel Provider Influenza Surveillance Program; (2) Monterey County hospital ERs; (3) Monterey County public health clinics; and (4) laboratory-confirmed, hospitalized cases of 2009 H1N1 in Monterey County. These four sets of data reflect four different populations.

The first population consists of patients seen by medical providers throughout the state of California who voluntarily conduct surveillance for ILI and report weekly to the Centers for Disease Control and Prevention (CDC). As described on the California Department of Public Health's website (California Department of Public Health, 2010), the case definition for ILI is any illness with fever greater than 100°F and cough and/or sore throat (in the absence of a known cause). As

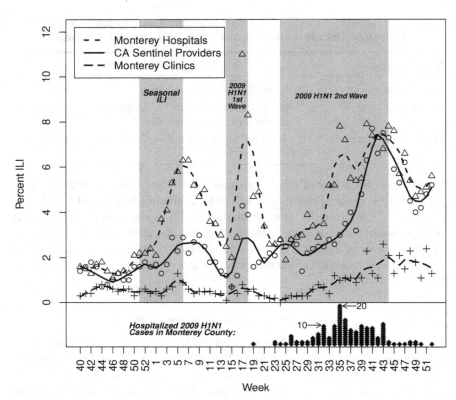

Figure 9.14. Percentage of patients classified with ILI from September 28, 2008 (week 40), to January 2, 2010 (week 52) for (1) the California Sentinel Provider system, (2) Monterey hospital ERs, and (3) Monterey public health clinics. The diamonds are laboratory-confirmed, hospitalized cases of 2009 H1N1 in Monterey County, where each diamond represents one person and is plotted for the week the individual first became symptomatic due to 2009 H1N1 infection. The arrows show that week 32 had 10 cases and week 35 had 20 cases.

such, the circles in Figure 9.14 are a measure of ILI activity throughout the entire state. The solid black line is locally weighted smoothing line to better show the underlying trends in the state-level data.

The second population, represented by the triangles and associated dashed line in Figure 9.14, are individuals who went to an ER of one of the four Monterey County hospitals and who were subsequently classified with ILI by EARS using the MCHD restricted definition. The third population, represented by the crosses and the associated dashed line, are individuals who went to one of six Monterey County public clinics and who were subsequently classified with ILI by EARS using the restricted definition.

Finally, the fourth population is the entire population of Monterey County, and the data are the laboratory-confirmed, hospitalized cases of 2009 H1N1 in Monterey County. These are shown as the black diamonds at the bottom of the plot, where each diamond represents one person and is plotted for the week the individual first became symptomatic due to 2009 H1N1 virus infection. A note about these data is in order: At the epidemic's onset, medical providers were required to report all laboratory-confirmed cases of 2009 H1N1 to their local health jurisdictions under Title 17 of the California Code of Regulations. In May 2009, the providers reporting requirements were restricted to fatal or hospitalized, laboratory-confirmed 2009 H1N1 cases. This allowed health officials to focus on the determinants of severe illness. Providers were encouraged to use clinical presentation rather than laboratory testing to guide management of patients. Widespread laboratory testing was not recommended. The reporting requirements were further restricted in May 2010 to laboratory-confirmed cases resulting in intensive care unit admission or death. Therefore, no centralized database of outpatient 2009 H1N1 cases, which represented the majority of 2009 H1N1 infections, exists with which we could compare ILI reports.

In looking at the smoothed curves in Figure 9.14, the MCHD hospital ER and clinic ILI syndrome trends tend to have patterns similar to each other and the California Sentinel Provider data. However, there are also some differences. For example, as highlighted by the left-most shaded region in Figure 9.14, the seasonal ILI pattern is visible with similar trends in both the sentinel provider and hospital data, starting late in week 50 and peaking in week 6, but in the clinic data, seasonal ILI is much less evident and seems to start later, showing up as a slight increase starting around week 2 and peaking in week 5. Furthermore, note that the statewide seasonal ILI pattern peaks from weeks 5 to 9, but the Monterey County hospital ERs and clinics have a much sharper peak around week 5 or 6 after which the ILI incidence decreases substantially. This pattern is consistent with the fact that the California Sentinel Provider data are for the whole state, where the longer peak likely reflects the outbreak occurring in different times and parts of the state. Monterey County is a small geographic location, and it appears the ILI had peaked early on in this location compared with the entire state.

As for the second outbreak period in Figure 9.14 (the "2009 H1N1 1st Wave"), there is consistency across all three time series, with the 2009 H1N1 pandemic starting in week 14 and peaking in week 18 of 2009. Subsequent to the first wave, a second wave of the H1N1 pandemic ("2009 H1N1 2nd Wave" in the figure) may have started as early as week 24 and peaked somewhere between weeks 35 and 44. This is where there is a bit of divergence between the three time series. The hospital ERs show an initial spike at weeks 34 and 35 followed by a larger peak around week 42 and then a subsequent decline. The California Sentinel Provider data and the clinic data are consistent with this later peak around weeks 42 to 44, but they both show a more gradual increase to the peak and no spike at weeks 34 and 35. Perhaps the difference is that the 2009 H1N1 virus spread slightly differently in the population served by the Monterey County hospitals or perhaps during the weeks 34 to 35 peak, people were more likely to go to the ER than to public clinics. These differences may also be due to how people use hospitals versus clinics and the severity of or worry about their symptoms. The laboratory-confirmed, hospitalized cases at the bottom show a combination of the two trends, where we see that weeks 26, 32, and 34 through 36 had spikes in cases,

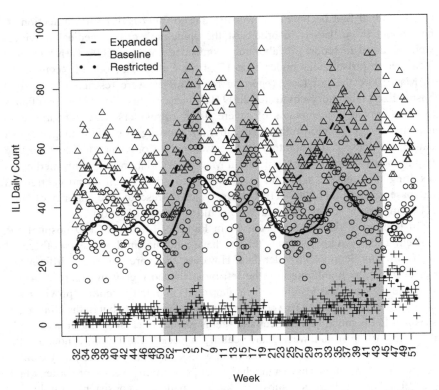

Figure 9.15. Comparison of the estimated ILI counts using the baseline, expanded, and restricted definitions. The shaded areas, which match those of Figure 9.14, show that the three outbreak periods are largely consistent across the different populations and ILI syndrome definitions.

but the entire "2009 H1N1 2nd Wave" period shows substantial 2009 H1N1 activity.

Figure 9.14 illustrates that the outbreak indications are quite similar across the three populations. However, it is important to note that the clinic and hospital percentages of ILI are based on the MCHD's restricted ILI syndrome definition. As such, it is not obvious that these observed trends will manifest in the same way in the raw daily count data and under the baseline and expanded ILI definitions. However, as shown in Figure 9.15, the dates do in fact match up fairly well. Thus, regardless of the definition used, Monterey County clinic ILI syndrome data followed the sentinel provider trends fairly closely, and "ground truth" will be taken to be the three periods of rising counts shown via the shaded areas in Figures 9.14 and 9.15. These correspond to:

- Seasonal ILI outbreak period: 12/12/2008 (week 50) to 2/13/2009 (week 6),
- First 2009 H1N1 pandemic outbreak period: 4/6/2009 (week 14) to 5/8/2009 (week 18), and

- Second 2009 H1N1 pandemic outbreak period: 6/15/2009 (week 24) to 11/6/2009 (week 44),

where the term "outbreak period" is defined as the period of time in which the syndrome counts were increasing from their nominal state up to some peak.

9.2.2 Assessing Performance

To assess how these definitional changes might affect EED performance, the standard EARS C1, C2, and C3 methods as defined in Chapter 7, Section 7.5.2 were used, as well as the CUSUM of Chapter 7, Section 7.3 applied to adaptive regression forecast errors (based on a 7-week sliding baseline). In so doing, current MCHD practice of not resetting the EED methods after each signal was followed. See the previous section and Fricker (2010) for additional discussion about the pros and cons of such practice. As with the previous section, the first 35 days of the clinic data were used to parameterize the EED methods and fit the adaptive regression, and then the methods were prospectively run on the rest of the data.

For the CUSUM, three variants are used – based on the values of k and h – to investigate a range of performance. As shown in Table 9.2, these are referred to as "aggressive," "moderate," and "routine." CUSUM1 is called aggressive because, based on $k = 0.5$, it will signal quickly for a 1–standard deviation increase in the forecast errors, and with $k = 0.5$ and $h = 0.365$, it has an ATFS of 5 days. Intuitively, one can think of small ATFS values giving the CUSUM a higher probability of detecting outbreaks but at the expense of a higher false-positive signal rate, where an ATFS of 5 days means that there will be a false-positive signal once a week on average (assuming the CUSUM is reset after each signal).

In comparison, CUSUM2 is called moderate because, based on $k = 1.0$, it will signal quickly for a 2–standard deviation increase in the forecast errors, and with $k = 1.0$ and $h = 0.695$, it has an ATFS of 20 days. Thus, CUSUM2 will be less sensitive than CUSUM1, but it will also have fewer false-positive signals, with only one per month on average (four times less than CUSUM1). Finally, CUSUM3 is called routine because although it will signal quickly for a 2–standard deviation increase in the forecast errors like CUSUM2, with $k = 1.0$ and $h = 1.2$, it has an ATFS of 60 days. Thus, CUSUM3 will be less sensitive than either CUSUM1 or

Table 9.2. Parameters for the three CUSUM variants used. CUSUM1 is designed to have a high probability of signaling an actual outbreak and, concomitantly, a higher false-positive signal rate. At the other extreme, CUSUM3 is designed to have a low false-positive rate as well as a lower probability of signaling an actual outbreak

Type	Label	k	h	ATFS
Aggressive:	CUSUM1	0.5	0.365	5
Moderate:	CUSUM2	1.0	0.695	20
Routine:	CUSUM3	1.0	1.200	60

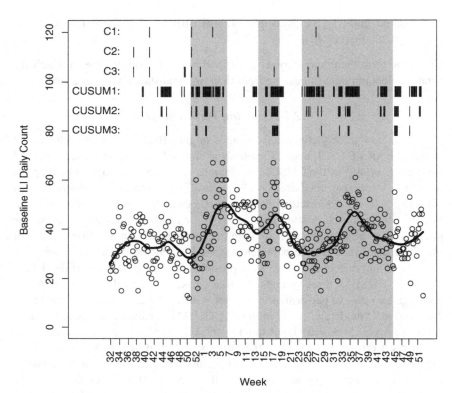

Figure 9.16. EED method signal times using the CDC baseline ILI syndrome definition. A signal on a particular day is denoted by a vertical line "|," and the heavier black bars indicate a sequence of daily signals. The black line is a locally weighted smoothing line to show the underlying trends.

CUSUM2, but it will also only have a false-positive signal of once per quarter on average.

Results Using Early Aberration Reporting System Baseline Influenza-Like Illness Definition

Figure 9.16 compares the results of the six EED methods under the CDC's baseline ILI syndrome definition. The circles show the aggregate daily ILI counts for Monterey County clinics, and the black line is a locally weighted smoothing line to show the underlying trends in the data. The shaded areas denote the three outbreak periods that were just defined: the seasonal ILI followed by the two 2009 H1N1 waves. Finally, at the top of the plot are the daily signals for the six EED methods. A signal on a particular day is denoted by a vertical line "|," where heavier black bars simply indicate a sequence of daily signals.

Figure 9.16 shows that right at the start of the seasonal ILI outbreak (i.e., at week 51 or December 15, 2008), all EED methods with the exception of CUSUM3 signaled (and, in fact, CUSUM1 signaled for three consecutive days). Subsequent to the initial signal, the EARS C1 and C3 methods each only signaled one additional time during the outbreak period. In comparison, the CUSUM methods continued to signal periodically throughout the outbreak period and in a manner consistent with their design. That is, CUSUM1 was designed to be the most sensitive, CUSUM2 less so, and CUSUM3 the least sensitive. Of course, this comes with the trade-off that the more sensitive the CUSUM, the more it also signals in the non-outbreak periods as well.

For the first 2009 H1N1 outbreak period (e.g., weeks 14–19), none of the methods signaled at the outset of the outbreak period although the fact that CUSUM1 signals 2 days prior and CUSUM2 signals 3 days prior might be an indication that the outbreak period started a few days earlier than the shading shows. What is clear is that the EARS C1 and C2 methods completely miss the outbreak, and the C3 only signals once at the peak of the outbreak. In contrast, the CUSUM methods all signal more consistently and regularly and, with the exception of CUSUM3, earlier than C3. Finally, for the second 2009 H1N1 outbreak period (weeks 24–44), CUSUM1 signals right at the outset of the outbreak period with CUSUM2 and C3 following 5 and 7 days later, respectively. In comparison, C2 fails to signal at all, C1 takes 16 days to signal, and CUSUM3 takes 22 days.

Results Using Monterey County Health Department Expanded Influenza-Like Illness Definition

Figure 9.17 compares the performance of the six EED methods under the MCHD expanded ILI syndrome definition. What is most striking in this plot is the complete lack of signals over all three outbreak periods for the C1 and C2 methods. In particular, note the large observation of $y = 100$ in week 52 (that occurred on December 22) where, for this particular day, the estimated standard deviations (S_t in Equation 7.19 and S_t^* in Equation 7.20) are so large that the resulting statistics are just below the signaling threshold. And although the C3 method does signal for the 2009 H1N1 outbreak periods, the initial signals are 17 and 18 days after the start of the outbreak, respectively, which is more than a 3-week delay. The CUSUM methods seem to do better, although CUSUM1 and CUSUM2 each have delays of 6 days for the first 2009 H1N1 outbreak and 7 days for the second 2009 H1N1 outbreak, and the CUSUM3 does not perform any better than the C3 in terms of delay.

Thus, the most important result is that all of the methods perform substantially worse using the MCHD expanded ILI syndrome definition compared with the CDC baseline definition. This is surprising because the motivation for this definition was to make the EARS system more sensitive to detecting outbreaks, yet at least for these three outbreak periods, the expanded definition does just the opposite. The explanation for this outcome, which is clear in hindsight, is that the expanded definition introduced excessive noise into the data. That is, it classifies individuals with ILI who should not have been and thus masks the outbreak signals with noise. This introduction of noise is evident in Figure 9.15, where the MCHD expanded

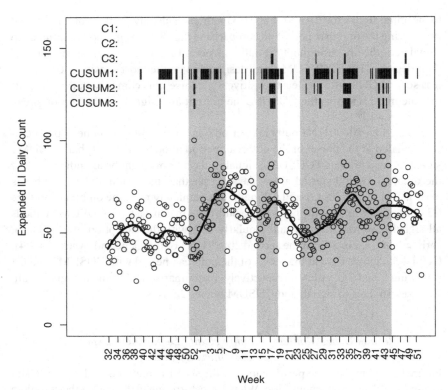

Figure 9.17. EED method signal times using the MCHD expanded ILI syndrome definition. A signal on a particular day is denoted by a vertical line "|," and the heavier black bars indicate a sequence of daily signals. The black line is a locally weighted smoothing line to show the underlying trends.

ILI syndrome curve essentially mirrors the CDC baseline curve except it is shifted upward.

Results Using Monterey County Health Department Restricted Influenza-Like Illness Definition

Figure 9.18 compares the performance of six EED methods under the MCHD restricted ILI syndrome definition. Here we see that the CUSUM methods perform better than the EARS methods using the other ILI definitions in the sense that they more regularly signal during the outbreak periods. Furthermore, many of the EARS and CUSUM methods' signals tend to align temporally, suggesting that all the methods are detecting similar aberrations in the restricted data.

Compared with Figure 9.16, with the exception of CUSUM3, it appears that all of the methods are slower at detecting the seasonal ILI outbreak. However, this conclusion is confounded by the fact that the shaded area better corresponds to when the baseline and expanded data show an uptick. The restricted data do not show an increase in ILI counts until week 52 or so, which is when the CUSUMs

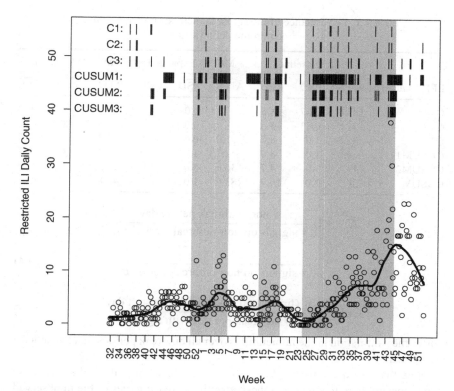

Figure 9.18. EED method signal times using the MCHD restricted ILI syndrome definition. A signal on a particular day is denoted by a vertical line "|," and the heavier black bars indicate a sequence of daily signals. The black line is a locally weighted smoothing line to show the underlying trends.

signal. Whether the outbreak actually began in week 50, 51, or 52 for the population served by the clinics is simply unknowable. It is clear, however, that the CUSUM methods signal the seasonal ILI earlier than the EARS methods.

Summarizing the Results

Visually, the restricted ILI syndrome definition seems to pretty clearly result in better EED performance, particularly for the EARS methods. To more formally and quantitatively compare between ILI syndrome definitions and EED methods, estimate the ATFS, PSD, and CED from the data as follows:

$$\widehat{\text{PSD}} = \frac{\text{\# outbreak periods with one or more signals}}{\text{\# outbreak periods}}$$

$$= \frac{\text{\# outbreak periods with one or more signals}}{3}. \tag{9.3}$$

Table 9.3. Performance of the six EED methods under the three ILI
syndrome definitions

EED Method	CDC Baseline			MCHD Expanded			MCHD Restricted		
	$\widehat{ATFS}$	$\widehat{PSD}$	$\widehat{CED}$	$\widehat{ATFS}$	$\widehat{PSD}$	$\widehat{CED}$	$\widehat{ATFS}$	$\widehat{PSD}$	$\widehat{CED}$
C1	183.0	0.67	8.5	–	0.0	–	45.8	1.0	9.7
C2	91.5	0.33	1.0	–	0.0	–	45.8	1.0	9.7
C3	45.8	1.0	8.7	61.0	0.67	11.5	15.3	1.0	9.7
CUSUM1	4.0	1.0	3.0	4.1	1.0	4.7	4.2	1.0	3.7
CUSUM2	14.1	1.0	4.7	36.6	1.0	6.3	18.3	1.0	7.0
CUSUM3	30.5	1.0	14.7	183.0	1.0	14.7	45.8	1.0	10.7

$$\widehat{ATFS} = \frac{\text{\# non-outbreak period days}}{\text{\# signals on non-outbreak period days}}$$

$$= \frac{183}{\text{\# signals on non-outbreak period days}}. \tag{9.4}$$

$$\widehat{CED} = \frac{\sum (\text{first signal day} - \text{outbreak start day})}{\text{\# outbreak periods with signals}}, \tag{9.5}$$

where the summation in the numerator is over all outbreak periods that had at least one signal.

Note that in Equations 9.3, 9.4, and 9.5, the "hats" on left-hand sides of the equations are there to stress that these quantities are *estimates* of the unobserved theoretical quantities, and only very crude estimates at that, based on limited data with a small number of outbreaks. For example, the PSD calculation is only based on three outbreaks and thus can only take on values 0, 1/3, 2/3, and 1.

In addition, these results are highly dependent on the particular observed time series, where without additional time series on other populations with different outbreaks it is impossible to know how generalizable these results may (or may not) be. Furthermore, these estimates are based on the assumption that the three outbreaks are the only outbreaks in the data and that their start and stop times have been correctly identified. These are all unverifiable, but questionable, assumptions that limit how much can be concluded from this one set of results. However, the goal here is to only gain some rough insight into how the the ILI definitions affect EED performance.

It is also important to note that Equation 9.4 is appropriate to apply to the CUSUM variants because in this analysis the CUSUMs were reset after each signal. If they had not been reset, then a more complicated calculation would need to have been done.

That all said, Table 9.3 shows the estimated PSD, ATFS, and CED values for each combination of EED method and ILI definition.

Table 9.3 clearly demonstrates the benefit of the MCHD restricted ILI definition. In particular, for the EARS methods, it improves PSD at a very modest cost to

ATFS and CED. In comparison, the expanded definition performed very poorly, particularly in conjunction with the EARS methods, where for the C1 and C2 methods there was not even enough information to estimate ATFS and CED. When comparing between the performance of the EARS and CUSUM methods, what is striking in Table 9.3 is that the CUSUM methods are more robust to the ILI syndrome definition, in the sense that the performance of each variant was fairly similar across all three ILI definitions.

When comparing among the CUSUM methods, CUSUM1 clearly had the best performance in terms of CED followed by CUSUM2 and then CUSUM3. This is not surprising because this is how the CUSUMs were defined: aggressive, moderate, and routine.

The speed-of-detection performance of the CUSUM1 does not come for free, however. The cost is in terms of the ATFS, which characterizes the false signal rate. In particular, we see that CUSUM1 signals roughly 1 day out of every 4 when there is no outbreak. This is likely to be unacceptably high. If so, then adjusting the CUSUM's parameters, such as with CUSUM2 and CUSUM3, can reduce the false signal rate, although this will come at the cost of additional delay and possibly reduced PSD.

For example, under the restricted ILI definition, switching from CUSUM1 to CUSUM2 will decrease the rate of false signals from one per 4 days to roughly one per 14 to 37 days (depending on the ILI definition), but it will also add an additional 2.3 days of delay on average (i.e., increase in the CED). Ultimately, these sorts of trade-offs should be made by the public health practitioner in the context of the public health threats being faced and the resources available to investigate biosurveillance signals.

9.3 Discussion and Summary

One benefit of biosurveillance systems designed for bioterrorism detection is that they can also be used to detect and monitor natural diseases. However, it does not follow that a system operated for detecting natural diseases will be most effective at detecting bioterrorism. As Shmueli and Burkom (2010) say,

> Determining whether an abnormality is present in the data requires defining normal behavior. One complication arises from the intended dual-use of biosurveillance systems for detecting natural and bioterror-related or pandemic disease outbreaks, because the data footprint of a seasonal influenza epidemic is a target signal in the former context but part of the background clutter in the latter. In the bioterrorism monitoring context, all usual seasonal influences should be removed for sensitivity even at the peak and aftermath of a usual influenza outbreak.

At issue is that if a system that is signaling during a natural disease outbreak is not reset, then it cannot detect a bioterrorism attack during that time. An analogy: The smoke alarm that goes off every time the oven is used is worthless for detecting a stovetop fire that occurs when a cake is being baked in the oven.

This suggests that additional emphasis needs to be placed on operational paradigms and EED method design. In particular, during natural disease outbreaks, systems must be designed to adjust for revised background incidence rates so the system can look for further anomalies. In addition, the current practice of not resetting EED methods after a signal and, in fact, using multiple sequential signals as evidence of an actual outbreak should be recognized as practices potentially detrimental to detecting a bioterrorism attack.

Of course, this begs the question of whether it is even possible to adjust for a transient disease outbreak in any reliable fashion that would then allow for further anomaly detection. If the main purpose of biosurveillance systems is bioterrorism protection, then this is an important area of future research. After all, when would a smart bioterrorist attack? During the flu season, of course.

Biosurveillance systems have great promise as a public health tool for improving population health and well-being. They also have the potential to improve public health response to natural disease outbreaks and bioterrorism. However, continuing research is necessary to better understand how to most effectively design and employ them.

For example, as these results have shown, biosurveillance system EED performance can be improved with changes in syndrome definitions. This idea is simple: To the extent that noise can be eliminated from the data, it will be easier for EED methods to identify anomalies in the data. To date, more research has been focused on developing complicated and sophisticated detection algorithms rather than improving the data upon which the algorithms are run.

However, arguably, better data are the "low-hanging fruit" with the potential to significantly improve biosurveillance performance. This suggests that greater emphasis should therefore be focused on improvements in the data, collection, management, text-searching logic, syndrome definitions, and so on. This is a nontrivial exercise, particularly for rarely occurring diseases and bioterrorism agents for which (thankfully) there is little to no data from which to assess detection performance.

10

Comparing Methods to Better Understand
and Improve Biosurveillance Performance

When I have fully decided that a result is worth getting I go ahead of it and make
trial after trial until it comes.

Thomas A. Edison (1847–1931)

This chapter builds on Chapter 9, synthesizing everything from the first eight chapters (and Appendix B) to demonstrate how to compare the performance of early event detection (EED) methods using simulation. Assessing EED performance via simulation is critical because, as shown in the last chapter, comparisons using real data are limited in a number of ways.

The first limitation is that real data are opaque and often unknowable. For example, it is virtually impossible to specify with certainty when a known outbreak starts and stops. It is similarly impossible to state with certainty that data for a given period is free of outbreaks. The entire point of EED methods and tools such as change point analysis is to find outbreaks, but failure to find an outbreak does not prove the absence of outbreaks.

The second limitation is that all real data are unique, both temporally and spatially. As a result, any analysis on one set of data is limited in terms of how generalizable the results might be for another time, or location, or under another set of circumstances. Given that EED methods will be broadly applied across many different populations, it is important that the performance of the methods is robust to such differences.

The third limitation is that outbreaks are (thankfully) scarce, as is the availability of real data sets (unfortunately). Hence, as shown in Section 9.2 of the last chapter, it is very hard to reliably estimate average time between false signals (ATFS), probability of successful detection (PSD), and condition expected delay (CED), because for any given set of data, the number of known or observable outbreaks will be small. The result is that comparisons between EED methods using real data will be inherently variable, and thus clear and clean conclusions will be hard (at best) to reach.

281

Simulation overcomes many of these limitations. For example, with simulation, the specifics of an outbreak can be precisely known, and hence the performance of EED methods can be precisely quantified. In addition, many simulations can be conducted over a wide variety of conditions, from which the robustness (or lack thereof) of various EED methods can be judged. Furthermore, simulated data can easily be shared, facilitating collaboration and allowing for replication of research results.

The major criticism of simulation is that simulated data cannot capture all of the complexity inherent in real data. But this is a strength as well as a weakness of simulation. It is a weakness if simulated data fail to mimic the important and salient features of real data, where it is important to note that not all real-world data complexity is necessarily relevant. However, it is also a strength in the sense that the appropriate abstraction often facilitates the identification of the specific conditions under which an EED method is more or less effective.[1]

This chapter contains two examples of using simulation to compare EED methods. The first compares the univariate cumulative sum (CUSUM) with the Early Aberration Reporting System (EARS) methods. It is drawn from joint research with Ben Hegler and Andy Dunfee (Fricker *et al.*, 2008a). The second compares the multivariate CUSUM (MCUSUM) and multivariate EMWA (MEWMA) methods and is drawn from joint research with Matt Knitt and Cecilia Hu (Fricker *et al.*, 2008b).

---

[1] This point brings the text full circle back to the quotes in the Preface on page xi.

Chapter Objective

The goal of this chapter is to demonstrate the use of simulation for comparing the performance of EED methods. Upon completion of the chapter, the reader should:

- Understand how to appropriately apply simulation to compare the performance of both univariate and multivariate EED methods.
- Have some insight into and an understanding of the utility of making such comparisons, including the pros and cons of comparing methods using simulated data versus actual data.

The results presented herein are meant to be illustrative, both of one simulation approach and of the utility of simulation for comparing EED performance. While the results are informative with respect to the performance of the particular EED methods compared herein, definitive conclusions should follow only after these results have been replicated and additional comparisons under other conditions have been made.

Mathematical Notation

A	Amplitude of the sinusoid simulating seasonal variation
c	Mean level of disease in univariate temporal method #1 (UTM1) simulation
C_t	CUSUM statistic for day t
D	Outbreak duration
$\mathbb{E}(Y)$	Expected value of random variable Y
h	EED method threshold
$\mathbf{I}$	Identity matrix
k	MCUSUM/CUSUM parameter
M	Outbreak magnitude
n	Length of sliding baseline
$N(\mu, \sigma^2)$	Univariate normal distribution with mean μ and variance σ^2
$N_5(\mathbf{0}, \sigma^2\mathbf{I})$	Five-dimensional multivariate normal distribution with mean vector $\mathbf{0}$ and covariance matrix $\sigma^2\mathbf{I}$
$o, \mathbf{o}$	Mean outbreak level
$U(a, b)$	Uniform distribution over the range a to b
y_t	Observation y on day t
$Y, \mathbf{Y}$	Random variable/vector representing a count before it is observed
$Z, \mathbf{Z}$	Random noise component in data simulations
$\delta, \boldsymbol{\delta}$	Day-of-the-week effect
$\gamma, \boldsymbol{\gamma}$	Seasonal deviation from annual mean
λ	MEWMA smoothing parameter
$\boldsymbol{\mu}$	Vector of mean disease in multivariate temporal method #1 (MTM1) simulation
σ_Z	Standard deviation of random variable Z
τ	Random day of outbreak start
$\theta, \boldsymbol{\theta}$	Within-season deviation

10.1 Performance Comparisons: A Univariate Example

This section illustrates how to conduct simulation comparisons among some of the univariate EED methods presented in Chapter 7. In so doing, it brings together many concepts discussed in previous chapters, including adaptive regression from Chapter 5, as well as methods for simulating biosurveillance data from Appendix B. In particular, this section compares the EARS C1, C2, and C3 methods with the CUSUM method applied to the forecast errors of an adaptive regression model.

10.1.1 Simulating Biosurveillance Data

To compare the EARS and CUSUM EED methods, background disease incidence was simulated and then various types of simulated bioterrorism attacks or natural disease outbreaks were overlaid. The background disease incidence data were simulated using the UTM1 of Appendix B as the sum of a mean disease incidence, a seasonal sinusoidal cycle, a systematic day-of-the-week effect, and random noise. Outbreaks, when they occurred, were incorporated as an additive term.

That is, a daily observation Y_t was simulated as

$$Y_t = \max(0, \lceil c + \gamma_t + \delta_t + o_t + Z_t \rceil), \quad t = 1, 2, 3, \ldots, \qquad (10.1)$$

where

- c is a constant level of disease incidence;
- γ is the seasonal deviation;
- δ is the day-of-the-week effect;
- Z is the random noise around the systematic component, $c + \gamma_t + \delta_t$;
- o_t is the mean outbreak level, which, when an outbreak is occurring, increases the disease incidence level as described below; and
- $\lceil x \rceil$ is the ceiling function, which rounds x up to the next largest integer.

The seasonal effect is calculated as $\gamma_t = A[\sin(2\pi t/365)]$, where A is the maximum deviation from c with $t = 1$ corresponding to October 1 on a 365-day per year calendar. For the random noise, the simulations use $Z \sim N(\mu, \sigma^2)$ when c is large and $Z \sim LN(\mu, \sigma^2)$ when c is small.

The day-of-the-week effect is the systematic deviation from $c + \gamma_t$, where $\delta_t = \delta_{t+7}$ for all t. It is defined in terms of σ, a parameter of Z: $\delta = -0.5\sigma$ on Sunday, $\delta = 0.1\sigma$ on Monday, $\delta = 0.2\sigma$ on Tuesday, $\delta = 0.3\sigma$ on Wednesday, $\delta = 0.4\sigma$ on Thursday, $\delta = 0$ on Friday, and $\delta = -0.3\sigma$ on Saturday.

Table 10.1 specifies parameter values for Equation 10.1 for 12 scenarios designed to span a range of possible underlying disease incidence patterns. Scenarios 1 to 6 are large-count scenarios, and Scenarios 7 to 12 are low-count scenarios. The parameters were selected to generate synthetic data that mimic disease incidence patterns similar to selected data sets published by the Centers for Disease Control and Prevention (http://www.bt.cdc.gov/surveillance/ears/datasets.asp).

Table 10.1. Parameters for Equation 10.1
that define 12 background disease
incidence scenarios

Scenario	c	A	μ	σ
1	90	80	0	30
2	90	80	0	10
3	90	20	0	30
4	90	20	0	10
5	90	0	0	30
6	90	0	0	10
7	0	6	1.0	0.7
8	0	6	1.0	0.5
9	0	2	1.0	0.7
10	0	2	1.0	0.5
11	0	0	1.0	0.7
12	0	0	1.0	0.5

In particular, $c = 90$, $A = 80$, $\mu = 0$, and $\sigma = 30$ or $\sigma = 10$ in Equation 10.1 result in disease incidence patterns similar to EARS data set S08. Setting $c = 90$, $A = 20$, $\mu = 0$, and $\sigma = 10$ results in disease incidence patterns similar to the S01 data set, as well as other patterns that are intermediate between S01 and S08. For Scenarios 7 to 12, combinations of the values in Table 10.1 result in disease incidence patterns similar to S03, S04, S15, and S34. Figure 10.1 shows one set of simulated data for Scenario 1.

For the low count scenarios, data set S04 is characteristic of hospital-level respiratory or influenza-like illness (ILI) chief complaint counts, S03 of hospital-level rash chief complaint counts, and S34 of hospital-level neurological chief complaint counts. For the high count scenarios, S08 is characteristic of state-level aggregate respiratory or ILI chief complaint counts, S45 of state-level aggregate gastrointestinal (GI) chief complaint counts, and S15 of state-level neurologic chief complaint counts.

Outbreaks were incorporated into Equation 10.1 as an additive term o_t representing the mean outbreak level. As with the simulated data themselves, the outbreak is an idealized form that could be parameterized simply. The parameters are the peak magnitude M, the outbreak duration D, and a random start day τ. Outbreaks increase linearly up to M and then linearly back down to zero:

$$
o_t = \begin{cases} M\left[2(t - \tau + 1)/(D + 1)\right], & \tau \leq t \leq \tau + D/2 - 1/2 \\ M\left[1 - (2(t - \tau) - D + 1)/(D + 1)\right], & \tau + D/2 - 1/2 < t \leq \tau + D - 1 \\ 0, & \text{otherwise.} \end{cases}
$$

The performance of the EED methods were assessed for outbreaks of various magnitudes and durations.

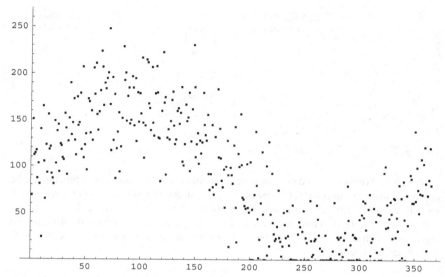

Figure 10.1. One year of simulated Scenario 1 data.

- Scenarios 1 to 6 used three magnitudes – small, medium, and large – defined as a fraction of the constant disease incidence c: $M = 0.1c$, $M = 0.25c$, and $M = 0.5c$, respectively, where $c = 90$ from Table 10.1.
- Scenarios 7 to 12 used four magnitudes – very small, small, medium, and large – defined as a fraction of the mean plus 3 standard deviations of the lognormally distributed random variable Z from Equation 10.1.
  - Large outbreaks: $M = \mathbb{E}(Z) + 3\sigma_Z$;
  - Medium outbreaks: $M = 0.5[\mathbb{E}(Z) + 3\sigma_Z]$;
  - Small outbreaks: $M = 0.25[\mathbb{E}(Z) + 3\sigma_Z]$; and
  - Very small outbreaks $M = 0.1[\mathbb{E}(Z) + 3\sigma_Z]$.

For Scenarios 7 to 12,

$$\mathbb{E}(Z) = \exp(\mu + \sigma^2/2)$$

and

$$\sigma_Z^2 = (e^{\sigma^2} - 1)e^{2\mu+\sigma^2},$$

where μ and σ are specified in Table 10.1 for the various scenarios.

For all the scenarios considered, durations ranged from short to long: $D = 3, 5, \ldots, 15$ days. The simulations were conducted in MatLab 7.1.0.246 using the randn function to generate random normal variates and lognrnd to generate log normal random variates.

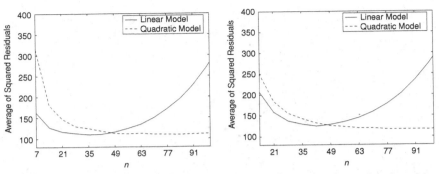

Figure 10.2. Average squared residuals for linear and quadratic models as a function of the amount of historical data – i.e., the size of the sliding baseline (n) – used to fit the regression models under Scenario 2. On the left are the results when there is no day effect in the data, and on the right, the data have day effects. From this, a linear model form for the adaptive regression, with an "optimal n" of about 30 days for no day effects and about 40 days with day effects, was chosen.

10.1.2 Determining the Cumulative Sum Parameters

To use the CUSUM EED method on the forecast errors of an adaptive regression, a number of choices need to be made. First, the form of the adaptive regression must be chosen (linear, quadratic, etc.), and the length of the sliding baseline (n) must be set. For the CUSUM, the reference value k must be chosen. How these choices were made are briefly discussed here. See Fricker *et al.* (2008a) for additional details.

All other factors being equal, adaptive regressions based on a shorter sliding baseline will less accurately estimate the underlying systematic trends in the data than those based on longer sliding baselines. However, although a longer sliding baseline should allow for a more detailed regression model and potentially a better prediction, often in biosurveillance the amount of available data are limited or the older data are of questionable relevance because of changing trends or phenomena. Hence, there is a trade-off to be made between the amount of historical data used in a particular model and the predictive accuracy of that model.

To assess this trade-off, for each of the 12 scenarios in Table 10.1, Dunfee and Hegler (2007) conducted detailed preliminary simulations to find the form of the adaptive regression that forecast best. Figure 10.2 is an example of how the form of the adaptive regression and size of the "optimal" sliding baseline for Scenario 2 ($c = 90$, $A = 80$, $\mu = 0$, $\sigma = 10$, with and without day-of-the-week effects) were determined. The optimal n was chosen by visual inspection with the criteria that the n be as small as possible but also as close to achieving the best forecast in terms of the minimum average squared residual.

Figure 10.2 shows that the linear model achieved almost the same minimum average squared residual as the quadratic model but with a smaller n. As described in Dunfee and Hegler (2007), this occurred consistently for all of the scenarios, leading them to choose a linear adaptive regression model in all of their evaluations. For the linear model, across all the scenarios without day-of-the-week effects, the optimal n values ranged from 15 to 40 days. For the scenarios with day-of-the-week effects, the optimal n values increased, with the largest being around 56 days – the size recommended by Burkom et al. (2006).

As discussed in Section 7.3, a common setting for the CUSUM reference value k is one-half the distance between the mean of the normal disease incidence and the level of incidence it is important to quickly detect. Here the CUSUM is not being applied to the raw data but rather to the standardized residuals from an adaptive regression, so the change in mean can be expressed in terms of some number of standard deviations increase in the standardized residuals. If a 1-standard deviation increase in the residuals is important to detect because there is also some effect of the length of the baseline (see Fricker et al. 2008a for details) for CUSUMs with larger sliding baselines (e.g., $30 \leq n \leq 60$), set $k = 1/2$; for the CUSUMs using a 7-day sliding baseline (designed to match the baseline used in the EARS methods), set $k = 0.65$.

10.1.3 Comparison Methodology

The usual metrics – ATFS, PSD, and CED – are used to compare performance. For each EED method and scenario in Table 10.1, the threshold for each method required to achieve an ATFS of 100 days was determined empirically. After the thresholds were set, the methods were then compared across all the scenarios specified in Table 10.1 for all the outbreak types just described.

The purpose of setting the thresholds to achieve equal time between false signals was to ensure a fair comparison among the methods. That is, it is always possible to improve a method's ability to detect an actual outbreak by lowering the threshold, but this comes at the expense of also decreasing the ATFS. Thus, by first setting the thresholds to achieve equal time between false alarms, it is then possible to make an objective judgement about which method is best at detecting a particular type of outbreak.

Across all the scenarios in Table 10.1, the CUSUM thresholds ranged from $h = 2.9$ to $h = 4.2$, including all combinations of c, A, μ, and σ and with and without day-of-the-week effects. For the EARS methods, across all of the scenarios in Table 10.1, the thresholds for C1: $2.7 \leq h \leq 8.2$; for C2: $2.6 \leq h \leq 7.4$; and for C3: $3.0 \leq h \leq 18.2$.

Having set the thresholds to achieve equal ATFS performance, the CED and PSD were calculated as follows. For each iteration i, the methods were run for 100 time periods (using data from $100 + n$ time periods so that the adaptive regression could be fit for period 1) without any outbreaks. If a method signaled during this time, it was reset and restarted, just as it would be in a real application. This allowed the CUSUM statistics to be in a steady-state condition at the time of the outbreak. Outbreaks began at time 101 and continued for the appropriate duration. If the method signaled at time t_i within the duration of the outbreak, the time to first outbreak signal was recorded as $t_i - 100$, and the steady-state CED was estimated as $\sum_{i=1}^{s}(t_i - 100)/s$ for the s iterations that signaled within the outbreak duration. The PSD was calculated as the number of iterations for which the method signaled during the outbreak divided by the total number of iterations run.

10.1.4 Results

Figure 10.3, in many ways, summarizes the results of all the evaluations conducted by Dunfee and Hegler (2007). In it, the plots on the left side show the CED versus various outbreak durations (D) for Scenario 2 starting with a small outbreak at the top ($M = 9$), a medium outbreak in the middle ($M = 22.5$), and a large outbreak at the bottom ($M = 45$). The plots on the right side show the PSD of an outbreak versus outbreak duration. Each plot gives the results for six methods, the C1, C2, and C3, as well as three CUSUMs using various sliding baseline lengths: 7, 15 (the "optimal" for Scenario 2), and 56 days.

Figure 10.3 shows that the C1, C2, and C3 methods do not perform as well as the CUSUM methods with the larger sliding baselines. Focusing for a moment just on the C1, C2, and C3 methods, note that the C1 and C2 methods perform somewhat similarly, with the C1 generally having a slightly lower CED than the C2 but at the expense of having a slightly lower PSD as well. However, when comparing the C1 and C2 with the CUSUMs, note that they all have similar CED performance but the CUSUMs with longer sliding baselines have much higher PSDs. This difference in performance is evident for all the outbreak magnitudes but is most striking with the larger magnitude outbreaks. For example, in the middle row of plots, the C1 and C2 CED can be up to a day or so shorter than the longer sliding baseline CUSUMs, but they only catch between about 20 to 30 percent of the outbreaks, but the 56-day sliding baseline CUSUM catches nearly 80 percent of the outbreaks of the longest duration. For this scenario, it is clear that the CUSUM with a 56-day sliding baseline is the preferred method.

A note about the CED plots is in order for those used to looking at graphs of average run lengths in the statistical process control (SPC) literature. Such readers may be surprised that the CED curves increase as outbreak duration increases. Remember in the biosurveillance problem that the time to first outbreak signal is constrained to the interval $[1, D]$. That is, the earliest a "true signal" can occur is on the first day of the outbreak and the latest is on the last day of the outbreak (D). Thus, for $D = 3$, the CED is constrained to be between 1 and 3 and, as shown in the plot, is about 2 for all the methods. On the other hand, for $D = 15$, the CED can be much larger and, in fact, falls anywhere from about 3.5 days to about 6.5 days for the various methods.

Also in Figure 10.3, the C1 and the CUSUM with a 7-day sliding baseline suffer from being contaminated by the outbreak data in the largest magnitude outbreak scenarios. That is, in the lower right plot, the PSD for these two methods actually *decreases* for longer duration outbreaks (as eventually do the C2 and C3, as well

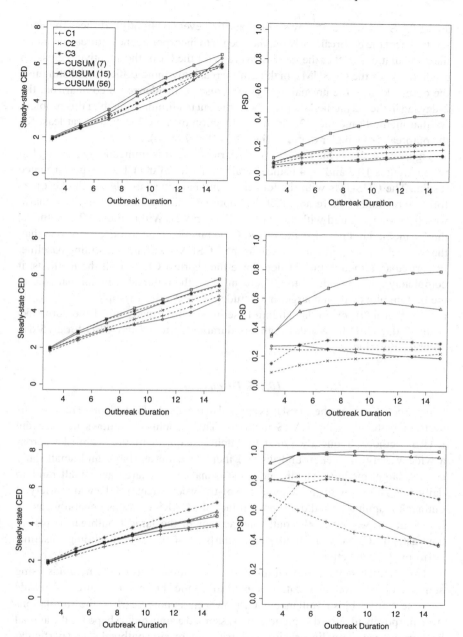

Figure 10.3. CED and PSD performance of the methods for Scenario 2 for three magnitudes of outbreaks – $M = 9$, $M = 22.5$, and $M = 45$, shown from top to bottom – versus various outbreak durations.

as the CUSUM with a 15-day sliding baseline ever so slightly). If these methods fail to detect the outbreak early on, they begin to incorporate the outbreak data into their calculations (either the moving average for the C1 or the adaptive regression predictions for the CUSUM), making it increasingly more difficult to distinguish the outbreak from the normal background disease incidence. In comparison, the 2-day lag in the C2 method seems to be sufficient to eliminate much of this problem for that method (and the C3 which is a function of the C2 statistics), at least for the outbreaks of smaller duration (i.e., $3 \leq D \leq 7$ or so).

Figure 10.4 shows the results for Scenario 7. What is immediately striking between Figures 10.3 and 10.4 is the overall similarity of the CUSUM performance results. The CUSUMs with the longer sliding baselines are clearly the best performing methods (where note that the "optimal" sliding baseline in this scenario was 30 days compared with 15 days for Scenario 2). Within the EARS methods, the C1 method not only has the lowest CED but also misses more outbreaks than the C2, and neither performs as well as the CUSUMs with longer sliding baseline. In particular, although the C1 does have the shortest CED of all the methods, it completely misses from 85 to 90 percent of all the outbreaks. In comparison, in the bottom plots with the larger magnitude outbreaks, for example, the CUSUMs using either a 30- or 56-day sliding baseline catch virtually all of the outbreaks with a 2-day CED for a 3-day outbreak duration up to a 4-day CED for a 15-day outbreak duration.

10.1.5 Discussion

In these comparisons, the CUSUMs applied to the residuals of adaptive regressions perform better than the EARS methods. This conclusion follows because the EARS methods frequently failed to catch a majority of the outbreaks across a wide variety of background disease incident patterns (large and small daily counts; large, medium, small, and no seasonal cycles; large and small random daily fluctuations; with and without day-of-the-week effects) and a wide variety of outbreak magnitudes and durations. In fact, the EARS methods generally caught less than 30 percent of the outbreaks except in the largest outbreak cases. In contrast, the CUSUM methods, particularly with the 8-week sliding baseline, performed much better.

These conclusions are based on extensive comparisons of the methods using simulated biosurveillance data designed to mimic the major features of a wide cross section of biosurveillance data. However, as noted earlier, the simulations were purposely idealized depictions that assumed a sinusoidal shape for the annual background variation, linearly increasing and decreasing outbreaks, and particular error term distributions. In addition, these analyses used a fixed ATFS of 100 days, which is a reasonable false alarm rate for a biosurveillance system, and a particular choice for the CUSUM reference interval parameter k. However, confirmation of whether these results hold more generally under other conditions requires further research.

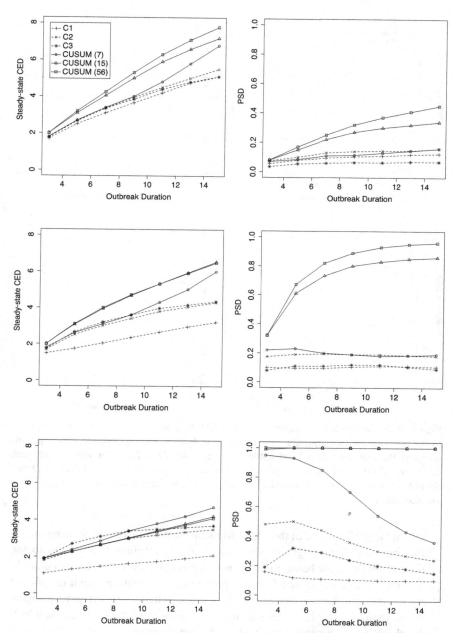

Figure 10.4. Performance of the methods for Scenario 7 for three magnitudes of outbreaks – $M = 4$, $M = 8$, and $M = 16$, shown from top to bottom – versus various outbreak durations.

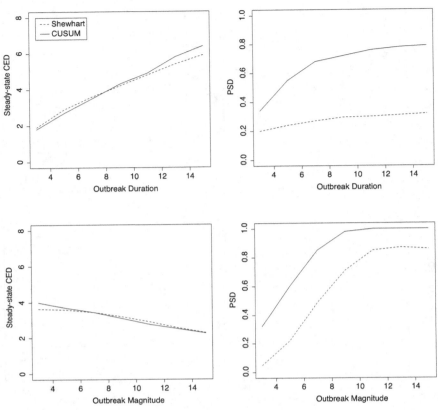

Figure 10.5. Performance comparison of the CUSUM versus Shewhart method applied to the residuals of an adaptive regression with an 8-week sliding baseline. The top plots compare the methods for a fixed outbreak magnitude ($M = 22.5$) for varying outbreak durations. The bottom plots compare the methods for a fixed outbreak duration ($D = 7$ days) for various outbreak magnitudes. The background disease incidence was generated via Scenario 2.

Given the performance of the CUSUM methods, particularly those using longer sliding baselines, one might be tempted to simply attribute the success to the additional information being used in the adaptive regressions. This is certainly part of the reason, but some additional preliminary simulations seem to indicate that is not the complete answer. Specifically, it seems that Shewhart and Shewhart-based methods may be less well suited for the biosurveillance problem in which outbreaks do not occur instantaneously and are transient.

For example, Figure 10.5 compares the performance of a CUSUM method and a Shewhart method, both applied to the residuals from an adaptive regression with a 56-day sliding baseline. Each day, the Shewhart method compares the standardized residual from the adaptive regression for that day with a threshold (chosen so that the ATFS is 100 days, the same as with the CUSUM). In Figure 10.5, the top plots compare the methods for a fixed outbreak magnitude ($M = 22.5$) for varying outbreak durations. The bottom plots compare the methods for a fixed outbreak duration ($D = 7$ days) for various outbreak magnitudes. The background disease incidence was generated via Scenario 2.

The top plots show that the CED is roughly equal between the two methods, with the Shewhart seeming to have a slight advantage for outbreaks of short duration and the CUSUM for outbreaks with long durations. This is consistent with the literature on the performance of these two methods in industrial SPC applications. However, the upper right plot shows that the Shewhart is much poorer at actually catching outbreaks than the CUSUM.

In the bottom two plots, the magnitude is varied rather than the outbreak duration. That is, the duration is fixed at $D = 7$ days, and then the performance of the two methods is compared as M varied from 10 to 70. In terms of CED, the Shewhart does slightly better than the CUSUM for smaller outbreaks and slightly worse for larger outbreaks. But again, it does significantly poorer in terms of PSD. From this, a conjecture is that the poorer performance of the EARS methods *may be* due both to the additional data used in the CUSUMs with the longer sliding baselines *and* to the Shewhart-like design of the C1 and C2 methods.

In summary, the CUSUM applied to residuals from an appropriately employed adaptive regression model with an 8-week sliding baseline outperformed the EARS methods in all the scenarios Dunfee and Hegler (2007) evaluated. These scenarios were chosen to mimic the major features of biosurveillance data over a wide variety of conditions. For standard biosurveillance systems using the EARS methods, this suggests biosurveillance systems may benefit from replacing the EARS methods with CUSUM methods and from setting the CUSUM thresholds appropriately to minimize the false alarm burden as much as appropriate.

Of course, the EARS methods were originally designed for a drop-in surveillance system with little or no baseline data available. In these situations, the use of an 8-week sliding baseline may be impossible, at least upon initiation of the drop-in system. However, the simulations show that a CUSUM with a 7-day sliding baseline performs about the same as the EARS methods, and as the length of the sliding baseline increases, the performance of the CUSUM quickly improves. This suggests a strategy for drop-in surveillance systems of starting with a CUSUM with a 7-day sliding baseline and, as time progresses and more data accumulate, allowing the baseline to increase until such time as enough data are accumulated so that baseline can be allowed to slide.

10.2 Performance Comparisons: A Multivariate Example

As with the previous section, this section illustrates how to conduct simulation comparisons between the multivariate EED methods presented in Chapter 8, specifically the MCUSUM and the MEWMA. In so doing, it brings together many concepts discussed in previous chapters, such as simulating biosurveillance data from Appendix B and adaptive regression from Chapter 5, as well as the multivariate methods from Chapter 8.

10.2.1 Simulating Multivariate Biosurveillance Data

To begin, using scenarios similar to those in Table 10.1, the MTM1 (see page 354) is used to simulate background disease incidence data for a biosurveillance system monitoring the GI syndrome from five hospitals. As with the univariate comparisons in the previous section, the goal is to assess how the multivariate methods perform over a range of outbreak magnitudes and durations.

To simulate the background data for Scenario 4, the parameters used in Equation B.8 are:

- $\mu = \{90, 90, 90, 90, 90\}$;
- $\gamma_t = \{\gamma_{t1}, \gamma_{t2}, \gamma_{t3}, \gamma_{t4}, \gamma_{t5}\}$;
- $\theta_t = \{0, 0, 0, 0, 0\}$; and
- $Z_t \sim N_5(0, \sigma^2 I)$, with $\sigma = 10$.

In this simulation day-of-the-week effects (δ) were omitted and $\gamma_{tj} = 20[\sin(2\pi(t + \tau_j)/365)]$ with $\tau_j \sim U(-30, 30)$ for $j = 1, \ldots, 5$. More realistic simulations would likely use μ and γ levels that vary among the hospitals, and they could incorporate day-of-the-week effects and other model terms, but the purpose here is to illustrate how to conduct a performance comparison under some relatively simple conditions. Given this background disease incidence, outbreaks (o) were simulated using Equation B.5 with $M = 5, 10$, and 20, and $D = 3, 4, \ldots, 14$, and 15 days.

10.2.2 Determining the MEWMA and MCUSUM Parameters

As discussed with the univariate methods, to use the MCUSUM and MEWMA EED methods on the forecast errors of an adaptive regression, a number of choices need to be made. Just like before, the form of the adaptive regression must be chosen (linear, quadratic, etc.), and the length of the sliding baseline (n) must be set. For the MCUSUM, the reference value k must be chosen, and for the MEWMA, the smoothing parameter λ must be chosen. How these choices were made is briefly discussed here. See Fricker *et al.* (2008b) for additional details.

In the standard statistical process control setting, it is well known that the standard univariate EWMA can be designed (through the appropriate choice of λ) to perform very similarly to the CUSUM. Furthermore, the way to choose the reference value k in the univariate CUSUM follows directly from its derivation, but the choice for k in Crosier's MCUSUM is not clear.

Very little research into these issues has been conducted in a biosurveillance context. Indeed, the literature only contains one attempt to address these questions, where Fricker *et al.* (2008b) found that (for $p = 4$) the MCUSUM detection

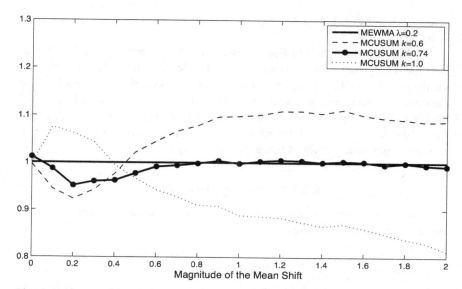

Figure 10.6. Comparison of the MCUSUM for various k to the MEWMA with $\lambda = 0.2$ in terms of the percent change from the MEWMA ATFS. The MCUSUM with $k = 0.74$ came closest to matching the MEWMA's performance over a wide range of mean shifts.

method with $k = 0.74$ performed very similarly to the MEWMA detection method with $\lambda = 0.2$.

Figure 10.6 shows the results they obtained where, to simplify their analysis, the evaluation was conducted using the standard statistical process control assumptions of *iid* observations and a sustained jump change in the mean. Then, comparing how well the MCUSUM detected the various sustained mean shifts for a four-dimensional standard multivariate normal, Figure 10.6 shows that $k = 0.74$ gives the closest performance to the MEWMA with $\lambda = 0.2$.

That is, Figure 10.6 shows the percent change in the ATFS for the MCUSUM for various k compared with the MEWMA. The plot shows that the MCUSUMs with $k < 0.74$ signal faster than the MEWMA for small mean shifts and signal slower as the mean shift increases. Conversely, as k increases from 0.74, the MCUSUM begins to signal slower than the MEWMA for small shifts and much faster as the mean shift increases. The MCUSUM with $k = 0.74$ has the closest performance over a wide range of shifts: it achieves almost precisely the same ATFS for shifts between about 0.6 and 2.0 and is at most about 5 percent off over the entire range of shifts considered, from 0 to 2.0.

Thus, for the purposes of these simulation comparisons, for the MEWMA, $\lambda = 0.2$ was used, and for the MCUSUM, $k = 0.7$ was used. In terms of setting thresholds, quantile-quantile plots of the residuals confirmed that they are reasonably normally distributed. Thus, the tables in Appendix C can be used to set the thresholds so that each detection method will achieve an ATFS of 100 days. From the tables for $p = 5$, the MCUSUM detection method with $k = 0.8$ for $h = 5$

gives ATFS = 103.1. For the MEWMA detection method with $\lambda = 0.2$ for $h = 12$ gives ATFS = 98.

Finally, the form of the adaptive regression and the optimal length of the sliding baseline was evaluated, much as was done by Dunfee and Hegler (2007) with very similar results. The linear form had smaller sliding baselines that achieved almost the same minimum average squared residuals. And for the linear model, across all the scenarios, the optimal ns ranged from 30 to 45 days. For other scenarios with day-of-the-week effects, not described here (see Fricker et al., 2008), the optimal ns were larger with the largest being around 56 days.

10.2.3 Comparison Methodology

The multivariate comparisons in this section were conducted the same way as the univariate methods in the previous section.

10.2.4 Results

Figures 10.7 and 10.8 summarize the main findings: the MEWMA and MCUSUM performed virtually identically, in terms of both CED and PSD, across all the scenario and outbreak combinations evaluated. Although the lines deviate slightly in Figures 10.7 and 10.8, the differences are not statistically significant. Thus, it seems that, just like for the univariate methods in the classical SPC situation, with an appropriate choice of parameters, the MCUSUM and MEWMA EED methods can be made to perform virtually identically for biosurveillance.

Specifically, the plots in Figure 10.7 show that there is no difference in MCUSUM and MEWMA performance for Scenario 4 across all the types of outbreaks, from small to large magnitudes and for all the durations. This result was also true for the other scenarios. For example, Figure 10.8 shows the results for Scenarios 1, 3, and 5 for an outbreak of medium magnitude. See Knitt and Hu (2007) for plots for all of the scenarios and types of outbreaks.

Figure 10.7 demonstrates how the procedures perform for the various types of outbreaks. For example, the CED plots show that outbreaks of small magnitude and of 3 days of duration will only be detected about 30 percent of the time and, when detected, it will take about 2 days on average for either the MCUSUM or MEWMA to signal. As the outbreak magnitude increases, the procedures detect virtually all of the outbreaks, and the CED decreases to about 1 day for the largest magnitude outbreak. In comparison, for durations of 15 days, the methods detect almost 70 percent of the small-magnitude outbreaks and again virtually all of the larger outbreaks. For the small-magnitude outbreaks, the average time to signal is about 6 days; for the medium magnitude, it is just under 5 days; and for the large-magnitude outbreak, it is about 2-1/2 days.

Furthermore, Figure 10.8 demonstrates that the adaptive regression with sliding baseline methodology does very well at removing the systematic component, at least for this synthetic biosurveillance data. Here the systematic component is the

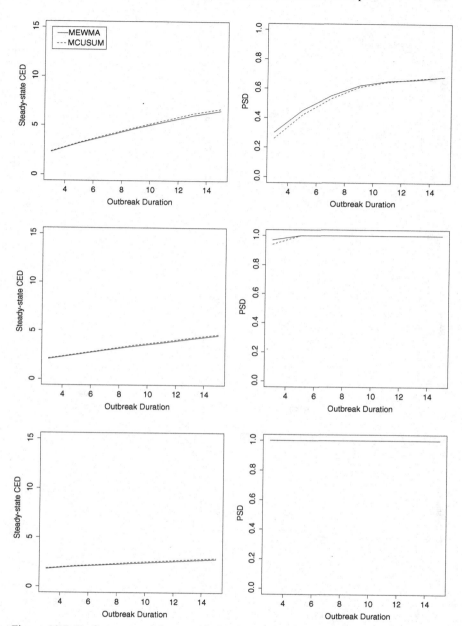

Figure 10.7. Performance of the MCUSUM and MEWMA under Scenario 4 for three magnitudes of outbreaks – $M = 9$, $M = 22.5$, and $M = 45$, shown from top to bottom – versus various outbreak durations.

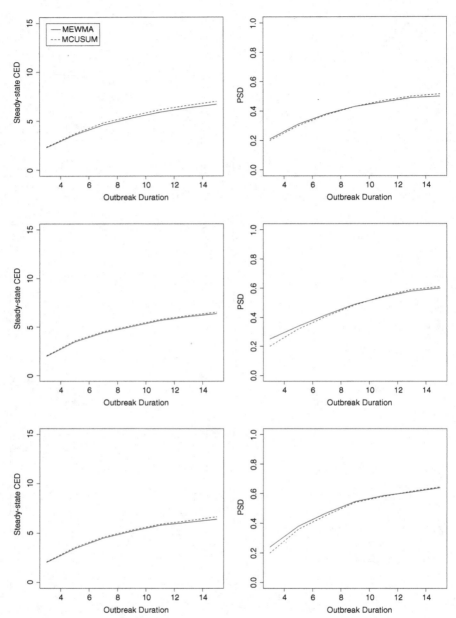

Figure 10.8. Performance of the MEWMA and MCUSUM for $m = 90$, $\sigma = 30$, and $M = 22.5$ for three magnitudes of amplitude – $A = 90$, $A = 20$, and $A = 0$, shown from top to bottom – versus various outbreak durations for $M = 22.5$.

seasonal sinusoid where at the top the sinusoid is large ($A = 90$); in the middle, it is medium sized ($A = 20$); and at the bottom, it is nonexistent ($A = 0$). In terms of CED, there is no visible difference between the three plots in Figure 10.8. In terms of percent of outbreaks missed, there is a slight degradation in the number of outbreaks caught as the amplitude increases. However, these plots demonstrate that overall, the adaptive regression is quite effective at accounting for the systematic trends in the data.

10.3 Discussion and Summary

Because the performance of most proposed methods is demonstrated on data that are not publicly available, it is very difficult and often impossible to compare the performance of the various detection methods across the biosurveillance literature. This is often driven by the public health community's desire to see methods demonstrated on real data. Yet precisely because the data are real, there is a lack of general availability of such data to the research community because of confidentiality and privacy concerns.

One solution is to make real data more widely available. Shmueli & Burkom (2010) say, "Currently syndromic data are only available to researchers affiliated with a particular biosurveillance system or research group, for reasons of data confidentiality and non-disclosure agreements. This a major obstacle in the way of scientific progress in both temporal and spatio-temporal biosurveillance, and hopefully some data will be made available to academic researchers."

However, seemingly unrecognized in this discussion is the fact that all real data are simply one realization of a stochastic process. When focusing only on a particular stream of data, one fails to recognize and account for the full randomness of the underlying phenomenon, which is a process involving the interaction of very complicated population and disease transmission dynamics.

In addition, even if some real data are made available, they will provide little to no information about what outbreaks look like, particularly those associated with bioterrorism-related events. The challenge, as Rolka *et al.* (2007) have said, ". . . is to develop improved methods for evaluating detection algorithms in light of the fact that we have little data about outbreaks of many potential diseases that are of concern."

Simulation is an alternative. Of course, it is very difficult to (stochastically) characterize, and thus simulate, all the detailed features characteristic of the normal or baseline state of disease incidence, as well as the various outbreak conditions. However, one could also make similar statements about industrial quality control problems. Yet that field, over time, has come to use various data abstraction conventions that facilitate simulation and, as a result, allow comparisons among methods and across the literature. As Rolka *et al.* (2005) say, "Reliance on the use of Monte Carlo simulation in the field of Statistics is well known. It has been this author's experience that the technique is undervalued in the field of Public Health because it has previously not been required."

As this chapter has demonstrated, simulation can be useful in evaluating the performance of EED methods, particularly their relative performance. In addition, simulation is useful for:

- evaluating methods across many scenarios;
- eliminating unnecessary or distracting real-world complexities;
- allowing clean and clear comparisons of methods; and
- making it easier to get at generalizable conclusions and results.

Part V

Appendices

A

A Brief Review of Probability, Random Variables, and Some Important Distributions

A pinch of probability is worth a pound of perhaps.
James Thurber (1984–1961)

Much of this text assumes a working knowledge of probability, sometimes at a fairly advanced understanding and insight, and a basic facility with the mathematics of probability. For those who may require a refresher, this appendix provides a brief review of probability, including:

- Rules for calculating the probability of various simple and compound events;
- Conditional probability and independence of events;
- Random variables, including the concepts of expected value and variance;
- Important discrete and continuous probability distributions; and
- Sampling distributions, standard errors, and the Central Limit Theorem.

Why is probability important to biosurveillance? As the rest of the text hopefully makes clear, disease is stochastic, which means that the transmission and progression of a disease or an outbreak through a population is subject to chance: the chance encounters of people; the chance transmission of disease between people (and perhaps animals); the chance progression of disease within a person; and the chance treatment of disease, including whether and how any particular individual seeks treatment (or not). All of these effects and more mean that the data observed in any biosurveillance system is the product of chance and thus must be addressed using the tools of probability.

Probability is particularly critical to the design and implementation of effective early event detection (EED) algorithms. Good implementation requires methods tailored to the probabilistic behavior of the statistics being monitored, and the EED methods require metrics from which to judge performance that account for the stochastic nature of the data. Furthermore, good EED method evaluation requires that one recognize that any particular observed set of data arises as a result of a stochastic process and thus it is generally insufficient to evaluate EED performance against any one longitudinal data set. Such an evaluation will almost certainly fail to capture all the variation that will occur in actual application.

This appendix begins by defining probability from a frequency point of view. It proceeds to develop and illustrate the basic rules for calculating the probability of various types of events. It then develops the notion of the random variable and introduces a number of discrete and continuous distributions used throughout the text. It concludes with a discussion of some important advanced concepts including sampling distributions and the Central Limit Theorem. For those who need additional refresher or who want to go beyond the material presented in this appendix, the Additional Reading section at the end provides further resources.

Mathematical Notation

A, B	Events
A^C	Complement of event A
Bin(n, p)	Binomial distribution with parameters n and p
Cov(X, Y)	Covariance of random variables X and Y
e	Euler's constant, $e = 2.71828\ldots$
$\mathbb{E}(Y)$	Expected value of random variable Y
$f_y(y)$	Probability density function (pdf) of Y evaluated at y
F	F distribution (with parameters m and n)
$F_y(y)$	Cumulative distribution function (cdf) of Y evaluated at y
n	Sample size
$N(A)$	Number of A events in the sample space
Nbin(r, p)	Negative binomial distribution with parameters r and p
$N(\mu, \sigma^2)$	Normal distribution with mean μ and variance σ^2
$\mathbb{P}(A)$	Probability of event A
Pois(λ)	Poisson distribution with parameter λ
$s.e.$	Standard error
t	t-distribution (with $n-1$ degrees of freedom)
U(a, b)	Uniform distribution on the interval a to b
Var(Y)	Variance of random variable Y
$x!$	Factorial function evaluated at integer x, which is $x \cdot (x-1) \cdot (x-2) \ldots 3 \cdot 2 \cdot 1$
Y	Random variable (single observation)
Y	Random variable vector (k observations)
y	Observed value of random variable Y
y	Vector of observed value of Y
Z	Observation from a standard normal distribution
χ_n^2	Chi-square distribution with parameter n
$\in$	Mathematical operator that means "is an element of"
$\Gamma(y)$	Gamma function evaluated at y, which is $(y-1)!$
∞	Infinity
μ, σ	Parameters of a normal distribution
Ω	Sample space
ρ	Correlation
$\sum$	Summation sign, variance-covariance matrix
$[a, b]$	Interval from a to b, inclusive
$\cap$	Intersection operator
$\cup$	Union operator

A.1 Probability

A *sample space*, often denoted by the Greek capital letter Ω, is a list of all possible outcomes of an event or an experiment. An *event* is one particular outcome in the sample space. For example, the sample space for one flip of a two-sided coin is the set consisting of "heads" and "tails." Mathematically, $\Omega = \{\text{heads, tails}\}$, or more succinctly, $\Omega = \{H, T\}$, where "H" stands for the event of the coin coming up heads. For the roll of one six-sided die, Ω would be the set of integers between 1 and 6, inclusive, so $\Omega = \{1, 2, 3, 4, 5, 6\}$. For a continuous measurement that could take on positive values only, say the weight of a person picked at random, then the sample space might be the positive, nonzero part of the real line: $\Omega = (0, \infty]$.

A *probability measure* on the sample space Ω is a function $\mathbb{P}$ from subsets of Ω to the real numbers that satisfy the following axioms. The notation $\mathbb{P}(A)$ stands for "the probability that event A occurs."

Probability Axioms

1. For each event $A \in \Omega$, $0 \leq \mathbb{P}(A) \leq 1$.
2. $\mathbb{P}(\Omega) = 1$.
3. If two events A and B are *disjoint* then $\mathbb{P}(A \cup B) = \mathbb{P}(A) + \mathbb{P}(B)$.

The first axiom says that probability of each event in the sample space occurring must be between 0 and 1 (inclusive). The second axiom says that the total probability in the sample space is equal to 1. The third axiom says that the probability of one of two events occurring that do not have anything in common is the sum of the probabilities of the two individual events. More about this axiom shortly.

Under the assumption that every event in Ω is equally likely to occur, the probability that one of the events occurs is defined as the number of that type of event in Ω divided by the total number of events in Ω. Using the notation $N(A)$ to mean "the number of events of type A in Ω," then

$$\mathbb{P}(A) = \frac{N(A)}{\text{total number of outcomes in } \Omega}. \tag{A.1}$$

So, for example, for a "fair" coin, the probability of getting heads is one-half because $N(H) = 1$ and there are a total of two events in Ω. On the other hand, the probability of getting heads on a two-headed coin is 1 (i.e., the coin is guaranteed to come up heads), because $N(H) = 2$. Of course, this is an idealized model of coin flipping because the event "the coin lands on its side" is not in the sample space.

A.1.1 Some Basic Rules for Calculating Probabilities

Union of Disjoint Events

Axiom 3 defines a rule for calculating the probability of the union of two disjoint events. *Union* means together, so the probability of the union of two events A and

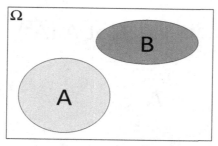

Figure A.1. A simple Venn diagram representing two *disjoint* events, A and B.

B means the probability that either A or B occurs. It is written as $A \cup B$. *Disjoint* means that A and B cannot happen at the same time.

In the Venn diagram of Figure A.1, the box represents the entire sample space, and the circles are the events A and B. The box has a total area of 1, corresponding to the probability that something in the sample space must happen (Axiom 2), and the size of the circles correspond to $\mathbb{P}(A)$ and $\mathbb{P}(B)$. Since the events are disjoint, the circles do not overlap, and because they do not overlap, the probability of $A \cup B$ occurring is simply the probability that A occurs plus the probability that B occurs:

$$\mathbb{P}(A \cup B) = \mathbb{P}(A) + \mathbb{P}(B). \qquad (A.2)$$

This is sometimes referred to as the *addition rule*. A single role of a six-sided die provides a simple example to illustrate this rule. To determine the probability of rolling either a 1 or a 2, since the event "roll a 1" is disjoint from the event "roll a 2" (they cannot both happen at the same time):

$$\mathbb{P}(\text{"roll a 1 or roll a 2"}) = \mathbb{P}(\text{"roll a 1"} \cup \text{"roll a 2"})$$
$$= \mathbb{P}(\text{"roll a 1"}) + \mathbb{P}(\text{"roll a 2"})$$
$$= 1/6 + 1/6 = 1/3.$$

Note that this rule applies for any number of disjoint events, not just two. For example, the addition rule can be used to determine the probability of rolling a 1, 2, or 3 on the die. It is

$$\mathbb{P}(\text{"roll a 1, 2, or 3"}) = \mathbb{P}(\text{"roll a 1 or 2"} \cup \text{"roll a 3"})$$
$$= \mathbb{P}(\text{"roll a 1 or 2"}) + \mathbb{P}(\text{"roll a 3"})$$
$$= \mathbb{P}(\text{"roll a 1"} \cup \text{"roll a 2"}) + \mathbb{P}(\text{"roll a 3"})$$
$$= \mathbb{P}(\text{"roll a 1"}) + \mathbb{P}(\text{"roll a 2"}) + \mathbb{P}(\text{"roll a 3"})$$
$$= 1/6 + 1/6 + 1/6 = 1/2.$$

Complementary Events

Using the axioms, additional useful rules for calculating probabilities can be defined. For example, consider an event A for which it is easy to calculate $\mathbb{P}(A)$,

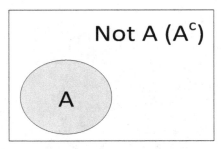

Figure A.2. A Venn diagram representing an event A and its complement "not A."

but perhaps what is of interest is calculating the probability that anything other than A happens. In other words, the event of interest is "not A," which is denoted A^c for the complement of A. Rather than calculating $\mathbb{P}(A^c)$ directly from the other events in the sample space, if $\mathbb{P}(A)$ is easy to calculate, then the rule $\mathbb{P}(\text{not } A) = \mathbb{P}(A^c) = 1 - \mathbb{P}(A)$ makes it easy to also calculate the complement of event A.

This rule follows directly from Axioms 1 and 2, and it is visually evident in the Venn diagram of Figure A.2. In the figure, the box represents Ω, and the circle is the event A. As before, the box has a total probability of 1, and the size of the circle corresponds to $\mathbb{P}(A)$, so it should be clear that $\mathbb{P}(A^c) + \mathbb{P}(A) = 1$, from which it follows that $\mathbb{P}(A^c) = 1 - \mathbb{P}(A)$.

A simple example illustrates the utility of this rule. Consider the problem of calculating the probability of *not* throwing a 4 on one roll of a fair die. Since $\mathbb{P}(\text{"roll a 4"}) = 1/6$, it follows that $\mathbb{P}(\text{"not rolling a 4"}) = 1 - \mathbb{P}(\text{"roll a 4"}) = 1 - 1/6 = 5/6$. This is a fairly trivial example, but this rule can be very useful when calculating the probability of "not A" is hard.

For example, imagine you want to determine the chance of getting a 4 on at least one of three rolls of a fair die. That would be complicated to calculate directly (since there are $6^3 = 216$ events in the sample space). However, recognizing that the complement to this is the probability of getting no 4s on all three rolls of the die simplifies the problem. On one roll, the probability of not getting a 4 is 5/6. Using another concept (independent events) to be defined shortly, it turns out that not getting a 4 on three rolls is just $5/6 \times 5/6 \times 5/6$. So, the probability of getting a 4 on at least one of three rolls is $1 - (5/6)^3 = 0.42$.

To put this in a biosurveillance context, imagine that during an outbreak, the probability of successful detection (PSD) on any particular day using some early event detection algorithm is p. Assuming detection is independent between days and constant at p, then the probability of failing to detect the outbreak on any one day is $1 - p$, and the failure to detect the outbreak for k days is $(1 - p)^k$. Thus, the probability of successfully detecting the outbreak over all k days is $1 - (1 - p)^k$.

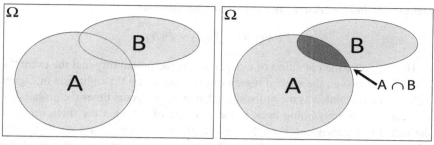

Figure A.3. Left side: The gray area in the Venn diagram is the union of two non-disjoint events, A and B: $A \cup B$. Right side: The dark gray area in the Venn diagram is the intersection of A and B: $A \cap B$.

Union of Events in General

There is a more general rule for events that may or may not be disjoint. The left Venn diagram of Figure A.3 illustrates the union of two events A and B that are not disjoint. The event "A and B" is the *intersection* of the two events, denoted $A \cap B$, and is depicted by the dark shaded region in the right Venn diagram of Figure A.3. Four possible events can now happen: A, B, "A and B," and "neither A nor B." The general rule for calculating $A \cup B$ is:

$$\mathbb{P}(A \cup B) = \mathbb{P}(A) + \mathbb{P}(B) - \mathbb{P}(A \cap B). \tag{A.3}$$

This rule says that, in general, the probability of the union of two events is the sum of their individual probabilities minus the probability of their intersection. The way to think about this is to see that the sum of their individual probabilities counts the intersection area twice, that area must be subtracted to make everything add up correctly.

Note that the previous rule for disjoint events is really a special case of the general rule. When events are disjoint, the probability of their intersection is zero (i.e., $\mathbb{P}(A \cap B) = 0$), so the expression in Equation A.3 simply reduces to the expression in Equation A.2. Also, note that the expression for the union of two events can be generalized to cases with more than two events.

Intersection of Independent Events

A very useful rule deals with the probability of the intersection of two independent events. Intuitively, two events are *independent* if knowing the outcome for one of the events provides no information about the outcome of the other event. For example, in two independent flips of a fair coin, knowing that a heads occurred on the first flip provides no information about what will happen on the second flip. Probabilistically, the condition that two events are independent is defined as follows.

Definition: *Independence.* *Two events are independent if*

$$\mathbb{P}(A \cap B) = \mathbb{P}(A) \times \mathbb{P}(B).$$

Hence, under the condition of independence, the probability that the event "*A* and *B*" occurs (i.e., the shaded region of the diagram on the right side of Figure A.3) can be calculated as the probability that event *A* occurs times the probability that event *B* occurs. Going back to the example of rolling a die three times, if the rolls are independent, then the probability of not getting a 4 on three rolls of the die is simply the probability of not getting a 4 on the first roll of the die times the probability of not getting a 4 on the second roll of the die times the probability of not getting a 4 on the third roll of the die: $5/6 \times 5/6 \times 5/6$.

A.1.2 Conditional Probability

If two events are *dependent*, then knowing the outcome of one event *does* provide information about the outcome of the other event. The notation is $\mathbb{P}(A \mid B)$, which is read "the probability of *A* given *B*," meaning the probability that *A* will occur given that *B* has occurred. Assuming $\mathbb{P}(B) \neq 0$, it is defined as

$$\mathbb{P}(A \mid B) = \frac{\mathbb{P}(A \cap B)}{\mathbb{P}(B)}. \tag{A.4}$$

The idea behind this definition is that, given the event *B* occurred, the relevant sample space becomes the events in *B* rather than Ω, and the relevant probability measure is now over *B*. Equation A.4 re-normalizes the probabilities from the entire sample space Ω to *B*, because it is now known that the event must be one of those in *B*.

Note that when *A* and *B* are independent, $\mathbb{P}(A \mid B) = \mathbb{P}(A)$. Why is this true? If *A* and *B* are independent, then $\mathbb{P}(A \cap B) = \mathbb{P}(A) \times \mathbb{P}(B)$, so substitute this result in Equation (A.4) to get the result. The interpretation, of course, is that if *A* and *B* are independent, then knowing what happened with event *B* provides no additional information about *A*.

A simple example to illustrate conditional probability is determining the probability of rolling a total of 4 on two dice. First imagine that two fair dice are rolled simultaneously so that their outcomes are independent. Then the probability of rolling a total of 4 is 3/36 (there are three ways to get a total of 4 out of 36 possible two-dice outcomes – write out the sample space if this is not obvious).

But now consider that it is known that the total of the two rolls is 4, and the question is to determine the probability that the first die came up a 2. Let *A* be the event that the first die shows a 2 and let *B* be the event that the total of the two dice is 4. Then the intersection of *A* and *B* has probability 1/36 (there is only one way to get a total of 4 with the first die showing a 2) and $\mathbb{P}(B) = 3/36$. So, $\mathbb{P}(A \mid B) = (1/36)/(3/36) = 1/3$.

To check this result, note that the event B consists of only three events from Ω: $\{1, 3\}$, $\{3, 1\}$, and $\{2, 2\}$. After the information is provided that B has occurred, the relevant probability calculation is then based on only these three possible outcomes. If the question is the probability that the first roll is a 2, then there is only one event out of three in B where that occurs, and thus the conditional probability is $1/3$.

Intersection of Events in General

Equation A.4 can be turned around to define a more general way to calculate the intersection of two events. Let A and B be events and assume $\mathbb{P}(B) \neq 0$. Then

$$\mathbb{P}(A \cap B) = \mathbb{P}(A \mid B)\mathbb{P}(B). \tag{A.5}$$

This is sometimes referred to as the *multiplication rule*.

Equation A.5 is often useful in finding the probabilities of intersections, such as the dark area in Figure A.3. For example, imagine a hat that contains the names of six people, four men and two women. Two names will be drawn at random from the hat, and the question is to determine the probability that two men's names are drawn. Let M_1 and M_2 denote the events of drawing a man's name on the first and second tries, respectively. From the multiplication rule, it follows that

$$\mathbb{P}(M_1 \cap M_2) = \mathbb{P}(M_1)\mathbb{P}(M_2 \mid M_1) = 4/6 \times 3/5 = 6/15.$$

If this is not obvious, write out all the possible unique pairs that can occur and then count how many of them consist of two men.

A.2 Random Variables

A *random variable* is a variable whose value is subject to variations due to chance (i.e., its value is *stochastic*). Compared with other mathematical variables that are typically fixed values (although perhaps unknown), a random variable by definition does not have a single, fixed value (even if unknown). Rather, a random variable can take on a set of possible different values (which may be finite or may be infinite). A random variable is either discrete, where it can take on any of a specified list of specific values, or continuous, where it can take on a value in an interval or a set of intervals.

For discrete random variables, the *probability mass function* (pmf) maps the possible values of a random variable to their associated probabilities. For example, let Y denote a discrete random variable that can take on one of two possible outcomes, y_0 and y_1. Then for some p, $0 \leq p \leq 1$, the probability mass function is:

$$\mathbb{P}(Y = y_i) = \begin{cases} p, & \text{if } i = 0 \\ 1 - p, & \text{if } i = 1. \end{cases} \tag{A.6}$$

Equation A.6 says that the probability random variable Y takes on the value y_0 is p, and the probability that Y takes on value y_1 is $1 - p$. Because, per probability Axiom 2, the total probability must add up to 1, this also implies that the probability that Y take on any value other than y_0 or y_1 is zero. In Equation A.6, Y is an example of a *Bernoulli random variable*. It is often the convention for a Bernoulli random variable to define $y_0 = 1$ and $y_1 = 0$.

Note the convention. Capital Roman letters are typically used to denote random variables, and small Roman letters are used to denote the values the random variable can take on. Thus, in Equation A.6, Y is a random variable whose value is not known. All that is known is that it can take on one of two values, y_0 or y_1.

To make this idea concrete, consider another random variable X that represents the outcome of a fair die. Prior to rolling the die, X can take on any one of six values: $i = 1, 2, 3, 4, 5,$ or 6. Then the probability mass function is

$$\mathbb{P}(X = i) = \begin{cases} 1/6, & \text{if } i = 1 \\ 1/6, & \text{if } i = 2 \\ 1/6, & \text{if } i = 3 \\ 1/6, & \text{if } i = 4 \\ 1/6, & \text{if } i = 5 \\ 1/6, & \text{if } i = 6. \end{cases} \tag{A.7}$$

From this, one can write probability statements such as $\mathbb{P}(X = 3) = 1/6$ to represent the statement "the probability of rolling a 3 with a fair, six-sided die is one-sixth." More generally, $\mathbb{P}(X = x)$ is the mathematical statement "the probability that random variable X takes on value x."

Continuous random variables have probability density functions. For a continuous random variable Y, the *probability density function* (pdf) is a non-negative function $f_Y(y)$ defined on the real line having the property that for any set A of real numbers

$$\mathbb{P}(Y \in A) = \int_A f_Y(y)dy. \tag{A.8}$$

The notation $f_Y(y)$ means that the probability density function f evaluated at the point y is for the random variable Y. When the random variable is understood, the notation can be abbreviated to $f(y)$.

Probability density functions must satisfy the property that

$$\mathbb{P}\{Y \in (-\infty, \infty)\} = \int_{-\infty}^{\infty} f(y)dy = 1 \tag{A.9}$$

and the probability that Y falls in some interval between two values a and b is

$$\mathbb{P}(a \le Y \le b) = \int_a^b f(y)dy. \tag{A.10}$$

Both discrete and continuous random variables have cumulative distribution functions. For random variable Y, the *cumulative distribution function* (cdf) is $F_Y(y) = \mathbb{P}(Y \leq y)$. That is, the cdf is a function that for every value y on the real line (i.e., for every $y \in \Re$), it gives the cumulative probability that Y is less than or equal to y. If Y is a discrete random variable, then the cdf is

$$F_Y(y) = \mathbb{P}(Y \leq y) = \sum_{y_i \leq y} \mathbb{P}(Y = y_i),$$

and if Y is a continuous random variable, then the cdf is

$$F_Y(y) = \mathbb{P}(Y \leq y) = \int_{-\infty}^{y} f_Y(y) dy.$$

A.2.1 Expected Value

The expected value of a random variable can be thought of as the average of a very large number (infinite, really) of observations of the random variable. Denote the expected value of a random variable Y as $\mathbb{E}(Y)$.

Calculation of the expected value of Y for discrete random variables is straight-forward: it is the sum of the products of each possible outcome times the probability of the outcome. That is, if Y can take on outcomes $y_1, y_2, y_3, \ldots$, then

$$\mathbb{E}(Y) = \sum_{i=1}^{\infty} y_i \mathbb{P}(Y = y_i). \qquad (A.11)$$

What is the expected value? Simply stated, it is the average value of a random variable. However, the word "average" here refers to a theoretical quantity that is different from the sample average defined in Chapter 4. Although it is useful intuition to think about the expected value as taking the average of a large number of observations, calculating an expected value does not require a sample of data like the calculation for the sample mean calculation does.

Returning to the Bernoulli random variable Y in Equation A.6, the expected value of Y in that case is

$$\mathbb{E}(Y) = \sum_{i=0}^{1} y_i \mathbb{P}(Y = y_i) = y_0 \times p + y_1 \times (1 - p) = y_1 + p(y_0 - y_1).$$

As previously mentioned, with Bernoulli random variables it is often the convention that $y_0 = 1$ and $y_1 = 0$. Using this convention, $\mathbb{E}(Y) = p$.

Similarly, calculating the expected value of Y in the die example of Equation A.7 is straightforward. It is simply the sum of each possible outcome (1, 2, 3, 4, 5, and 6) times their individual probabilities of occurrence which, in the case of a fair die, is always 1/6. That is:

$$\mathbb{E}(Y) = \sum_{i=1}^{6} i\,\mathbb{P}(X = i)$$

$$= \sum_{i=1}^{6} (i \times 1/6)$$

$$= 1/6 + 2/6 + 3/6 + 4/6 + 5/6 + 6/6 = 21/6 = 3.5.$$

The result: $\mathbb{E}(Y) = 3.5$, which can be interpreted as, if a fair die was rolled an infinite number of times, then the resulting average of all those rolls would be 3.5. Note that the expected value of Y is not an integer nor even one of the possible outcomes.

The expected value of Y for continuous random variables uses calculus to do the calculation analogous to the discrete case:

$$\mathbb{E}(Y) = \int_{-\infty}^{\infty} y f(y)\,dy.$$

The calculations for the continuous case will become clearer in the next section after specific pdfs are introduced.

A.2.2 Variance

The variability of a random variable is measured via its variance (and standard deviation). The general definition for the variance in Equation A.12 is a bit more complicated than the one for the expected value – in fact, it uses the expected value within it:

$$\text{Var}(Y) = \mathbb{E}\left([Y - \mathbb{E}(Y)]^2\right). \tag{A.12}$$

For a discrete random variable, substituting the definition of the expectation in the outermost expression gives:

$$\text{Var}(Y) = \sum_{i=1}^{\infty} (y_i - \mathbb{E}(Y))^2\,\mathbb{P}(Y = y_i). \tag{A.13}$$

Equation A.13 is not as complicated as it may first appear. Starting inside the left set of parentheses, the expression $y_i - \mathbb{E}(Y)$ is simply the difference between each possible value of the random variable and the random variable's expected value. It is simply how far each observation is from the expected value of Y. These differences are all then squared to make everything positive, multiplied by the probability that y_i occurs, and summed over all possible values of y_i.

So, the variance is just the average squared distance of a random variable from its expected value. The larger the variance, the more one should expect to see observations far from the expected value. The smaller the variance, the more such observations are likely to be closer the expected value and thus closer together.

Returning to Chapter 4 and the definition of the sample variance, the above description should seem very similar. That is because the sample variance is calculating the variance for a sample of data while this is calculating an equivalent quantity for a random variable.

Equations A.12 and A.13 are mathematically equivalent to

$$\text{Var}(Y) = \mathbb{E}(Y^2) - (\mathbb{E}(Y))^2, \tag{A.14}$$

which is sometimes easier to use to calculate the variance. For example, using Equation A.14, the variance of the Bernoulli random variable Y in Equation A.6 is calculated as follows. First,

$$\mathbb{E}(Y^2) = \sum_{i=0}^{1} y_i^2 \mathbb{P}(Y = y_i)$$

$$= y_0^2 \times p + y_1^2 \times (1 - p) = y_1^2 + p(y_0^2 - y_1^2).$$

Then,

$$\begin{aligned}
\text{Var}(Y) &= \mathbb{E}(Y^2) - (\mathbb{E}(Y))^2 \\
&= y_1^2 + p(y_0^2 - y_1^2) - [y_1 + p(y_0 - y_1)]^2 \\
&= y_1^2 + p(y_0^2 - y_1^2) - y_1^2 - 2py_1(y_0 - y_1) - p^2(y_0 - y_1)^2 \\
&= p(y_0^2 - y_1^2) - 2py_1(y_0 - y_1) - p^2(y_0 - y_1)^2 \\
&= p(y_0 - y_1)^2 - p^2(y_0 - y_1)^2 \\
&= p(1 - p)(y_0 - y_1)^2.
\end{aligned}$$

Using the convention that $y_0 = 1$ and $y_1 = 0$, the variance of a Bernoulli random variable Y is $\text{Var}(Y) = p(1 - p)$.

To give a numeric example, the variance of Y in the die example of Equation A.7 is calculated as follows.

$$\mathbb{E}(Y^2) = \sum_{i=1}^{6} i^2 \mathbb{P}(Y = i)$$

$$= 1^2/6 + 2^2/6 + 3^2/6 + 4^2/6 + 5^2/6 + 6^2/6 = 91/6.$$

Then,

$$\begin{aligned}
\text{Var}(Y) &= \mathbb{E}(Y^2) - (\mathbb{E}(Y))^2 \\
&= 91/6 - (21/6)^2 \\
&= 546/36 - 441/36 = 105/36 \approx 2.92.
\end{aligned}$$

For a continuous random variable, the variance is calculated as

$$\begin{aligned}
\text{Var}(Y) &= \mathbb{E}[Y - \mathbb{E}(Y)]^2 \\
&= \mathbb{E}(Y^2) - [\mathbb{E}(Y)]^2 \\
&= \int_{-\infty}^{\infty} y^2 f(y) dy - \left(\int_{-\infty}^{\infty} y f(y) dy \right)^2.
\end{aligned}$$

As with sample statistics, the standard deviation of a random variable is simply the square root of the variance. For example, in the die example, the standard deviation is $\sqrt{2.92} = 1.71$.

A.2.3 Covariance and Correlation

The sample covariance is defined in Equation 4.11 in Chapter 4. The equivalent concept for random variables is

$$\text{Cov}(X, Y) = \mathbb{E}[(X - \mathbb{E}(X))(Y - \mathbb{E}(Y))]. \qquad (A.15)$$

A mathematically equivalent expression to Equation A.15 is

$$\text{Cov}(X, Y) = \mathbb{E}(XY) - \mathbb{E}(X)\mathbb{E}(Y).$$

For any two random variables X and Y,

$$\text{Var}(X + Y) = \text{Var}(X) + \text{Var}(Y) + 2\text{Cov}(X, Y),$$

and

$$\text{Var}(X - Y) = \text{Var}(X) + \text{Var}(Y) - 2\text{Cov}(X, Y). \qquad (A.16)$$

However, if X and Y are independent, then $\text{Cov}(X, Y) = 0$.

Covariance is a measure of both the strength and direction of the *linear* relationship between X and Y. However, it is often much easier to work with the correlation, ρ, defined as

$$\rho = \frac{\text{Cov}(X,Y)}{\sqrt{\text{Var}(X)\text{Var}(Y)}}, \qquad (A.17)$$

because $-1 \leq \rho \leq 1$.

A.3 Some Important Probability Distributions

A.3.1 Discrete Distributions

Although there are many important and useful probability distributions for discrete random variables, this section describes just three: the binomial, Poisson, and negative binomial.

Binomial

In an experiment with n independent trials, each of which results in either a "success" with probability p or a "failure" with probability $1 - p$, the number of successes follows a *binomial distribution* with parameters n and p, often abbreviated $\text{Bin}(n,p)$. For example, imagine flipping a coin n times, where the random variable Y is the number of heads observed out of the n flips. As long as the probability of getting a heads is constant for each flip, with probability p, then Y has a binomial distribution. The shorthand notation is $Y \sim \text{Bin}(n,p)$.

The probability mass function of a binomial random variable with parameters n and p is

$$\mathbb{P}(Y = y) = \binom{n}{y} p^y (1 - p)^{n-y}, \quad y = 0, 1, 2, \ldots, n \quad (A.18)$$

where $\binom{n}{y} = n!/(n - y)!y!$ equals the number of different groups of y objects that can be chosen from the set of n objects. For the parameters, n is a positive, non-zero integer, and $0 < p < 1$. For $n = 1$, the distribution reduces to the Bernoulli. The expected value of a binomial random variable is $\mathbb{E}(Y) = np$, and the variance is $\mathrm{Var}(Y) = np(1 - p)$.

Figure A.4 shows a variety of binomial probability mass functions for select values of n and p.

An example should help illustrate the application of this distribution. Imagine that a fair coin is flipped four times, each flip being independent of the others. What is the probability of obtaining two heads and two tails? The solution is as follows: Let Y denote the number of heads that occur on four flips of the coin, so that Y is a binomial random variable with parameters $n = 4$ and $p = 1/2$. Then by Equation A.18,

$$\mathbb{P}(Y = 2) = \binom{4}{2} \left(\frac{1}{2}\right)^2 \left(\frac{1}{2}\right)^2 = \frac{4 \cdot 3 \cdot 2 \cdot 1}{2 \cdot 1 \cdot 2 \cdot 1} \left(\frac{1}{2}\right)^4 = \frac{3}{8}.$$

To verify this manually, write out all the possible combinations of heads and tails that can occur on four flips of a coin. There are $2 \times 2 \times 2 \times 2 = 16$ possible ways, and six of them have two heads and two tails. For this example, $E(Y) = np = 4 \times 1/2 = 2$, so if this experiment was conducted a large number of times, on average two heads will be observed. The variance is $\mathrm{Var}(Y) = np(1 - p) = 4 \times 1/2 \times 1/2 = 1$. So, the variance is 1 and thus the standard deviation is also 1.

Poisson

The *Poisson distribution* is often useful for modeling the probability of a given number of events occurring in a fixed interval of time or space. To apply, the events occur with a constant average rate and independently of the time since the last event.

The probability mass function for the Poisson distribution, with parameter λ, is

$$\mathbb{P}(Y = y) = \frac{\lambda^y e^{-\lambda}}{y!}, \quad (A.19)$$

for $\lambda > 0$ and $y = 0, 1, 2, 3, \ldots$, and where e is the base of the natural logarithm ($e = 2.2.7182\ldots$). The notation is $\mathrm{Pois}(\lambda)$ and for $Y \sim \mathrm{Pois}(\lambda)$ $\mathbb{E}(Y) = \mathrm{Var}(Y) = \lambda$.

Figure A.5 shows a variety of Poisson probability mass functions for select values of λ.

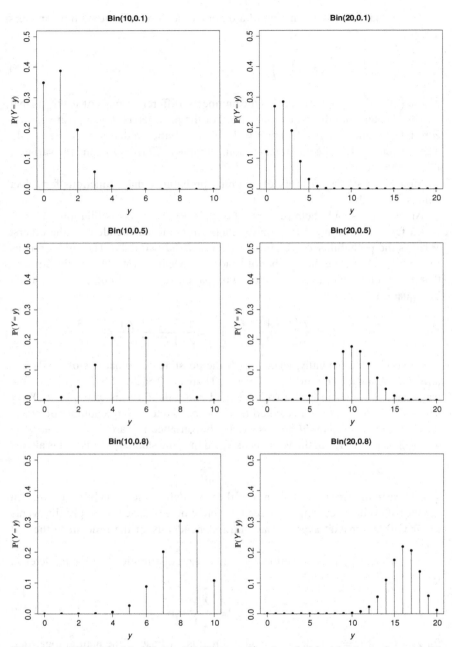

Figure A.4. Illustrative binomial probability mass functions for combinations of $n = 10, 20$, and $p = 0.1, 0.5, 0.8$.

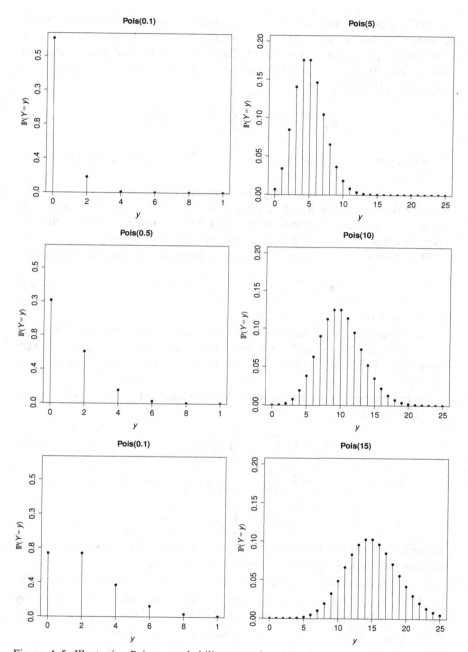

Figure A.5. Illustrative Poisson probability mass functions for $\lambda = 0.1, 0.5, 1, 5, 10, 15$. (Note the change in y-axis scale between the left and right columns of pmfs.)

To illustrate the application of the Poisson distribution, imagine it is reasonable to assume that during the summer when there is no outbreak, the daily influenza-like illness (ILI) syndrome counts Y follow a Poisson distribution with mean of five per day. That is, $Y \sim \text{Pois}(5)$. Given this, the probability that a daily count greater than 10 is observed is

$$\mathbb{P}(Y > 10) = 1 - \sum_{y=0}^{10} \frac{5^y e^{-5}}{y!} = 0.014, \tag{A.20}$$

so there is only a 1.4 percent chance of observing an ILI daily count of 11 or larger.

Negative Binomial

With the Poisson distribution, it must be that $\mathbb{E}(Y) = \text{Var}(Y)$. However, biosurveillance data are often *overdispersed*, meaning $\mathbb{E}(Y) < \text{Var}(Y)$. A distribution for count data that allows for overdispersion is the *negative binomial*.

The negative binomial distribution has two parameters, r and p, and its pmf is

$$\mathbb{P}(Y = y) = \binom{y+r-1}{r-1} p^r (1-p)^y, \tag{A.21}$$

where $r > 0$, $0 < p < 1$, and $y = 0, 1, 2, \ldots$.

The negative binomial is a probability distribution on the number of failures (y) until observing r "successes," where each "trial" has a Bernoulli distribution with probability of success p. For $Y \sim \text{NBin}(r, p)$, $\mathbb{E}(Y) = r(1-p)/p$ and $\text{Var}(Y) = r(1-p)/p^2$.

An alternative parameterization of the binomial pmf, setting $p = r/(r+l)$ with $l = r(1-p)/p$, is

$$\begin{aligned}
\mathbb{P}(Y = y) &= \binom{y+r-1}{r-1} \left(\frac{r}{r+l}\right)^r \left(1 - \frac{r}{r+l}\right)^y \tag{A.22}\\
&= \frac{\Gamma(y+r)}{y!\Gamma(r)} \left(\frac{r}{r+l}\right)^r \left(1 - \frac{r}{r+l}\right)^y \\
&= \frac{l^y}{y!} \left(\frac{r}{r+l}\right)^r \frac{\Gamma(y+r)}{\Gamma(r)(r+l)^y},
\end{aligned}$$

where the second line follows because $(y-1)! = \Gamma(y)$ and the third line is just an algebraic rearrangement of the terms from the second line.

With this parameterization, as $r \to \infty$, $\left(\frac{r}{r+l}\right)^r \to e^{-l}$. This follows from the fact that $\lim_{n\to\infty} \left(1 + \frac{x}{n}\right)^n = e^x$. Furthermore, if $r \to \infty$ and $p \to 1$ in such a way that $r(1-p)$ converges to a constant, then $\frac{\Gamma(y+r)}{\Gamma(r)(r+l)^y} \to 1$. Under these conditions, the limiting distribution of the negative binomial is the Poisson:

$$\lim f(y) = \frac{l^y e^{-l}}{y!}.$$

Figure A.6 shows a variety of negative binomial probability mass functions, using the definition in Equation A.21, for select values of r and p.

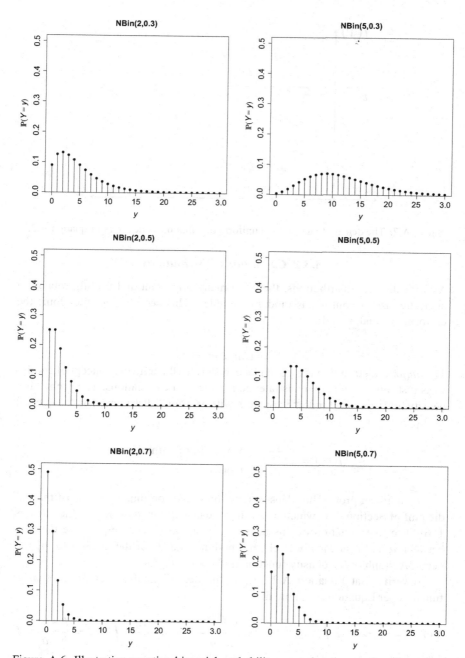

Figure A.6. Illustrative negative binomial probability mass functions, using the pmf as defined in Equation A.21, for combinations of $r = 2, 5$ and $p = 0.3, 0.5, 0.7$.

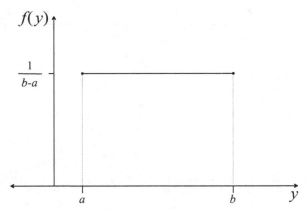

Figure A.7. The density function for a uniform distribution as defined in Equation A.23.

A.3.2 Continuous Distributions

As with discrete distributions, there are many important and useful probability distributions for continuous random variables. This section describes four: the uniform, normal, t, and F.

Uniform

The *uniform* distribution is a good place to start to illustrate the concept of continuous distributions and demonstrate their associated calculations. The probability density function for a random variable Y with a uniform distribution on the interval $[a, b]$, is

$$f_Y(y) = \begin{cases} \frac{1}{b-a}, & \text{for } y \in [a, b] \text{ with } b > a \\ 0, & \text{otherwise.} \end{cases} \tag{A.23}$$

The uniform probability density function is the continuous analog of the fair die pmf of Section A.1 (which was a discrete uniform distribution on the integers 1–6). The interpretation of this density is that every set of equal size that lies between a and b is equally likely, but nothing outside of the interval $[a, b]$ can occur. A graph of the density function is shown in Figure A.7.

To verify that Equation A.23 meets the definition of a probability density function per Equation A.9, note that

$$\mathbb{P}\{Y \in (-\infty, \infty)\} = \int_{-\infty}^{\infty} f_Y(y)dy = \int_{-\infty}^{\infty} \frac{1}{b-a}dy = \frac{1}{b-a} \int_a^b dy = \frac{b-a}{b-a} = 1.$$

The expected value of a uniform random variable is

$$\mathbb{E}(y) = \int_{-\infty}^{\infty} y f_Y(y)dy = \frac{1}{b-a} \int_a^b ydy = \frac{1}{b-a} \cdot \frac{y^2}{2}\Big|_a^b = \frac{b+a}{2}.$$

Then, by calculating $\mathbb{E}(Y^2)$ as

$$\mathbb{E}(Y^2) = \int_{-\infty}^{\infty} y^2 f_Y(y)dy = \frac{1}{b-a} \int_a^b y^2 dy = \frac{1}{b-a} \cdot \frac{y^3}{3}\Big|_a^b = \frac{b^3 - a^3}{3(b-a)},$$

the variance is

$$\text{Var}(Y) = \mathbb{E}(Y^2) - (\mathbb{E}(Y))^2 = \frac{b^3 - a^3}{3(b-a)} - \left(\frac{b+a}{2}\right)^2.$$

Thus, for example, if Y has a continuous uniform distribution on the interval $[0, 1]$, denoted as $Y \sim U(0, 1)$, then $\mathbb{E}(Y) = \frac{1}{2}$ and $\text{Var}(Y) = \frac{1}{12}$.

Normal

The *normal distribution* is an important distribution in statistics, perhaps the most important distribution. Many natural physical phenomena and statistics follow a normal distribution. This happens for a very good reason described more fully in Section A.3.3: the *Central Limit Theorem* (CLT).

The univariate normal distribution is described by two parameters: μ (Greek letter "mu") and σ (Greek letter "sigma"). For $Y \sim N(\mu, \sigma^2)$, the probability density function is

$$f_Y(y) = \frac{1}{\sigma\sqrt{2\pi}} \exp\left(\frac{-(y-\mu)^2}{2\sigma^2}\right). \tag{A.24}$$

For the parameters of the normal distribution, $-\infty < \mu < \infty$ and $\sigma^2 > 0$. For $Y \sim N(\mu, \sigma^2)$, $\mathbb{E}(Y) = \mu$ and $\text{Var}(Y) = \sigma^2$.

It is conventional to use the letter Z to represent a random variable from a "standard normal" distribution. A standard normal distribution has $\mu = 0$ and $\sigma^2 = 1$. The symbol $\Phi(z)$ represents the cumulative probability that Z is less than or equal to some number z: $\Phi(z) = \mathbb{P}(Z \leq z)$.

The probability density function for the standard normal is plotted in Figure A.8, and Figure A.9 compares the density functions for the standard normal with a normal distribution $\mu = 0$ and $\sigma^2 = 2$, a $N(0, 2)$.

Note that the normal distribution is symmetric about μ, meaning if pdf is "folded in half" along the vertical line at μ, then the two halves would line up exactly. This is evident in Figure A.8, where the left and right halves of the curve on either side of $z = 0$ look exactly alike. The normal distribution is also the canonical "bell-shaped curve."

The normal distribution also has "thin tails," meaning that the curve drops quite sharply as you move away from the mean. This property of thin tails is in particular reference to the t-distribution described in the next section. Note that the name "normal" does not imply that random variables following other distributions are abnormal – they are simply not normally distributed.

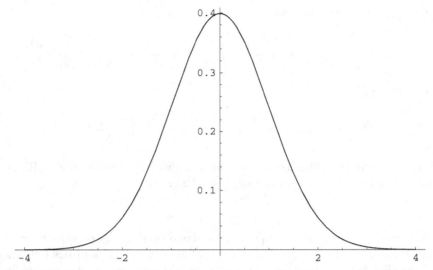

Figure A.8. The probability density function for a standard normal distribution.

Standardizing

An observation from any normal distribution, $N(\mu, \sigma^2)$, is standardized by subtracting off the mean and dividing by the standard deviation. That is, if Y comes from a $N(\mu, \sigma^2)$ distribution, then $Z = (Y - \mu)/\sigma$ has a $N(0, 1)$ distribution.

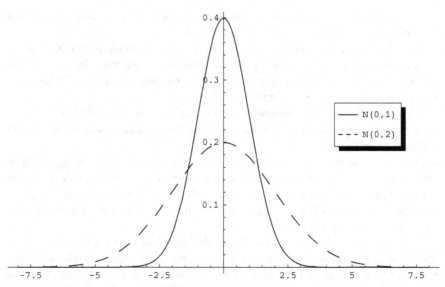

Figure A.9. Comparison of the standard normal distribution probability density function, $N(0,1)$, versus a $N(0,2)$ pdf.

Table A.1. The probability that a random variable with a
standard normal distribution falls between $-z$ and z:
$\mathbb{P}(-z \leq Z \leq z)$. The bold numbers show the probabilities for
falling with one, two, and three standard deviations of the mean

z	$\mathbb{P}(-z \leq Z \leq z)$	z	$\mathbb{P}(-z \leq Z \leq z)$
0.100	0.0797	1.400	0.8385
0.200	0.1585	1.439	0.8500
0.300	0.2358	1.500	0.8664
0.400	0.3108	1.600	0.8904
0.500	0.3829	1.645	0.9000
0.600	0.4515	1.700	0.9109
0.700	0.5161	1.800	0.9281
0.800	0.5763	1.900	0.9426
0.900	0.6319	1.960	0.9500
1.000	**0.6827**	**2.000**	**0.9545**
1.100	0.7287	2.500	0.9876
1.200	0.7699	2.576	0.9900
1.282	0.8000	**3.000**	**0.9973**
1.300	0.8064	4.000	0.9999

That is,

$$\mathbb{P}(a < Y < b) = \mathbb{P}\left(\frac{a - \mu}{\sigma} < Z < \frac{b - \mu}{\sigma}\right)$$

$$= \Phi\left(\frac{b - \mu}{\sigma}\right) - \Phi\left(\frac{a - \mu}{\sigma}\right)$$

This is very useful because it allows us to relate any normal distribution to the standard normal. Table A.1 provides values for the $\mathbb{P}(-z \leq Z \leq z)$, when Z is a random variable with a standard normal distribution.

Bivariate and Multivariate Normal Distributions

The bivariate normal distribution is the *joint distribution* of two variables, Y_1 and Y_2, each of which individually is normally distributed. The bivariate normal distribution is described by five parameters: the means of each variable, μ_1 and μ_2; the variances of each variable, σ_1^2 and σ_2^2; and the correlation between the two variables. The correlation is denoted as ρ, $-1 \leq \rho \leq 1$. The probability density function is

$$f_{Y_1,Y_2}(y_1, y_2) = \frac{1}{2\pi\sigma_1\sigma_2\sqrt{1 - \rho^2}} \exp\left(\frac{-z}{2(1 - \rho^2)}\right), \qquad (A.25)$$

where

$$z = \frac{(y_1 - \mu_1)^2}{\sigma_1^2} - \frac{2\rho(y_1 - \mu_1)(y_2 - \mu_2)}{\sigma_1\sigma_2} + \frac{(y_2 - \mu_2)^2}{\sigma_2^2}.$$

If $\rho = 0$, then Y_1 and Y_2 are independent. If, in addition, $\mu_1 = \mu_2$ and $\sigma_1 = \sigma_2$, then Y_1 and Y_2 are *iid*.

Now, let $\mathbf{Y}$ denote a vector of k observations, $\mathbf{Y} = \{Y_1, Y_2, \ldots, Y_k\}$. $\mathbf{Y} \sim N(\boldsymbol{\mu}, \boldsymbol{\Sigma})$ denotes that $\mathbf{Y}$ has a multivariate normal distribution with mean vector $\boldsymbol{\mu}$ and covariance matrix $\boldsymbol{\Sigma}$. The multivariate normal pdf is

$$f_{\mathbf{Y}}(y_1, \ldots, y_k) = \frac{1}{(2\pi)^{k/2} \mid \Sigma \mid^{1/2}} \exp\left(-\frac{1}{2}(\mathbf{y} - \boldsymbol{\mu})' \, \Sigma^{-1} (\mathbf{y} - \boldsymbol{\mu})\right), \quad (A.26)$$

where $|\Sigma|$ denotes the determinant of Σ.

For $k = 2$, Equation A.26 is equivalent to Equation A.25 with $\boldsymbol{\mu} = \{\mu_1, \mu_2\}$ and

$$\Sigma = \begin{pmatrix} \sigma_1^2 & \rho\sigma_1\sigma_2 \\ \rho\sigma_2\sigma_1 & \sigma_2^2 \end{pmatrix}.$$

For $k = 1$, Equation A.26 reduces to the univariate normal distribution with the pdf shown in Equation A.24, where Σ is a 1×1 matrix (i.e., it is a real number).

t-Distribution

When standardizing a normally distributed observation, it is often the case that the population standard deviation must be estimated from data. Under such circumstances, when the sample variance is used in the standardization calculation in place of the population variance, the standardized value then follows a *t-distribution* with $n - 1$ "degrees of freedom."

The density function for the t-distribution with n degrees of freedom is

$$f(y) = \frac{\Gamma[(n+1)/2]}{\sqrt{n\pi}\,\Gamma(n/2)} \left(1 + \frac{y^2}{n}\right)^{-(n+1)/2}, \quad (A.27)$$

where $n > 0$.

The t-distribution is symmetric and bell shaped, like the normal distribution, but has "heavier tails," meaning that it is more likely to produce values that fall further from its mean (compared with the normal distribution). When standardizing, the heavier tails account for the extra uncertainty that is introduced into the standardized value because of the use of the sample variance.

Figure A.10 shows four different t-distributions, corresponding to four different degrees of freedom, compared with a standard normal distribution. When looking at the tails of the curves, the curve with the largest tails (corresponding to "$t(2)$") is a t-distribution with 2 degrees of freedom; the curve with the next largest tails (corresponding to "$t(3)$") is a t-distribution with 3 degrees of freedom, followed by a t-distribution with 5 degrees of freedom; and the curve with the smallest tails is a t-distribution with 10 degrees of freedom.

This graph shows that the fewer degrees of freedom, the heavier the tails. Conversely, the more degrees of freedom, the closer the t-distribution gets to the normal. With an infinite number of degrees of freedom, the t-distribution is the normal distribution.

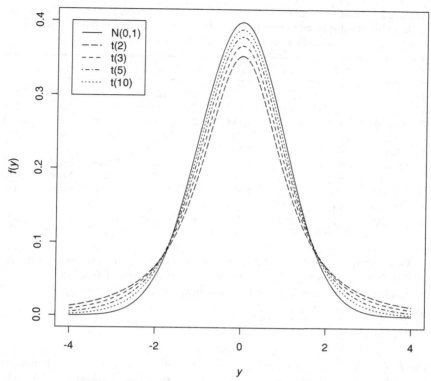

Figure A.10. Examples of the t-distribution for 2, 3, 5, and 10 degrees of freedom compared with the standard normal distribution.

Table A.2 gives selected quantiles from the t-distribution for various degrees of freedom. Most statistics textbooks provide more detailed tabulations, and various statistical software packages can also be used to look up the quantiles for any number of degrees of freedom or tail probabilities.

Chi-Square (χ^2) Distribution

The χ^2 (chi-square) distribution is another important statistical distribution. The sum of the squares of n standard normal random variables follows a χ^2 distribution with n "degrees of freedom." That is, for $Y = Z_1^2 + Z_2^2 + \cdots + Z_n^2$, $Y \sim \chi_n^2$ with $\mathbb{E}(Y) = n$ and $\mathrm{Var}(Y) = 2n$. Hence, the χ_n^2 distribution is characterized by n, the number of degrees of freedom.

The density function for $Y \sim \chi_n^2$ is

$$f_Y(y) = \begin{cases} \frac{1}{2^{n/2}\Gamma(n/2)} y^{n/2-1} e^{(-y/2)}, & y > 0 \\ 0, & \text{elsewhere,} \end{cases} \tag{A.28}$$

where n is a positive integer and Γ is the gamma function: $\Gamma(\alpha) = \int_0^\infty y^{\alpha-1} e^{-y} dy$.

Table A.2. Quantiles from the t-distribution for various degrees of freedom, where the quantiles displayed are for the probability that a random variable T with a t-distribution is greater than t_α: $\mathbb{P}(T > t_\alpha) = \alpha$

df	$t_{0.10}$	$t_{0.05}$	$t_{0.025}$	$t_{0.01}$	df	$t_{0.10}$	$t_{0.05}$	$t_{0.025}$	$t_{0.01}$
1	3.078	6.314	12.706	31.821	15	1.341	1.753	2.131	2.602
2	1.886	2.920	4.303	6.965	20	1.325	1.725	2.086	2.528
3	1.638	2.353	3.182	4.541	25	1.316	1.708	2.060	2.485
4	1.533	2.132	2.776	3.747	30	1.310	1.697	2.042	2.457
5	1.476	2.015	2.571	3.365					
6	1.440	1.943	2.447	3.143	40	1.303	1.684	2.021	2.423
7	1.415	1.895	2.356	2.998	60	1.296	1.671	2.000	2.390
8	1.397	1.860	2.306	2.896	120	1.289	1.658	1.980	2.358
9	1.383	1.833	2.262	2.821					
10	1.372	1.812	2.228	2.764	∞	1.282	1.645	1.960	2.326

As shown in Figure A.11, when the number of degrees of freedom is small, the χ^2 distribution is asymmetric. As the number of degrees of freedom increases, the resulting distribution becomes more symmetric (as a direct result of the CLT discussed in Section A.3.3).

F Distribution

The *F distribution* is related to the χ^2 distribution. Let W and X be independent χ^2 random variables with m and n degrees of freedom, respectively. Then the

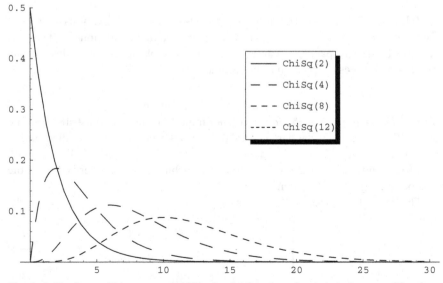

Figure A.11. Some chi-square probability density functions for various degrees of freedom.

random variable

$$Y = \frac{W/m}{X/n}$$

has an F distribution with m and n degrees of freedom. Note that the order of m and n is important. The density function for the F distribution is

$$f_Y(y) = \frac{\Gamma[(m+n)/2]}{\Gamma(m/2)\Gamma(n/2)} \left(\frac{m}{n}\right) y^{m/2-1} \left(1 + \frac{m}{n}y\right)^{-(m+n)/2}. \quad (A.29)$$

As shown in Figure A.12, a wide variety of probability density function shapes are possible with the F distribution depending on how the degrees of freedom (m and n) are varied.

A.3.3 Sampling Distributions, Standard Errors, and the Central Limit Theorem

A function of a set of random variables is itself a random variable with its own distribution referred to as the *sampling distribution*. For example, the sum of n *iid* normally distributed random variables, $X_i \sim N(\mu, \sigma^2)$, $i = 1, \ldots, n$, is also normally distributed with mean 0 and variance $n \times \sigma^2$. That is, if $Y = X_1 + \cdots + X_n$, then $Y \sim N(\mu, n\sigma^2)$. Similarly, for $\bar{Y} = \frac{1}{n}\sum_{i=1}^{n} X_i$ then $\bar{Y} \sim N(\mu, \sigma^2/n)$.

The term *standard error* (often abbreviated s.e.) is another name for the standard deviation of a statistic. Thus, in the previous example, the standard error of $\bar{Y}$ is $\sigma/\sqrt{n}$. Note that the standard error of the mean is smaller than the standard deviation of the individual observations, so the sampling distribution of the mean is narrower than the distribution of the individual observations. One consequence of this result is that as the sample size increases it becomes more likely that $\bar{Y}$ will be close to μ. When using a statistic to estimate some population quantity, the standard error is used to quantify the uncertainty in the estimate. For example, "The estimated ATFS is 4.3 days (s.e. $= 0.2$)."

Note the use of capital letters in the foregoing is purposeful. Capital letters represent random variables, and lowercase letters represent numbers. Hence, $\bar{Y}$ denotes the average of a set of random variables. Because the random variables are random, so is $\bar{Y}$, and thus $\bar{Y}$ has a probability density function, which is referred to as the sampling distribution of $\bar{Y}$. In contrast, $\bar{y}$ is a sample average, which is a number and hence does not have a distribution.

It turns out that the sums and averages of normally distributed random variables are themselves distributed normally. Thus, for example, the sampling distribution of the mean of normally distributed random variables with mean μ and variance σ^2 is itself normally distributed with mean μ and variance σ^2/n (and thus standard error $\sigma/\sqrt{n}$). Furthermore, even if the distribution of individual observations is not normally distributed, the sampling distribution will be approximately normal via the CLT.

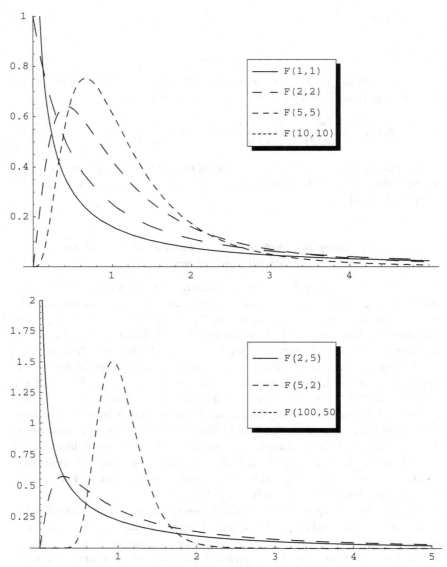

Figure A.12. Some F distribution probability density functions for various degrees of freedom.

The CLT says that the distribution of sums of random variables tends toward a normal distribution as the sum gets large even if the random variables are not themselves normally distributed. Formally:

Theorem A.1 (*Central Limit Theorem*) Let $X_1, X_2, \ldots, X_i, \ldots$ be a sequence of independent random variables having mean 0, variance σ^2, and a common

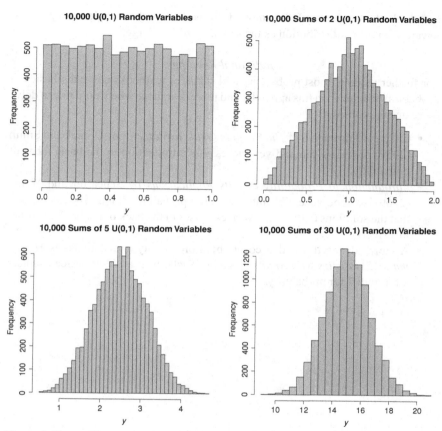

Figure A.13. An illustration of the CLT applied to sums of uniformly distributed random variables. The upper left plot is a histogram resulting from 10,000 draws from a $U(0, 1)$. The plot to the right is 10,000 sums of two draws from the same distribution. The bottom left plots 10,000 sums of five $U(0, 1)$ random variables, and the bottom right is 10,000 sums of 30.

distribution function. Then,

$$\lim_{n \to \infty} \mathbb{P} \left(\frac{\bar{X}_n}{\sigma / \sqrt{n}} \leq x \right) = \Phi(x), \ -\infty < x < \infty.$$

Furthermore, because the mean is just the sum of random variables renormalized by dividing by the number of random variables being summed, the mean also has an approximate normal distribution.

The Central Limit Theorem applies to both discrete and continuous random variables. Figure A.13 illustrates the CLT for data with a uniform distribution. In the figure, the upper left plot is a histogram resulting from 10,000 draws from a $U(0, 1)$. The plot to the right is 10,000 sums of two draws from the same distribution. The bottom left plots 10,000 sums of five $U(0, 1)$ random variables, and the bottom right is 10,000 sums of 30. Note how the sample average tends toward the normal distribution as the sample size gets large.

Additional Reading

For further reading, most probability and statistics textbooks cover the basics of probability discussed in this appendix and more. For those who would like to delve more deeply, consider:

- Chapters 3 through 6 of *The Cartoon Guide to Statistics* by Gonick and Smith (2009) provide a fun and very accessible introduction to the basic ideas of probability.
- *Introduction to Probability and Its Applications* by Scheaffer and Young (2009) is a good, accessible introduction to probability (though be forewarned that the solutions to the homework exercises in the back of the book are often incorrect).
- A more advanced text that covers both probability and statistics is *Mathematical Statistics with Applications* by Wackerly et at. (2007). See chapters 2 through 7 for probability.

B

Simulating Biosurveillance Data

It [the computer] is a medium that can dynamically simulate the details of any other medium, including media that cannot exist physically.

Alan Kay (1984, p. 59)

Although there is no substitute for actual data, there are times when simulated data can be very useful, particularly for evaluating how systems and methods will perform under conditions other than that which has already been observed. In addition, simulation gives researchers and practitioners control that is simply not achievable with real data. For example, in real data, it is very difficult – often impossible – to determine whether a particular data stream contains one or more outbreaks. And even when the existence of an outbreak is known, it is generally impossible to definitively determine when it started and ended.

Thus, although some reject simulated data under the assumption that they cannot mimic all the features of real biosurveillance data, the use of simulation – which must be based on idealizations of the real world to some degree – is useful precisely because:

- it permits definitive performance evaluations and comparisons under known conditions, and
- it can often allow one to assess how the various data features affect performance.

Indeed, it is often desirable to employ purposely idealized depictions of both background disease incidence and outbreaks that capture the main features of biosurveillance data but ignore some real-world complications so that specific effects can be isolated and understood.

This appendix discusses some methods for simulating biosurveillance data. Because there are so many ways biosurveillance simulations can be and have been conducted, this appendix is not a comprehensive survey of all possible simulation techniques. Rather, it focuses on (1) demonstrating how to characterize biosurveillance data stochastically and (2) illustrating some relatively simple simulation approaches that can be used to effectively simulate real biosurveillance data.

335

Mathematical Notation

A	Amplitude of the sinusoid simulating seasonal variation
B	Amplitude of the sinusoid simulating within-season variation
b	Length of within-season cycle
D	Duration of outbreak
$\mathbb{E}(Y)$	Expected value of random variable Y
f	Lowess parameter
M	Magnitude of outbreak
N_t	Total number of observations on day t
$N!$	N factorial $(1 \times 2 \times 3 \times \cdots \times (N-1) \times N)$
$N(0, 25)$	Univariate normal distribution with mean 0 and variance 25
$N_m(\mathbf{0}, \Sigma)$	Multivariate normal distribution of dimension m with mean vector $\mathbf{0}$ and covariance matrix Σ
$o, \mathbf{o}$	Mean outbreak level
p, r	Parameters of the negative binomial distribution
$\hat{p}, \hat{r}$	Estimated parameters of the negative binomial distribution
p_{tj}	Parameter of the multinomial distribution
$\mathrm{Pois}(\lambda)$	Poisson distribution with parameter λ
s	Sample standard deviation
s^2	Sample variance
t	Time index
$U(a, b)$	Uniform distribution the interval a to b
$\mathrm{Var}(Y)$	Variance of random variable Y
y, y_t	Observed count
$\bar{y}$	Sample mean
$Y, \mathbf{Y}$	Random variable/vector representing a count before it is observed
$Z, \mathbf{Z}$	Random noise component in data simulations
$\delta, \boldsymbol{\delta}$	Day-of-the-week effect
$\gamma, \boldsymbol{\gamma}$	Seasonal deviation from annual mean μ
λ	Parameter of the Poisson distribution
$\mu, \boldsymbol{\mu}$	Annual mean level of disease incidence
$\hat{\mu}_t$	Estimated annual mean level of disease incidence on day t
$\theta, \boldsymbol{\theta}$	Within-season deviation from $\mu + \gamma$
$\hat{\Sigma}$	Estimated covariance matrix
τ, ν	Random start day for seasonal and within-season variation

B.1 Types of Simulation

Simulations of biosurveillance data can be categorized in three dimensions:

- **Temporal vs. spatio-temporal simulations.** Temporal simulations only model how the data occur over time, whereas spatio-temporal simulations model the data in both space and time. The former is relevant for biosurveillance systems that, for example, only observe daily syndrome counts from a facility or region and do not have any information about location. The latter is relevant for systems that also observe and utilize information about the location of the data, whether it is aggregate count data from health care facilities in different locations or information about the location of sick individuals.

- **Aggregate vs. individual-level data simulations.** As the name implies, aggregate simulations model the data aggregated to some level, such as daily counts of individuals with a particular syndrome or the number of individuals diagnosed with a particular disease by, say, home zip code. In contrast, individual-level simulations model individual entities, usually people. For example, a simulation might model the aerosol release of a bioagent, down to how much each individual in a region is exposed, whether they develop symptoms and seek treatment, and so on.

- **Completely synthetic vs. partially synthetic simulations.** Completely synthetic simulations are those that use Monte Carlo simulation to generate both the background disease incidence rate, say of the flu or flu-like symptoms, as well as outbreaks. In contrast, partially synthetic simulations may make some aspects of the simulation deterministic, perhaps deriving the deterministic components from actual data, often for the purpose of mimicking an actual data set. "Outbreak-only" simulations typically use actual data to characterize the background disease incidence rate and then insert (or "inject") simulated outbreaks into the actual data.

Authors in the literature have used other categorization taxonomies and terminology. In particular, Buckeridge *et al.* (2005) classify biosurveillance data sets into those that are "wholly authentic" or "wholly simulated" and those that superimpose simulated outbreaks onto actual data. Lotze *et al.* (2007) refer to partially synthetic simulations as "semi-simulated."

The choice of conducting aggregate versus individual-level simulations should be driven by the system or technique being analyzed. In general, individual-level simulations are larger in scope and more difficult to execute because they require more involved modeling. On the other hand, individual-level simulations are useful for determining how an outbreak might manifest in a population, particularly when there is little or no data on what an outbreak would look like for a particular bioagent.

Temporal simulations tend to also be aggregate simulations because there is generally little added value in modeling at the individual level (except when simulating how outbreaks manifest in a population, as previously discussed).

Spatio-temporal simulations can be simulated at either the aggregate or individual level, depending on the requirements of the analytical technique. If the technique being analyzed uses aggregate measures, say daily counts by zip code in a region, then it is likely to be easier to use aggregate simulation. On the other hand, if the technique requires the location of individuals, then an individual-level simulation will be necessary.

Outbreak-only simulations are based on an historical set of data, so there is no randomness in the background disease incidence data. Thus, when using an actual historical set of data to evaluate performance, the data represent just one "past reality" which, although it contains all the complications of the real world, may not reflect what might happen in the future or even what could have happened in the past under the same conditions. In contrast, completely synthetic simulations allow biosurveillance system performance evaluation across many "possible realities." This provides insight into a system's general performance and mitigates the chance that a particular finding will be too closely tied to or the result of one particular data set.

When conducting completely synthetic simulations, one must think of observed data as arising from some random process.[1] This is reasonable because the observed data are the result of a complicated series of events and interactions, and small changes in those events and interactions would likely have resulted in a different set of observed data. Thus, to appropriately simulate biosurveillance data, it is critical to probabilistically characterize the underlying random process so that the data it produces reasonably represent reality. The first step in constructing such simulations is to determine which probability distributions best characterize actual biosurveillance data.

B.1.1 Fitting Distributions to Count Data

Before biosurveillance data are observed, they can be thought of as random variables Y_t, $t = 1, 2, 3, \ldots$, each eventually resulting in an observation y_t generated according to some probability distribution. The most commonly used distribution for modeling counts is the Poisson. A Poisson random variable has the property that its expected value is equal to its variance, $\mathbb{E}(Y) = \text{Var}(Y) = \lambda$, so data that do not have this property cannot have come from a Poisson distribution. (See Section A.3.1 of Appendix A for a review of the Poisson distribution.)

In general, biosurveillance count data are overdispersed, meaning $\text{Var}(Y) > \mathbb{E}(Y)$, which would make the Poisson distribution inappropriate for modeling the data. For example, Example B.1 illustrates that the clinic daily counts for influenca-like illness (ILI) and gestrointestinal (GI) syndromes are overdispersed. As discussed in Appendix A, the negative binomial distribution

---

[1] The phrase "random process" does not mean events occur arbitrarily or without reason. Rather, it means that outcomes are stochastic and thus governed by the rules of probability. As Democritus said more than two millennia ago, "Everything existing in the universe is the fruit of chance."

allows for overdispersion. (See Section A.3.1 of Appendix A for additional information.)

Example B.1. The table below illustrates overdispersion in biosurveillance data. It shows the sample means and variances for the clinic data divided up into four 63-day intervals. For both syndromes and all 63-day intervals except the first interval for GI, $s^2 > \bar{y}$, significantly so for ILI.

Syndrome	Days 1–63 $\bar{y}$	s^2	Days 64–126 $\bar{y}$	s^2	Days 127–189 $\bar{y}$	s^2	Days 190–252 $\bar{y}$	s^2
ILI	20.7	28.7	25.1	112.9	33.6	79.5	23.8	83.9
GI	6.0	5.7	6.0	7.8	7.8	11.6	6.0	7.1

Figures B.1 and B.2 compare the empirical distributions of the clinic data versus fitted Poisson and negative binomial distributions for the data divided into four 63-day periods. The Poisson was fit using the usual estimator for λ, $\hat{\lambda} = \bar{y}$ (which can be derived using either method of moments or maximum likelihood, both assuming the observations are independent). The negative binomial was fit using the method of moments estimators for the parameters p and r, which are $\hat{p} = \bar{y}/s^2$ and $\hat{r} = \bar{y}^2/(s^2 - \bar{y})$. Because the estimator for r is defined only when $s^2 > \bar{y}$, for cases where $s^2 \leq \bar{y}$ (e.g., the days 1–63 for the GI syndrome in Example B.1), it is reasonable to assume the limiting form applies and thus fits a Poisson distribution.

The figures show, not unexpectedly given the preceding discussion, that the negative binomial distribution visually fits the overdispersed ILI data better. On the other hand, for the GI syndrome, the Poisson distribution looks quite reasonable even in cases in which the data show some evidence of overdispersion. Chi-square goodness-of-fit tests fail to reject both the Poisson and negative binomial distributions for the GI syndrome data, but the Poisson distribution is nearly rejected for days 1 to 63 in the ILI data ($p = 0.09$) and strongly rejected for the other three periods of data ($p \approx 0$); the negative binomial is not rejected for any of the periods ($0.55 \leq p \leq 0.83$).

As discussed in Jackson (1972), overdispersion in count data can arise for many reasons, including when events occur in clusters, when they are the result of mixing, and when the underlying distribution is not stationary. In biosurveillance, contagious diseases are likely to lead to clusters because when one individual in a household or neighborhood gets sick, then it is likely that his or her family members and neighbors will, too. Similarly, mixing can occur if two or more groups of individuals present at different rates with symptoms corresponding to the same chief complaint. And as demonstrated, in Chapter 2, biosurveillance data tend to be autocorrelated, and the underlying distribution is unlikely to be stationary. Hence, there are multiple reasons to expect biosurveillance data to be overdispersed.

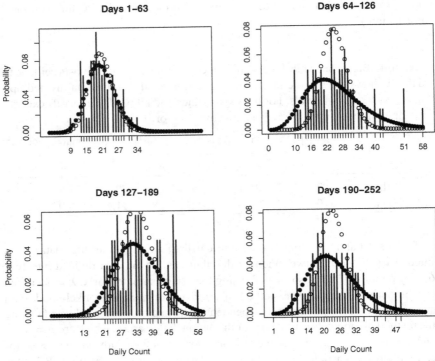

Figure B.1. Distribution of ILI syndrome counts for the clinic data. The heights of the vertical lines represent the fraction of days with that count out of the total number of days in the group (63) – an empirical estimate of the probability of that count occurring. The white dots are the probability of each count based on a fitted Poisson distribution, and the black dots are the probability of each count based on a fitted negative binomial distribution.

Table B.1 uses county-level ILI and GI data to illustrate how non-stationarity can lead to overdispersion. The table is based on simulated daily counts, where each day's count was a random draw from a Poisson distribution with λ_t estimated for each day using a moving average calculated from the real data. In the simulated data, the means match reasonably well to the actual sample means in Example B.1 and ILI do show overdispersion. However, the resulting variation in ILI is too small compared with the actual variation, suggesting that the actual overdispersion observed in Example B.1 arose as a result of more than just nonstationarity.

B.1.2 Fitting Distributions to Residuals

An alternative to fitting distributions to the raw data is to first remove the systematic effects from the data and then fit distributions to the residuals. Doing so provides some insight into the stochastic nature of the "noise" in the data. Figure B.3 shows normal quantile-quantile (Q-Q) plots for the residuals from the ILI and GI syndrome clinic data. Note that the residuals look reasonably normally distributed,

Table B.1. The mean and variance of simulated daily counts for four consecutive 63-day periods. The statistics were calculated from simulated daily counts, where each day's count was a random draw from a Poisson distribution with λ_t estimated for each day using a moving average calculated from the real data

Syndrome	Days 1–63		Days 64–126		Days 127–189		Days 190–252	
	$\bar{y}$	s^2	$\bar{y}$	s^2	$\bar{y}$	s^2	$\bar{y}$	s^2
ILI	19.9	22.8	25.0	59.7	34.4	48.8	24.5	65.5
GI	5.6	5.1	6.9	9.4	6.8	6.0	5.7	6.1

perhaps with a few larger outliers, but such outliers are to be expected if the data contain naturally occurring outbreaks such as the flu.

Formal tests of normality using the Shapiro-Wilks test show that a normal distribution cannot be rejected for both syndromes and all time periods except the ILI syndrome for days 64 to 126 and that is rejected only because of the large outlier that occurred on day 98. This was the next to the last day the clinics

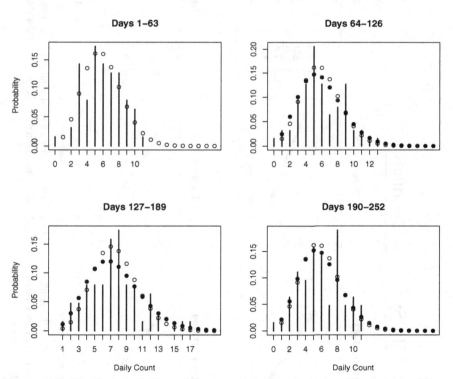

Figure B.2. Distribution of GI syndrome counts for the clinic data. The heights of the vertical lines represent the fraction of days with that count out of the total number of days in the group (63) – an empirical estimate of the probability of that count occurring. The white dots are the probability of each count based on a fitted Poisson distribution, and the black dots are the probability of each count based on a fitted negative binomial distribution.

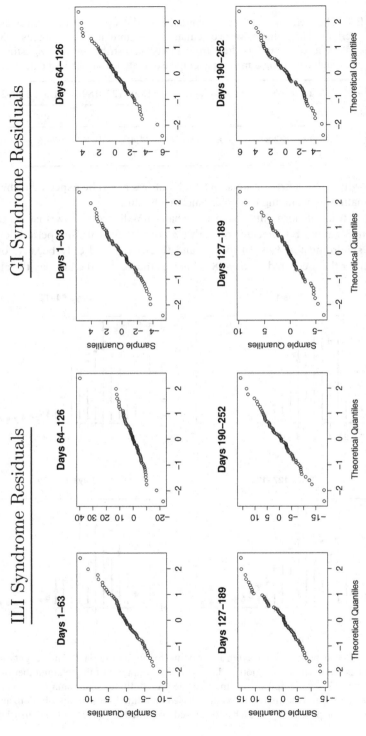

Figure B.3. Q-Q plots of the residuals from the ILI syndrome data and GI syndrome data showing the residuals are reasonably normally distributed. The residuals were calculated by subtracting the locally smoothed estimate of the mean (calculated using a lowess smoother with $f = 0.1$) and the appropriate average day effect from each count.

342

were open before Christmas, and that particular day had a count of 58 for the ILI syndrome, suggesting an outbreak perhaps combined with a holiday effect.

Now, of course, these specific examples do not prove that residuals are normally distributed for all biosurveillance data. For example, Lotze *et al.* (2008) give examples of non-normal residuals in biosurveillance data. However, it does demonstrate that residuals from count data can sometimes be modeled using a continuous distribution. That, combined with the residuals having minimal autocorrelation as shown in the correlograms of Figures 5.1 and 5.2 in Chapter 5, suggests that some count data can reasonably be modeled as the sum of systematic effects and independent error terms.

B.2 Simulating Biosurveillance Data

This section explores some methods for simulating temporal data and spatiotemporal data. As mentioned in the chapter introduction, the methods presented are neither comprehensive nor even representative of what is being done in the current state of practice. Rather, they are examples of useful techniques and approaches that effectively simulate biosurveillance data and that are relatively easy to implement.

B.2.1 Univariate Temporal Data Simulations

To simulate aggregate univariate temporal data, this section starts with methods that explicitly model the various systematic effects present in biosurveillance data. It then proceeds to simulation methods based on fitting a probability distribution to the data that are used to generate random observations. This is followed by a discussion about simulating outbreaks, and the section concludes with the often-used approach of "injecting" artificial outbreaks into actual biosurveillance data.

Explicitly Modeling Data Features
Univariate Temporal Method #1 (UTM1) is a completely synthetic method that explicitly models the main systematic effects in the disease incidence data and then overlays on this simulated outbreaks. As Chapter 2 demonstrates, biosurveillance data can contain an annual or season cycle, resulting, for example, from a winter flu season, a systematic day effect, and then random variation. A simple model of this process simulates a daily observation Y_t as

$$Y_t = \max(0, \lceil \mu + \gamma_t + \delta_t + o_t + Z_t \rceil), \quad t = 1, 2, 3, \ldots, \tag{B.1}$$

where

- μ is the annual mean level of disease incidence;
- γ is the seasonal deviation;
- δ is the day-of-the-week effect;
- o is the mean outbreak level, which, when an outbreak is occurring, increases the disease incidence level;

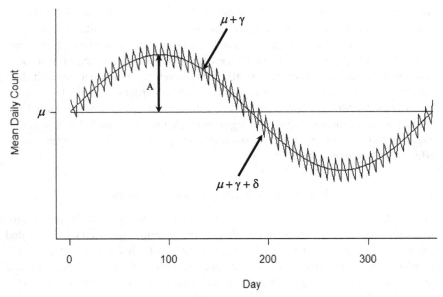

Figure B.4. The systematic effects, μ, γ, δ, and A, for UTM1 as parameterized in Equation B.1.

- Z is the random noise around the systematic component, $(\mu + \gamma_t + \delta_t)$; and
- $\lceil x \rceil$ is the ceiling function, which rounds x up to the next largest integer because the data are daily counts.

Assuming the seasonal effect is a simple sinusoid, set $\gamma_t = A[\sin(2\pi i/365)]$, where A is the maximum deviation from μ and $t = 1$ corresponds to the first day in the sinusoidal cycle that $\gamma > 0$ (so the maximum occurs at $t = 365/4 = 91.25$). The day effect is the systematic average deviation from $\mu + \gamma_t$, where $\delta_t = \delta_{t+7}$ for all t. For the random component, based on Figure B.3, assume $Z \sim N(0, \sigma^2)$.

The systematic effects, μ, γ, δ, and A are illustrated in Figure B.4.

Example B.2. Using UTM1 construct a simulation to mimic the GI syndrome daily counts for Hospital #7, which Figure 2.7 shows to be quite cyclical, for one year.

Solution: To estimate the parameters of the model in Equation B.1, the obvious choice for estimating the average level of disease incidence is $\mu = \bar{x} = 16.75$, where the sample average is calculated from the counts for the year. To estimate A, fit a locally smoothed mean to the data, such as was used to draw the lines in Figure 2.7, and then take half the difference between the minimum and the maximum. Doing this for the Hospital #7 data gives $A = 6.4$. For the day

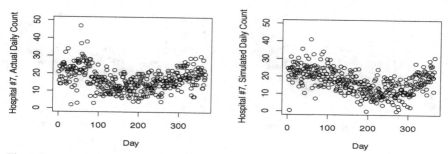

Figure B.5. A comparison of 1 year of Hospital #7 GI syndrome data versus 1 year of data simulated using UTM1 with γ estimated using a sinusoid function.

effects, use the mean day residuals, as calculated in Figure 2.9. And estimate σ as the standard deviation of the residuals calculated by subtracting the locally smoothed mean and the estimated day effects from the daily counts. For the hospital data, this gives $s = 5.3$. Rounding to 5 to account for a seeming outbreak in the winter that slightly inflated the background disease incidence variation gives $Z \sim N(0, 25)$.

Plugging the estimates into Equation B.1, the results from one simulation are shown in Figure B.5, where the simulated data seem to visually match quite closely the actual data. To match the cycle in the data, $t = 1$ was set to a day in mid-November. To add further realism, the simulation might make the date when $t = 1$ random, say with a uniform distribution, so that the peak of the sinusoid could occur over some range of months in the winter.

Now, modeling the seasonal component γ using a sinusoid has the advantage of a simple parameterization (requiring only the choice of A and the date when $t = 1$), but it may be too simple to appropriately reflect real-world complexity. A partially synthetic simulation alternative is to estimate some of the systematic effects in the actual data and then fix these as deterministic components in a simulation. This type of simulation still allows the exploration of "alternate realities" while keeping some of the inherent complexity of the way the actual average background disease incidence behaved.

Univariate temporal method #2 (UTM2) is one variant of this approach that uses a lowess line fitted to the actual data in place $\mu + \gamma$. Then the daily observations Y_t are simulated as

$$Y_t = \max(0, \lceil \hat{\mu}_t + \delta_t + o_t + Z_t \rceil), \quad t = 1, 2, 3, \ldots, \tag{B.2}$$

where δ, o, and Z are as defined in Equation B.1, and $\hat{\mu}_t$ is the value of the lowess line (with degree 0 and $f = 0.1$) for day t.

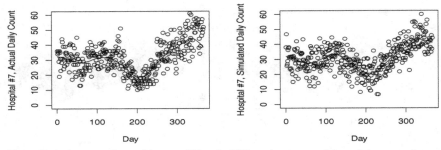

Figure B.6. A comparison of 1 year of Hospital #7 respiratory syndrome data versus 1 year of data simulated using UTM2 with $\mu + \gamma$ estimated using a locally smoothed mean. The lowess line fit to the actual data is visible in the left plot. This line was used in the simulation of the "data" in the right plot, and the lowess line subsequently fit to the simulated data in the right plot mimics the line from the left plot.

Example B.3. Using UTM2, simulate the more complex cyclical behavior of Hospital #7 daily respiratory syndrome counts (see Fig. 2.8).

Solution: After fitting a lowess line to the data and estimating the day effects, Equation B.2 was used to simulate data. Figure B.6 shows the actual data compared with the realization from this partially synthetic simulation.

An issue with this type of partially synthetic modeling, however, is the possibility of the system or algorithm being overfit to the deterministic components of the simulation (e.g., the lowess line in Example B.3), particularly if those deterministic components are likely to vary in the future. To use a completely synthetic approach while retaining some of complexity, the challenge is to stochastically generate realistic trend lines. One approach is to add a within-season sinusoid to the original UTM1 model, as in:

$$Y_t = \max(0, \lceil \mu + \gamma_t + \theta_t + \delta_t + o_t + Z_t \rceil), \quad t = 1, 2, 3, \ldots, \qquad \text{(B.3)}$$

where μ, γ, δ, Z, and o are defined as in Equation B.1, and $\theta_t = B[\sin(2\pi(t + \tau)/91.25)]$, where B is the maximum deviation from $\mu + \gamma$ and τ corresponds to a random starting day for the within-season sinusoidal cycle: $\tau \sim U(1, 91.25)$.

Example B.4. Use UTM1 with a within-season sinusoid term to add complexity to the Example B.2 simulation.

Solution: Figure B.7 shows one realization of a simulation using Equation B.3, with $\mu = 16.75$, $A = 6.4$, $B = 3$, $\sigma = 5$, and with the day effects as they were as in Example B.2.

Of course, Equations B.1 through B.3 can be further extended to incorporate other data features, such as the following:

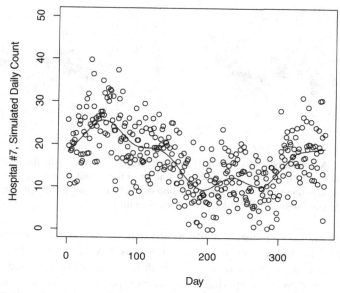

Figure B.7. One simulation realization for Hospital #7 GI syndrome data from Example B.4.

1. *Linear trends.* Growing or shrinking populations or changes in health conditions could result in linear (or other) trends in the disease incidence. If trends are of interest, a trend term could also be included in Equations B.1 through B.3.
2. *Holidays or other such effects.* Holiday and other types of systematic effects are often present in real syndromic surveillance data. Although these effects are not included in Equation B.1, they could be with the addition of the appropriate terms.

That said, there is a fine line between the realism of the simulation model and the utility and interpretability of the results. As previously discussed, the characterization of disease incidence in Equations B.1 to B.3 is purposely idealized. The idea is to mimic the most salient and important features of syndromic surveillance data in a simulation environment where what has occurred can be known precisely so that the biosurveillance system's performance can be definitively assessed.

Modeling Distributional Parameters

Univariate Temporal Method #3 (UTM3) is a partially synthetic method that uses data to estimate the parameters of a sequence of probability distributions. After the parameters of the distributions are estimated, the UTM3 method then draws random observations from those probability distributions to simulate the data. Given a particular distributional form (e.g., Poisson or negative binomial), the question is how to appropriately estimate the parameters of the distribution, which can be a challenge because of the lack of stationarity. Assuming the distributional

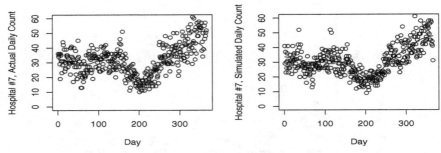

Figure B.8. A comparison of 1 year of Hospital #7 respiratory syndrome data versus 1 year of data simulated using UTM3. The lowess line fit to the actual data is visible in the left plot. The lowess line was used in the simulation of the "data" in the right plot, where each day t is a random draw from a Poisson distribution with $\lambda_t = \hat{\mu}_t$.

form stays the same, nonstationarity means that the parameter or parameters of the distribution change over time, and that means they cannot be estimated once using all of the data. One way around this difficulty is to use a neighborhood of data around any given time period to estimate the parameters for that time period.

Given that the Poisson distribution only has one parameter λ, which is its mean, and that the Poisson probability distribution is a discrete distribution on the non-negative integers, it seems like a logical place to begin. In particular, assuming a lowess line fit to some historical data is a reasonable estimate of the mean, each day t in the simulated data is a random draw from a Poisson distribution with $\lambda_t = \hat{\mu}_t$, where $\hat{\mu}_t$ is the value of the lowess line on day t.

To illustrate, consider the Hospital #7 respiratory syndrome data. Returning to Figure B.6, remember that the right plot is partially synthetic data generated via Equation B.2, which assumes a constant variance over time. Yet the variability of the actual data in the left plot of Figure B.6 does seem to change over time. In fact, it seems to change with the mean daily count, with the variability increasing with larger means and decreasing with smaller means.

In comparison, Figure B.8 is a plot of the actual data on the left plot versus partially synthetic data venerated using UTM3 with Poisson data randomly drawn with $\lambda_t = \hat{\mu}_t$ on the right. Here the partially synthetic data have the same property as the actual data, with the variability changing according to the mean count. This follows from the property of the Poisson distribution, where $\mathbb{E}(Y) = \text{Var}(Y) = \lambda$.

In Figure B.8, to capture as much of the underlying systematic variation in the actual data, the lowess line was fit with a very small f parameter ($f = 0.02 \approx 7/365$). The goal was for the $\hat{\mu}_t$ to capture the day effects as well as the larger seasonal effects. However, Figure B.8 does seem to show (as did other simulations) that the resulting partially synthetic data still are less variable than the original data. This is consistent with the results in Table B.1 and the associated discussion in the previous section.

However, as shown in Section B.1.1, the negative binomial distribution can be a good fit for biosurveillance count data because it allows for overdispersion.

The negative binomial has two parameters, p_t and r_t, where the subscript on the parameters is now used to denote that they change from time period to time period. The method-of-moments estimators for these parameters are based on the sample mean and variance. Thus, letting k denote the number of neighbors before time period t to include in the estimate, as well as the number of neighbors after time period t to include, estimate the sample mean and variance as:

$$\bar{y}_t = \frac{1}{2k+1} \sum_{j=t-k}^{t+k} y_j$$

and

$$s_t^2 = \frac{1}{2k} \sum_{j=t-k}^{t+k} \left(y_j - \bar{y}_t\right)^2.$$

Then, for day t, assume $Y_t \sim \text{NBin}(r_t, p_t)$, where the method-of-moments estimators are $\hat{p}_t = \bar{y}_t / s_t^2$ and $\hat{r}_t = \bar{y}_t^2 / (s_t^2 - \bar{y}_t)$. Because the estimator for r_t is defined only when $s_t^2 > \bar{y}_t$, when $s_t^2 \leq \bar{y}_t$, assume the data were generated from a Poisson distribution: $Y_t \sim \text{Pois}(\lambda_t)$ with $\hat{\lambda}_t = \bar{y}_t$.

The choice of k drives the smoothness in the sample mean and variance estimates. The larger k is set, the less they can change from time period to time period, the most extreme case being when k is set so that all the data are used to estimate $\bar{y}_t$ and s_t^2 for all t so that the estimates are all the same. On the other hand, the smaller k is set, the more variation is allowed between time periods. Of course, it must be that $k > 0$ so that the sample variance can be estimated. But it is also important to make k large enough so that the sample mean and sample variance are not overly affected by the period-to-period variation inherent in the data.

Figure B.9 plots the sample mean and variance for $k = 14$ along with two years of Hospital #7 data. Note that the sample mean estimate is reasonably smooth and the sample variance, although more variable, seems to appropriately reflect the underlying variability in the data, particularly in what look to be periods of increased GI activity, perhaps attributable to winter flu seasons. Choosing k as a multiple of 7 was purposeful and follows from the day effects seen in Section 2.2.2; the intention is to help ensure estimates are not biased up or down as a result of the inclusion or exclusion of certain days of the week in a given estimate. It is also possible to set $k = 7$, but an equivalent plot of Figure B.9 shows that at $k = 7$, the estimates of the mean start to get excessively variable. Similarly, $k = 21$ is possible, but the resulting simulated data look a little too oversmoothed. Thus, $k = 14$ seems to be the best choice for these data.

Note that in Figure B.9, there are periods when $s_t^2 \leq \bar{y}_t$ intermittently, particularly between days 400 and 500 or so, but additional smoothing results in $s_t^2 \approx \bar{y}_t$, and thus a Poisson distributional assumption seems like a reasonable choice for these periods. However, also note that for these data, although overdispersion is evident during periods when the mean incidence is high, which corresponds to winters and is likely the result of seasonal flu, there are also times when the mean

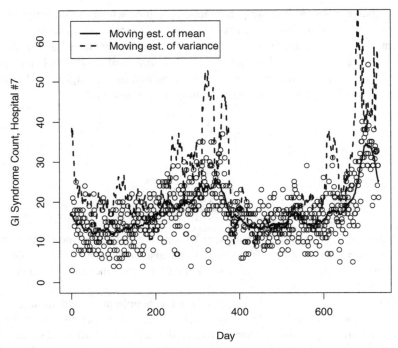

Figure B.9. Two years of Hospital #7 GI syndrome data with sample mean and variance overlayed. Sample means and variances for each day calculated using the data from the 2 weeks before and after (i.e., with $k = 14$).

rate is low and the data are still overdispersed (e.g., between days 1 and 150 or so). So, at least for this particular data, it does not seem reasonable to assume the data follow a Poisson distribution in the absence of outbreaks.

Given the estimates for the sample mean and variance for each day, it is now possible to fit the appropriate distribution with its estimated parameters and then randomly draw an observation for each day. Figure B.10 shows the results from one such simulation compared with the actual data. Note that the main features of the data, meaning the overall trends in the data, as well as the dispersion around the trends, look to be preserved. Unfortunately, one feature that is not preserved in this particular simulation is the day effects, which are essentially smoothed away because of the choice of $k = 14$.

Modeling Outbreaks

Given a preferred simulation methodology for the background incidence, outbreaks must also be modeled. If the form of the outbreak curve for a particular bio-agent is known, it can be incorporated into simulations based on Equations B.1 through B.3 by appropriately calculating the additive o_t terms from the outbreak curve for each day of the outbreak.

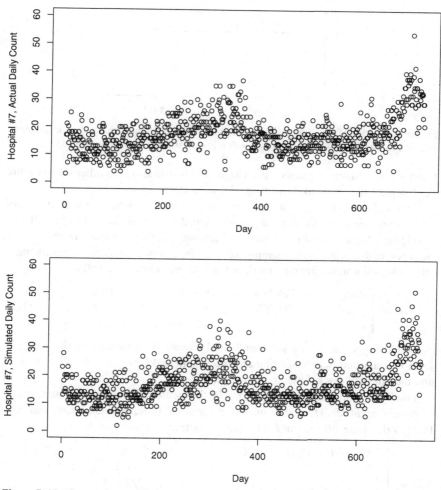

Figure B.10. Comparison of the actual data with one set of simulated data, where the data were simulated from a negative binomial with parameters based on the sample means and variances from Figure B.9.

Often, however, the outbreak curve is not known. In that case, the simulation may need to use a proxy functional form, the simplest of which is a jump increase in the mean for some duration of time. Assuming the outbreak is an additive term such as o_t in Equations B.1 through B.3, representing the mean outbreak level, define o_t as

$$o_t = M \times I\{\tau \leq t < \tau + D\}, \qquad (B.4)$$

where M is the average magnitude of the outbreak, D is the duration of the outbreak, τ is the starting time of the outbreak, and I is the indicator function.

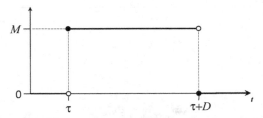

Figure B.11. Plot of the outbreak form from Equation B.4 where the outbreak is a jump increase in the mean of magnitude M for duration D starting on random day τ.

(An indicator function equals 1 if its argument is true and zero otherwise.) Figure B.11 depicts the outbreak form from Equation B.4.

Although jump changes in the mean are commonly assumed in statistical process control simulations, they are often viewed as unrealistic in biosurveillance simulations because outbreaks tend to increase and then decrease over time. To incorporate this feature most simply, keeping the parameterization of a peak magnitude M, a duration D, and a random start day τ, define o_t as follows:

$$
o_t = \begin{cases}
2M(t - \tau + 1)/(D + 1), & \tau - 1 < t \leq \tau + D/2 - 1 \\
2M(D + \tau - t)/(D + 1), & \tau + D/2 - 1 < t < \tau + D \\
0, & \text{otherwise.}
\end{cases} \tag{B.5}
$$

Although Equation B.5 looks complicated, Figure B.12 shows that the outbreak form is triangular, where starting at time τ, outbreaks increase linearly up to M and then linearly back down to zero at time $\tau + D$.

Finally, to combine these two forms, let the mean outbreak linearly increase up to some magnitude M, stay at that level for some time, denoted by m, and then linearly decrease, all for some duration D starting on a random day τ:

$$
o_t = \begin{cases}
2M(t - \tau + 1)/(D - m + 1), & \tau - 1 < t \leq \tau + (D - m)/2 - 1 \\
M, & \tau + (D - m)/2 - 1 < t \leq \tau \\
 & \quad + (D + m)/2 - 1 \\
2M(D + \tau - t)/(D - m + 1), & \tau + (D + m)/2 - 1 < t < \tau + D \\
0, & \text{otherwise.}
\end{cases}
$$

$$\tag{B.6}$$

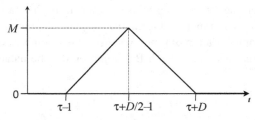

Figure B.12. Plot of the outbreak form from Equation B.5, where starting at time τ, the outbreak mean increases linearly up to M and then linearly back down to zero at time $\tau + D$.

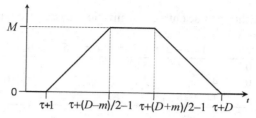

Figure B.13. Plot of the outbreak form from Equation B.6, where the outbreak mean linearly increases up to some magnitude M, stays at that level for some period m, and then linearly decreases, all for some duration D starting on a random day τ.

Figure B.13 depicts the form of the outbreak.

Of course, the form of the outbreak can be further modified and made more complex as desired.

Injecting Outbreaks in Actual Data

In biosurveillance research, outbreaks are often inserted into actual data (which is sometimes referred to as "injecting" outbreaks into data in the literature), generally by adding additional counts to an existing set of data, with the goal of analyzing the resulting combined data set to see how well one can find the injected outbreak. The point of this partially synthetic simulation approach is to preserve the real-world complexity of the actual data. Thus, a daily observation y_t^* is calculated as

$$y_t^* = y_t + o_t, \quad t = 1, 2, 3, \ldots, \tag{B.7}$$

where y_t is the observed (real) data and o_t is the injected outbreak for day t, and where $y_t^* = y_t$ except during an outbreak period.

Two types of outbreak insertions are possible, deterministic and stochastic. For deterministic outbreaks, a functional form for the outbreak is assumed (e.g., Equations B.4 through B.6, with the values rounded as necessary to produce integers), an outbreak start day is selected, perhaps randomly, and the outbreak values are added to the appropriate data values as in Equation B.8. For stochastic outbreaks, a functional form is assumed with some parameter or parameters of the outbreak distribution, and then for each day of the outbreak a random observation is drawn from the outbreak distribution.

Example B.5. Simulate three outbreaks for which Equation B.6, with $M = 4$, $m = 3$, and $D = 10$, appropriately models the mean of the outbreak distribution, where the outbreak counts follow a Poisson distribution.

Solution: Plugging the parameters into Equation B.6 gives:

t:	$\tau - 1$	τ	$\tau+1$	$\tau+2$	$\tau+3$	$\tau+4$	$\tau+5$	$\tau+6$	$\tau+7$	$\tau+8$	$\tau+9$
o_t:	0	1	2	3	4	4	4	3	2	1	0

The table below shows three outbreak realizations based on random draws from a Poisson, where $\lambda_t = o_t$.

t:	$\tau-1$	τ	$\tau+1$	$\tau+2$	$\tau+3$	$\tau+4$	$\tau+5$	$\tau+6$	$\tau+7$	$\tau+8$	$\tau+9$
$o'_t\#1:$	0	0	3	4	5	3	6	4	2	0	0
$o'_t\#2:$	0	0	4	3	2	3	7	5	0	3	0
$o'_t\#3:$	0	1	1	5	2	9	5	7	1	1	0

B.2.2 Multivariate Temporal Data Simulations

In the absence of correlation between, say, m time series,[2] then an appropriate simulation approach is to apply one of the univariate methods separately to each time series. However, if there is correlation between the time series, then this approach will not preserve the correlation, meaning it will tend to result in correlations between the time series that are less than what is in the actual data. In this situation, the correlation in the data must be accounted for and, as with the univariate simulations, this can be accomplished either by explicitly modeling the data features or by modeling the distributional parameters. This section begins by generalizing the UTM1 method for multivariate data and then proceeds through generalizations of the UTM2 and UTM3 simulation methods.

Explicitly Modeling Data Features

As with the univariate methods, a completely synthetic approach is to construct a model with terms for each of the structural components of the data (e.g., seasonal cycle, day effects). A generalization of the UTM1 method, it will be referred to as the *Multivariate Temporal Method #1* (MTM1). Alternatively, *Multivariate Temporal Method #2* (MTM2) is a generalization of UTM2, using smoothing splines calculated from real data to capture the underlying general trends and features.

MTM1 proceeds as follows. Simulate a daily observation $\mathbf{Y}_t = \{Y_{t1}, \ldots, Y_{tm}\}$ as

$$\mathbf{Y}_t = \max(0, \lceil \boldsymbol{\mu} + \boldsymbol{\gamma}_t + \boldsymbol{\theta}_t + \boldsymbol{\delta}_t + \mathbf{o}_t + \mathbf{Z}_t \rceil), \quad t = 1, 2, 3, \ldots, \quad \text{(B.8)}$$

where, as in the univariate case,

- $\boldsymbol{\mu}$ is the vector of mean level of disease incidence;
- $\boldsymbol{\gamma}$ is the vector of seasonal deviations;
- $\boldsymbol{\theta}$ is the vector of within-season or other such periodic deviations;
- $\boldsymbol{\delta}$ is the vector of day-of-the-week effects;
- $\mathbf{o}$ is the vector of mean outbreak levels; and

---

[2] The generic term "time series" is used because the data may be of various types. For example, each time series could be for the same syndrome but from different locations (e.g., hospitals, clinics) or each time series could be a different syndrome from the same location.

- Z is the vector of random noise around the systematic component,

where the ceiling and maximum functions are taken componentwise.

Assuming the seasonal effect is a sinusoid, set $\gamma_{tj} = A_j[\sin(2\pi(t + \tau_j)/365)]$ and $\theta_{tj} = B_j[\sin(2\pi(t + \nu_j)/b_j)]$, where A_j is the maximum deviation from μ_j for the jth time series and B_j is the maximum deviation from $\mu_j + \gamma_{tj}$. So that all the time series are not on exactly the same cycle (which would induce very high correlation between them), τ_j and ν_j are random integers drawn according to some distribution, perhaps uniform. Assume $Z_t \sim N_m(0, \Sigma)$, where Σ may be estimated from some actual data or assumed as desired. As before, the day effect is the systematic deviation from $\mu_j + \gamma_{tj} + \theta_{tj}$, where $\delta_{tj} = \delta_{tj+7}$ for all t and j.

Example B.6. Using MTM1, simulate the GI hospital syndrome data.

Solution: The following model parameters were estimated from the data

	μ	A	B	b
Hospital #1	22.9	2.4	0.8	120
Hospital #2	3.4	0.0	0.3	183
Hospital #3	6.8	0.0	0.5	150
Hospital #4	13.3	0.0	0.6	91.25
Hospital #5	11.9	2.4	0.8	100
Hospital #6	9.5	0.0	0.5	183
Hospital #7	17.5	10.1	3.0	50

and $\hat{\Sigma}$ was estimated using residuals from univariate lowess smoothing splines. Then the data were generated according to Equation B.8 using random start times $\tau_j \sim U(-50, 50)$ and $\nu_j \sim U(-30, 30)$ (whose distributions were chosen essentially for convenience) and random noise $Z_t \sim N_m(0, \hat{\Sigma})$.

Figure B.14 compares the results of one simulation using smoothing splines fit to the simulated data (bottom plot) with the actual data (top plot), where the resulting simulated data have general features and trends similar to the original data. Also, the correlations between hospitals in the simulated data, as shown in Table B.2, are similar to the actual correlations as shown in Table B.3.

As the example shows, this approach can be used to simulate data that are similar to actual data, but it also gives the modeler the flexibility to explore excursions, such as if the annual cycles are greater or smaller, for example. In addition, note that the sinusoids were used because they can be defined with a small number of parameters; however, their functional shape may be too simplistic for some modelers. If that is the case, nothing in this approach precludes the modeler from substituting in some other function, such as using smoothing splines to replace the $\mu + \gamma_t + \theta_t$ term.

Gastrointestinal Syndrome

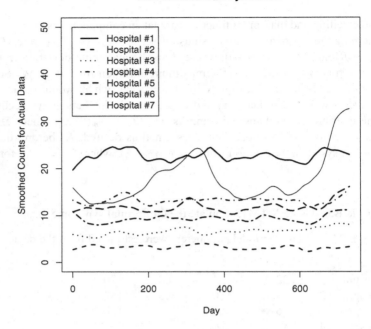

Gastrointestinal Syndrome

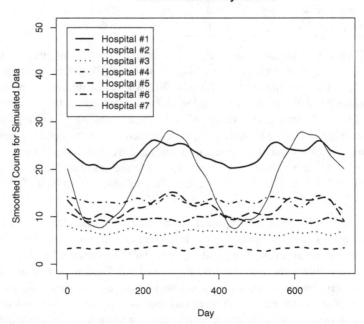

Figure B.14. Results of a multivariate simulation of the hospital GI syndrome data using MTM1. The general features and trends in the actual data (top plot) are preserved in the simulation (bottom plot).

Table B.2. Simulated GI syndrome daily count correlation matrix for the seven metropolitan hospitals. Comparing the simulation results with the actual correlations (see Table B.3) shows that this implementation has increased the pairwise correlations compared with the original data

	Hospital #1	Hospital #2	Hospital #3	Hospital #4	Hospital #5	Hospital #6	Hospital #7
Hospital #1	1.00	0.05	0.02	0.15	0.16	0.10	0.33
Hospital #2		1.00	−0.03	0.11	0.03	0.12	0.00
Hospital #3			1.00	0.05	0.07	0.06	0.05
Hospital #4				1.00	0.10	0.06	0.03
Hospital #5					1.00	0.02	0.37
Hospital #6						1.00	0.08
Hospital #7							1.00

MTM2 is a partially synthetic simulation method. As with the UTM2, the first step is to model the daily means using some type of smoothing spline, such as lowess. Let $\hat{\mu}_{tj}$ denote the estimated mean on day t for time series j, $t = 1, \ldots, n$ and $j = 1, \ldots, m$. For each day and each time series, also calculate the estimated residuals, $\hat{\epsilon}_{tj} = y_{tj} - \hat{\mu}_{tj}$, and calculate the sample covariance matrix of the residuals, $\hat{\Sigma}$. Then, for $\hat{\boldsymbol{\mu}}_t = \{\hat{\mu}_{t1}, \ldots, \hat{\mu}_{tm}\}$, simulate new observations $\mathbf{Y}_t = \{Y_{t1}, \ldots, Y_{tm}\}$ as

$$\mathbf{Y}_t = \max\left(\mathbf{0}, \lceil\hat{\boldsymbol{\mu}}_t + \mathbf{Z}_t\rceil\right), \tag{B.9}$$

where $\mathbf{Z}_t \sim N_m(\mathbf{0}, \hat{\Sigma})$.

This approach is very much like the univariate approach. However, the smoothing splines generated from the data preserve whatever general features and trends are present in the original data, including whatever correlation between the time series that is attributable to how these trends occurred over time. In addition, the simulated random errors $\mathbf{Z}_t$ preserve the data correlation structure. Not preserved in this approach are structural features that occur on a time scale smaller than the smoothing constant.

Table B.3. Actual GI syndrome daily count correlation matrix for the seven metropolitan hospitals

	Hospital #1	Hospital #2	Hospital #3	Hospital #4	Hospital #5	Hospital #6	Hospital #7
Hospital #1	1.00	0.08	0.04	0.15	0.09	0.09	0.13
Hospital #2		1.00	−0.05	0.04	0.04	0.06	0.03
Hospital #3			1.00	0.06	0.17	0.07	0.19
Hospital #4				1.00	0.05	0.09	0.07
Hospital #5					1.00	0.06	0.25
Hospital #6						1.00	0.16
Hospital #7							1.00

Gastrointestinal Syndrome

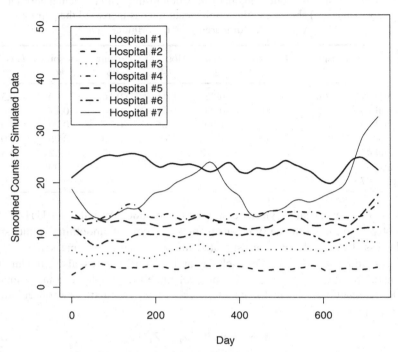

Figure B.15. Results of a multivariate simulation of the hospital GI data using Equation B.9. The general features and trends in the actual data are preserved in the simulation compared with the actual data (see the top plot of Figure B.14).

Example B.7. Returning to the hospital data to simulate two years of GI syndrome data, simulate the data using Equation B.9.

Solution: To simulate, proceed first by fitting a lowess smoothing spline (with $f = 0.1$) to each of the time series, calculating the residuals and their associated covariance matrix, and then simulating the data per Equation B.9. Figure B.15 summarizes the results of one simulation and shows that the resulting simulated data have preserved the general features and trends of the original data (compare with the top plot in Fig. B.14). In addition, the correlations between the hospitals are preserved, as shown in Table B.4 (compare with the table of actual correlations in Table B.3).

Modeling Distributional Parameters

MTM3, as with the UTM3 method, models distributional parameters from which random observations are drawn to simulate the data. One approach is to model the joint distribution of data, but that will likely prove to be too difficult. Instead,

Table B.4. Simulated GI syndrome daily count correlation matrix for the seven metropolitan hospitals. Comparing the simulation results with Table B.3 shows that the correlation structure in the simulated data is similar to the correlation structure of the actual data

	Hospital #1	Hospital #2	Hospital #3	Hospital #4	Hospital #5	Hospital #6	Hospital #7
Hospital #1	1.00	0.10	0.08	0.14	0.08	0.10	0.07
Hospital #2		1.00	−0.11	0.00	0.03	0.09	0.01
Hospital #3			1.00	0.11	0.20	0.05	0.19
Hospital #4				1.00	0.06	0.09	0.02
Hospital #5					1.00	0.02	0.19
Hospital #6						1.00	0.14
Hospital #7							1.00

the MTM3 retains the correlation in the data by conducting the simulation in two stages: first, simulate the aggregate number of individuals who get sick on a given day and then appropriately randomly apportion them to the hospitals.

Think about the approach as follows: Imagine a region for which there are m locations each reporting data on the population, so there are m time series being monitored. For example, consider the hospital data where seven GI syndrome time series are being monitored, one at each hospital. These hospitals are all collecting data from one large metropolitan area, from which on any given day (t), some number of individuals (N_t) in the population come down with GI syndrome symptoms of sufficient severity that they seek medical attention. Of these N_t, some fractions go to each hospital. Thus, the data are correlated by the total number of individuals with GI syndrome.

So, begin much as in the univariate case, except that first a distribution is fit to the total number of observations per period. That is, first add all the time series together by time period to create an aggregate time series, $N_1, \ldots, N_n$, $N_t = \sum_{j=1}^{m} y_{tj}$, where y_{tj} is the count for day t and time series j. Given the aggregate time series, fit a negative binomial distribution for each time period, as was done in Section B.2.1 for the univariate time series, and draw a random observation for each day. This then is the simulated aggregate time series for that syndrome: $(\hat{N}_1, \ldots, \hat{N}_n)$.

In the second step, use the multinomial distribution to apportion the aggregate count to the individual hospitals. The multinomial probability mass function for day t is

$$\mathbb{P}(Y_{t1} = y_{t1}, \ldots, Y_{tm} = y_{tm}) = \frac{N_t!}{y_{t1}! \cdots y_{tm}!} p_{t1}^{y_{t1}} \cdots p_{tm}^{y_{tm}}, \qquad (\text{B}.10)$$

for $y_{t1}, \ldots, y_{tm}$ non-negative integers with $\sum_{j=1}^{m} y_{tj} = N_t$. To implement this, first estimate $p_{t1}, \ldots, p_{tm}$, the daily probabilities that a sick individual goes to each hospital. For some smoothing constant k, estimate the probabilities for day t

as

$$\hat{p}_{tj} = \frac{\sum_{s=t-k}^{t+k} y_{sj}}{\sum_{s=t-k}^{t+k} \sum_{j=1}^{m} y_{sj}}, \quad j = 1, \ldots, m.$$

Finally, using $\hat{N}_t$ and $\hat{p}_{t1}, \ldots, \hat{p}_{tm}$ in Equation B.10, use a software package to generate the simulated counts for day t.

If a multinomial function is not available, the counts can be generated as a series of random draws from appropriate binomial distributions as follows. First, draw $\hat{N}_{t1}$, the simulated aggregate number of individuals on day t for Hospital #1, according to a Bin($\hat{N}_t$, $\hat{p}_{t1}$), and then recursively for $j = 2, \ldots, m$ draw $\hat{N}_{tj}$ according to a Bin $\left(\hat{N}_t - \sum_{s=1}^{j-1} \hat{N}_{ts}, \hat{p}_{tj} / \left(1 - \sum_{s=1}^{j-1} \hat{p}_{tj} \right) \right)$.

Example B.8. Using MTM3, simulate 2 years of the hospital GI syndrome data, 1 year of which is shown in Chapter 2 and that demonstrates mild positive correlation between the hospitals.

Solution: Using the MTM3 with $k = 14$, Figure B.16 shows the smoothed counts for the actual data (top) and the smoothed counts from one simulation (bottom). Note how the simulation preserved the general features and trends in the data. In addition, comparing the correlations from the simulated data in the table below with the correlation of the actual correlations in Table B.3 shows that the correlation structure is very similar.

	Hospital #1	Hospital #2	Hospital #3	Hospital #4	Hospital #5	Hospital #6	Hospital #7
Hospital #1	1.00	0.12	0.05	0.20	0.06	0.11	0.06
Hospital #2		1.00	−0.02	0.08	0.04	0.06	0.00
Hospital #3			1.00	0.03	0.07	0.07	0.16
Hospital #4				1.00	0.11	0.12	0.11
Hospital #5					1.00	0.21	0.22
Hospital #6						1.00	0.14
Hospital #7							1.00

So, as with the UTM1, UTM2, and UTM3 methods, the MTM1, MTM2, and MTM3 methods provide a continuum of simulation approaches, from completely synthetic to partially synthetic that mimics many of the features of an actual data set. Depending on the purpose of the simulation, the way MTM2 and MTM3 simulation methods explicitly reproduce the trends and features of the actual data may or may not be desirable. For example, closely mimicking the data may be desirable if the goal is to assess how a particular early event detection (EED) algorithm would work for under conditions that are similar to, but not precisely the same as, an actual set of data. Mimicking can also be useful for sharing data sets with specific features, particularly when the actual data cannot be shared. On the other hand, if the goal is to assess the performance of an EED algorithm

Gastrointestinal Syndrome

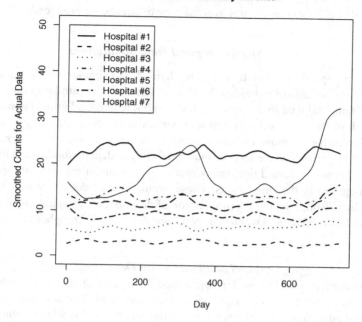

Gastrointestinal Syndrome

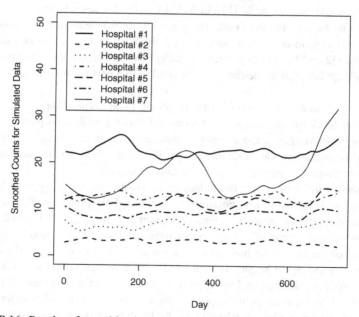

Figure B.16. Results of a multivariate simulation based on the modeling distributional parameters approach. The general features and trends in the actual data (top plot) are preserved in the simulation (bottom plot).

under a wide set of conditions, then one might prefer a simulation method such as MTM1 that allows more control over the type of data being produced.

B.2.3 Spatio-temporal Data Simulations

Spatio-temporal data simulations can be divided into simulations of aggregated data and simulations of individual-level data. The former is similar to the simulations of temporal data in the previous sections but with the additional complexity that each of the time series is tied to a particular location and the spatial configuration of the locations imparts a structure to the data. In contrast, simulating spatio-temporal data at the level of individual entities departs fundamentally from the simulations discussed thus far, particularly in terms of the level of modeling detail required in the simulations. These simulations model entire populations, person by person, tracking the progression of disease through space and time and tracking how, where, and when symptoms are manifested throughout the population.

Aggregate-Level Spatio-temporal Data Simulations

Spatio-temporal simulations for aggregated data can use the same techniques as the multivariate temporal methods already discussed. The fundamental issue that must be addressed in choosing an appropriate method is whether the spatial locations of the aggregated data are manifested only in the correlation of the residuals or whether the systematic components are also associated in some way. If it is both, then either the MTM2 or MTM3 method is appropriate because they both mimic the correlation in both the systematic components of the original data and the correlation in the residuals. Indeed, the hospital GI syndrome data used in the MTM2 and MTM3 examples are really an example of spatio-temporal data because each hospital in the data is associated with a particular location.

Individual-Level Spatio-temporal Data Simulations

Individual-level simulations attempt to model entire populations person by person. For biosurveillance, these types of simulations generally involve a series of detailed simulation models that interact to, ultimately, quantify the outcomes of a bioterrorist attack or natural disease outbreak in space and time.

As shown in Figure B.17, individual-level simulations begin by modeling the location and behavior of a population. Such a simulation may involve modeling how the population moves and interacts over time, either at the individual person level or by some type of group aggregation. The simulation also models the dispersal of the disease or bio-agent in space and time. For example, the aerosol release of a bio-agent might be simulated with a plume model that takes into account specific weather and wind patterns to estimate the dispersal of the bio-agent and thus the amount of exposure each member of the population has to the bio-agent. The dispersal model will vary by the type of disease or bio-agent and the specific scenario governing how it is distributed among the population.

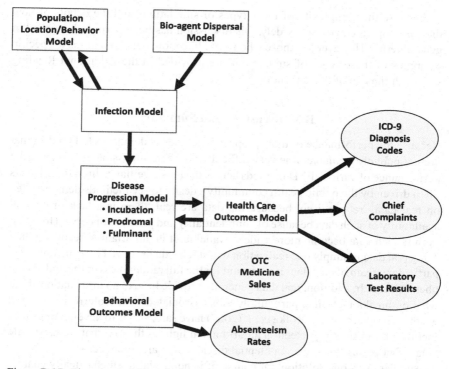

Figure B.17. Flowchart of the major steps in an individual-level spatio-temporal biosurveil-lance simulation. OTC, over-the-counter.

These two model outputs are then inputs into an infection model that estimates the dosage received by various members of the population and thus who is infected. For a contagious disease or bio-agent, the infection model must iterate with the population location and behavior model to simulate the spread of infection among the population as it moves and interacts over time. After infection, the disease progression model simulates how the disease or bio-agent manifests in each member of the population, and the treatment and health care outcomes model simulates each individual's health care–seeking behavior and the outcomes of their interaction with the health care system. Assuming medical treatment has an impact on disease progression, the treatment and health care outcomes model should interact with the disease progression model.

Ultimately, the simulation results in the quantification of various health outcomes, such as the number and types of diagnoses, chief complaints, and laboratory results, over time and location. Again, this could be at the level of each individual in the population or at some aggregate level, say by hospital or other health care facility. The simulation may also simulate other outcomes such as OTC medicine sales or absenteeism.

Because the complexity of these types of simulations and the details of how they are implemented vary widely, this discussion has been purposed couched in general terms. However, for those who would like more detail, citations to specific examples of these types of simulations are provided in the Additional Reading section at the end of this appendix.

B.3 Discussion and Summary

Because the performance of most proposed methods is demonstrated on data that are not publicly available, it is very difficult and often impossible to compare the performance of various EED methods across the biosurveillance literature. This is often driven by the public health community's desire to see methods demonstrated on real data. Yet precisely because the data are real, there is a lack of general availability of such data because of confidentiality and privacy concerns. However, even if such data become more widely available, it is important to recognize that using real data is simply one realization of a stochastic process. Focusing only on a particular stream of data does not account for the full randomness of the underlying phenomenon. In addition, real data generally provide little to no information about what outbreaks look like, particularly those associated with bioterrorism-related events. The challenge, as Rolka *et al.* (2007) have said, ". . . is to develop improved methods for evaluating detection algorithms in light of the fact that we have little data about outbreaks of many potential diseases that are of concern."

Simulation is one solution. Of course, it is nontrivial to stochastically characterize, and thus simulate, all the detailed characteristics of the normal or baseline state of disease incidence, as well as the various outbreak conditions. However, this appendix has demonstrated simulation techniques that are able to mimic aggregate biosurveillance data well. These types of simulations are useful for:

- evaluating biosurveillance systems and algorithms across many scenarios;
- allowing clean and clear comparisons between systems and algorithms; and
- making it easier to get at generalizable conclusions or results.

This appendix also described the steps in simulations that model at the individual person or entity level. These simulations can be useful in situations where little is known about how an outbreak will manifest in the population. In addition, modeling at the individual level is often attractive because the added detail makes the simulation seem more accurate. However, a couple of cautions are in order. First, more detail in a simulation does *not* necessarily result in a more accurate or more realistic simulation. This is because assumptions must be made at each step in a simulation – the more steps in the simulation, the more assumptions, some of which may be based on little information or made for computational convenience. These assumptions can potentially interact and compound in ways that result in simulation output that may be less accurate or realistic than a simpler simulation's results. Second, in simulations with excessive detail, it can be hard (sometimes virtually impossible) to determine how the simulation results are affected by or related to the simulation inputs. In such cases, it can be difficult to reach definitive conclusions about the cause of an observed effect, and that is often the whole point in doing the simulation in the first place.

B.3.1 Additional Reading

The papers listed below discuss various aspects of biosurveillance simulation or describe other simulation approaches.

- "Generating Synthetic Syndromic-Surveillance Data for Evaluating Visual-Analytics Techniques" (Maciejewski et al., 2009) describes a methodology using lowess to model annual, seasonal, and day-of-the-week systematic components from syndromic surveillance data. It also describes a kernel density estimation-based method for simulating spatio-temporal data.
- "Simulating Multivariate Syndromic Time Series and Outbreak Signatures" (Lotze et al., 2007) proposes a simulation method similar in spirit to MTM2 but differing in implementation details.

Below are examples of biosurveillance-related simulations published in the literature.

- Completely synthetic temporal simulations: Fricker et al. (2008a) and Hutwagner et al. (2005)
- Partially synthetic temporal simulations: Maciejewski et al. (2009) and Lotze et al. (2007)
- Evaluations based in injecting outbreaks into actual data: Burkom et al. (2006), Stoto et al. (2006), and Goldenberg et al. (2002).
- Aggregate-level multivariate or spatio-temporal simulations: Fricker et al. (2008b)
- Individual-level spatio-temporal simulations: Maciejewski et al. (2009), Clarke et al. (2007), Buckeridge et al. (2006), Coberly et al. (2006), Buckeridge et al. (2004), and Kleinman et al. (2005)

C

Tables

The scientist has a lot of experience with ignorance and doubt and uncertainty, and this experience is of very great importance, I think. When a scientist doesn't know the answer to a problem, he is ignorant. When he has a hunch as to what the result is, he is uncertain. And when he is pretty darn sure of what the result is going to be, he is in some doubt. We have found it of paramount importance that in order to progress we must recognize ignorance and leave room for doubt. Scientific knowledge is a body of statements of varying degrees of certainty – most unsure, some nearly sure, none absolutely certain.

Richard P. Feynman (1918–1988)

This appendix contains tables of thresholds (h) to achieve various average times between false signal (ATFS) for the χ^2, multivariate cumulative sum (MCUSUM), and multivariate exponentially weighted moving average (MEWMA) detection methods. See Chapter 8 for descriptions of the methods.

Hotelling's χ^2 Detection Method Tables

The following tables provide thresholds to achieve the specified ATFS values for the χ^2 detection method with dimensions $p = 3, 4, \ldots, 10, 15$, and 20. See Table 8.2 on page 225 for $p = 2$. The thresholds in these tables are for data distributed $N_p(\mathbf{0}, \boldsymbol{\Sigma})$, where

$$
\boldsymbol{\Sigma} = \begin{pmatrix} 1 & \rho & \rho & \cdots \\ \rho & 1 & \rho & \cdots \\ \rho & \rho & 1 & \\ \vdots & \vdots & & \ddots \end{pmatrix}.
$$

To read the tables, enter with the desired ATFS and value of ρ that most closely matches the data and then read off the threshold value h. The thresholds achieve the specified ATFS values with standard errors of less than 0.1.

HOTELLING χ^2 THRESHOLDS (h) FOR $p = 3$

ρ	0.0	0.1	0.2	0.3	0.4	0.5	0.6	0.7	0.8	0.9
ATFS										
30	8.4	8.4	8.3	8.2	8.2	8.1	8.0	7.9	7.8	7.6
60	9.9	9.9	9.8	9.8	9.7	9.6	9.5	9.4	9.3	9.1
91	10.9	10.8	10.7	10.7	10.6	10.5	10.4	10.3	10.2	10.1
182	12.3	12.3	12.2	12.2	12.1	12.0	11.9	11.8	11.7	11.6
273	13.2	13.2	13.1	13.0	13.0	12.9	12.8	12.7	12.6	12.4
365	13.9	13.8	13.7	13.7	13.6	13.5	13.4	13.3	13.2	13.1

HOTELLING χ^2 THRESHOLDS (h) FOR $p = 4$

ρ	0.0	0.1	0.2	0.3	0.4	0.5	0.6	0.7	0.8	0.9
ATFS										
30	10.3	10.2	10.2	10.1	10.0	9.9	9.8	9.7	9.6	9.4
60	11.9	11.9	11.8	11.7	11.7	11.6	11.5	11.4	11.2	11.0
91	12.9	12.9	12.8	12.7	12.6	12.6	12.5	12.3	12.2	12.0
182	14.5	14.5	14.4	14.3	14.2	14.1	14.1	13.9	13.8	13.6
273	15.4	15.4	15.3	15.2	15.1	15.1	15.0	14.9	14.7	14.5
365	16.1	16.0	15.9	15.9	15.8	15.7	15.6	15.5	15.4	15.2

HOTELLING χ^2 THRESHOLDS (h) FOR $p = 5$

ρ	0.0	0.1	0.2	0.3	0.4	0.5	0.6	0.7	0.8	0.9
ATFS										
30	12.0	12.0	11.9	11.8	11.7	11.6	11.5	11.4	11.2	11.0
60	13.8	13.7	13.7	13.6	13.5	13.4	13.3	13.2	13.0	12.8
91	14.8	14.7	14.6	14.6	14.5	14.4	14.3	14.2	14.0	13.8
182	16.5	16.4	16.4	16.3	16.2	16.1	16.0	15.9	15.7	15.5
273	17.4	17.3	17.3	17.2	17.2	17.1	17.0	16.8	16.7	16.4
365	18.1	18.1	18.0	17.9	17.8	17.8	17.7	17.5	17.4	17.2

HOTELLING χ^2 THRESHOLDS (h) FOR $p = 6$

ρ	0.0	0.1	0.2	0.3	0.4	0.5	0.6	0.7	0.8	0.9
ATFS										
30	13.6	13.6	13.5	13.5	13.4	13.3	13.2	13.0	12.8	12.6
60	15.5	15.4	15.4	15.3	15.2	15.1	15.0	14.8	14.7	14.4
91	16.5	16.5	16.4	16.4	16.3	16.2	16.1	15.9	15.8	15.5
182	18.3	18.3	18.2	18.1	18.0	17.9	17.8	17.7	17.5	17.3
273	19.3	19.2	19.2	19.1	19.1	18.9	18.8	18.7	18.5	18.3
365	20.0	19.9	19.9	19.8	19.7	19.7	19.5	19.4	19.3	19.0

HOTELLING χ^2 THRESHOLDS (h) FOR $p = 7$

ρ	0.0	0.1	0.2	0.3	0.4	0.5	0.6	0.7	0.8	0.9
ATFS										
30	15.2	15.2	15.1	15.0	15.0	14.8	14.7	14.6	14.4	14.1
60	17.1	17.1	17.0	16.9	16.9	16.8	16.6	16.5	16.3	16.0
91	18.2	18.2	18.1	18.1	18.0	17.9	17.8	17.6	17.4	17.2
182	20.0	20.0	19.9	19.9	19.8	19.7	19.6	19.5	19.3	19.0
273	21.1	21.0	21.0	20.9	20.8	20.7	20.6	20.5	20.3	20.1
365	21.8	21.8	21.7	21.6	21.6	21.5	21.4	21.2	21.1	20.8

HOTELLING χ^2 THRESHOLDS (h) FOR $p = 8$

ρ	0.0	0.1	0.2	0.3	0.4	0.5	0.6	0.7	0.8	0.9
ATFS										
30	16.7	16.7	16.6	16.6	16.5	16.4	16.3	16.1	15.9	15.6
60	18.7	18.6	18.6	18.5	18.5	18.4	18.2	18.1	17.9	17.6
91	19.8	19.8	19.7	19.7	19.6	19.5	19.4	19.2	19.1	18.8
182	21.7	21.7	21.6	21.6	21.5	21.4	21.3	21.1	21.0	20.7
273	22.8	22.7	22.7	22.7	22.6	22.5	22.4	22.2	22.1	21.8
365	23.5	23.5	23.5	23.4	23.4	23.2	23.1	23.0	22.8	22.5

HOTELLING χ^2 THRESHOLDS (h) FOR $p = 9$

ρ	0.0	0.1	0.2	0.3	0.4	0.5	0.6	0.7	0.8	0.9
ATFS										
30	18.2	18.1	18.1	18.0	18.0	17.9	17.7	17.5	17.3	17.0
60	20.2	20.2	20.1	20.1	20.0	19.9	19.8	19.6	19.4	19.1
91	21.4	21.4	21.3	21.3	21.2	21.1	21.0	20.8	20.6	20.3
182	23.3	23.3	23.3	23.2	23.1	23.0	22.9	22.8	22.6	22.3
273	24.4	24.4	24.4	24.3	24.3	24.2	24.0	23.9	23.7	23.4
365	25.2	25.2	25.2	25.1	25.0	24.9	24.8	24.7	24.5	24.2

HOTELLING χ^2 THRESHOLDS (h) FOR $p = 10$

ρ	0.0	0.1	0.2	0.3	0.4	0.5	0.6	0.7	0.8	0.9
ATFS										
30	19.6	19.6	19.5	19.5	19.4	19.3	19.2	19.0	18.8	18.4
60	21.7	21.7	21.6	21.6	21.5	21.4	21.3	21.1	20.9	20.6
91	22.9	22.9	22.9	22.8	22.8	22.7	22.5	22.4	22.2	21.9
182	24.9	24.9	24.9	24.8	24.7	24.7	24.5	24.4	24.2	23.9
273	26.1	26.0	26.0	25.9	25.9	25.8	25.7	25.5	25.3	25.0
365	26.8	26.8	26.8	26.8	26.7	26.6	26.5	26.4	26.1	25.8

HOTELLING χ^2 THRESHOLDS (h) FOR $p = 15$

ρ	0.0	0.1	0.2	0.3	0.4	0.5	0.6	0.7	0.8	0.9
ATFS										
30	26.5	26.5	26.5	26.4	26.3	26.2	26.1	25.9	25.7	25.3
60	28.9	28.9	28.8	28.8	28.8	28.7	28.5	28.4	28.1	27.7
91	30.3	30.3	30.2	30.2	30.1	30.0	29.9	29.8	29.5	29.2
182	32.5	32.5	32.5	32.5	32.4	32.3	32.2	32.0	31.8	31.5
273	33.8	33.8	33.8	33.7	33.7	33.6	33.5	33.3	33.1	32.7
365	34.7	34.7	34.7	34.6	34.6	34.4	34.3	34.2	34.0	33.7

HOTELLING χ^2 THRESHOLDS (h) FOR $p = 20$

ρ	0.0	0.1	0.2	0.3	0.4	0.5	0.6	0.7	0.8	0.9
ATFS										
30	33.1	33.0	33.0	33.0	32.9	32.9	32.7	32.5	32.3	31.8
60	35.7	35.7	35.7	35.6	35.6	35.5	35.4	35.2	34.9	34.5
91	37.2	37.2	37.2	37.2	37.1	37.0	36.9	36.8	36.5	36.1
182	39.7	39.7	39.7	39.6	39.6	39.5	39.4	39.2	39.0	38.5
273	41.1	41.1	41.1	41.0	41.0	40.9	40.8	40.6	40.4	40.0
365	42.0	42.0	42.0	42.0	41.9	41.9	41.8	41.6	41.3	41.0

Multivariate Exponentially Weighted Moving Average Detection Method Tables

The following tables provide estimated thresholds to achieve various ATFS as a function of λ and h for the MEWMA detection method for dimensions $p = 3, 4, \ldots, 10, 15$, and 20. See Table 8.4 on page 238 for $p = 2$. As with the χ^2 detection method, the thresholds in these tables are for data distributed $N_p(\mathbf{0}, \mathbf{I})$.

To use the tables, read down the chosen λ column until an ATFS value close to that desired is reached. Then read across to the left to find the threshold h. The thresholds achieve the specified ATFS values with standard errors of less than 0.1.

MEWMA ATFS FOR $p = 3$

λ	0.1	0.2	0.3	0.4	0.5	0.6	0.7	0.8	0.9
h									
1.0	5.1	3.5	2.9	2.6	2.4	2.3	2.3	2.2	2.2
2.0	9.4	6.1	5.0	4.3	3.9	3.8	3.6	3.6	3.6
3.0	15.0	9.6	7.8	6.8	6.3	5.8	5.7	5.7	5.8
4.0	22.4	14.6	11.6	10.4	9.5	9.1	8.9	9.1	9.3
5.0	32.7	21.4	17.4	15.5	14.5	14.0	14.0	14.3	15.0
6.0	46.9	31.3	25.9	23.4	22.1	21.6	21.9	22.6	24.0
7.0	67.6	45.5	38.5	35.3	34.0	33.7	34.2	35.8	38.5
8.0	97.5	67.5	58.0	53.8	52.3	52.4	53.9	57.0	61.8
9.0	142.2	100.3	87.4	82.7	81.5	82.4	85.5	91.0	99.6
10.0	208.8	150.4	133.4	127.9	127.7	130.6	136.3	145.7	160.6
11.0	308.6	227.6	205.3	199.6	201.3	207.6	217.9	234.1	259.4
12.0	460.9	347.3	318.2	312.9	318.9	330.9	349.2	376.8	419.0

MEWMA ATFS FOR $p = 4$

λ	0.1	0.2	0.3	0.4	0.5	0.6	0.7	0.8	0.9
h									
1.0	4.0	2.7	2.3	2.1	1.9	1.8	1.8	1.8	1.7
2.0	7.1	4.6	3.7	3.1	3.0	2.8	2.7	2.7	2.7
3.0	10.8	7.1	5.6	4.9	4.5	4.2	4.1	4.1	4.1
4.0	15.4	10.1	8.0	7.1	6.4	6.1	6.0	6.0	6.2
5.0	21.7	14.1	11.4	10.1	9.4	9.1	9.0	9.1	9.5
6.0	30.2	19.8	16.3	14.6	13.7	13.4	13.4	13.8	14.6
7.0	41.7	27.9	23.2	21.1	20.1	19.8	20.2	21.1	22.7
8.0	57.7	39.6	33.5	30.7	29.7	29.8	30.6	32.3	35.0
9.0	80.7	56.0	48.4	45.3	44.7	45.1	47.0	50.1	54.8
10.0	113.1	80.8	71.0	67.7	67.2	68.8	72.1	77.6	86.0
11.0	160.7	117.1	105.0	101.5	102.3	105.8	111.8	121.0	135.2
12.0	230.6	172.0	156.7	154.0	156.9	163.8	174.3	189.8	213.4
13.0	334.1	254.9	236.2	235.4	242.0	254.7	272.7	298.6	337.4
14.0	489.2	381.3	359.2	361.7	376.2	398.3	428.4	470.9	534.4

MEWMA ATFS FOR $p = 5$

λ	0.1	0.2	0.3	0.4	0.5	0.6	0.7	0.8	0.9
h									
1.0	3.3	2.2	1.9	1.8	1.6	1.6	1.6	1.5	1.5
2.0	5.7	3.8	3.0	2.6	2.4	2.3	2.2	2.1	2.1
3.0	8.4	5.5	4.3	3.7	3.5	3.2	3.1	3.1	3.1
4.0	11.8	7.6	6.1	5.2	4.8	4.6	4.5	4.4	4.5
5.0	16.1	10.4	8.3	7.3	6.8	6.5	6.4	6.4	6.6
6.0	21.5	14.1	11.4	10.2	9.5	9.2	9.2	9.4	9.9
7.0	28.9	19.1	15.7	14.2	13.4	13.2	13.3	13.8	14.7
8.0	38.6	26.0	21.8	19.9	19.2	19.1	19.5	20.5	22.3
9.0	51.9	35.6	30.5	28.3	27.6	27.8	28.7	30.7	33.6
10.0	70.6	49.5	43.0	40.5	40.2	41.1	43.0	46.4	51.5
11.0	96.5	69.2	61.3	59.0	59.2	61.2	64.8	70.3	79.3
12.0	133.6	98.0	88.6	86.6	88.1	91.8	98.2	107.4	121.7
13.0	186.8	140.4	129.3	127.9	131.3	139.0	149.8	165.3	188.1
14.0	263.9	203.3	190.5	191.4	199.1	212.0	229.7	254.8	292.1
15.0	376.8	297.1	282.9	288.2	303.0	324.7	353.8	394.4	455.1

MEWMA ATFS FOR $p = 6$

λ	0.1	0.2	0.3	0.4	0.5	0.6	0.7	0.8	0.9
h									
1.0	2.7	2.0	1.6	1.5	1.4	1.4	1.4	1.4	1.4
2.0	4.8	3.1	2.5	2.2	2.0	1.9	1.8	1.8	1.8
3.0	6.9	4.5	3.5	3.1	2.8	2.6	2.5	2.5	2.5
4.0	9.5	6.1	4.9	4.2	3.8	3.6	3.5	3.5	3.5
5.0	12.6	8.1	6.5	5.7	5.2	4.9	4.8	4.8	5.0
6.0	16.6	10.7	8.7	7.6	7.1	6.8	6.7	6.9	7.2
7.0	21.6	14.2	11.5	10.3	9.7	9.4	9.4	9.8	10.4
8.0	28.1	18.7	15.5	14.1	13.4	13.2	13.4	14.1	15.2
9.0	36.8	24.7	20.9	19.2	18.6	18.7	19.4	20.5	22.6
10.0	48.2	33.4	28.5	26.7	26.4	26.7	27.9	30.2	33.3
11.0	64.2	45.2	39.5	37.5	37.6	38.7	40.9	44.3	50.0
12.0	85.7	61.9	55.4	53.6	54.1	56.4	60.5	66.1	75.3
13.0	116.1	85.8	78.1	77.0	78.9	83.1	90.0	99.6	114.0
14.0	158.9	120.7	112.1	111.9	116.1	123.8	134.6	150.2	173.4
15.0	219.8	171.0	161.7	163.9	172.2	185.3	203.0	228.1	264.9

MEWMA ATFS FOR $p = 7$

λ	0.1	0.2	0.3	0.4	0.5	0.6	0.7	0.8	0.9
h									
1.0	2.4	1.8	1.5	1.4	1.3	1.3	1.3	1.3	1.2
2.0	4.1	2.6	2.2	1.9	1.8	1.6	1.6	1.6	1.6
3.0	5.8	3.8	3.0	2.6	2.4	2.2	2.1	2.1	2.1
4.0	7.9	5.1	4.0	3.5	3.2	3.0	2.8	2.8	2.9
5.0	10.4	6.7	5.3	4.6	4.2	4.0	3.8	3.8	3.9
6.0	13.4	8.6	6.9	6.0	5.6	5.3	5.2	5.3	5.5
7.0	17.0	11.1	9.0	8.0	7.4	7.2	7.1	7.3	7.7
8.0	21.7	14.2	11.7	10.5	9.9	9.8	9.8	10.2	11.0
9.0	27.7	18.5	15.5	14.0	13.4	13.4	13.8	14.4	15.8
10.0	35.4	24.1	20.5	18.9	18.5	18.7	19.4	20.8	23.0
11.0	45.8	31.7	27.6	25.8	25.7	26.1	27.7	29.9	33.6
12.0	59.6	42.6	37.3	35.8	35.9	37.2	39.9	43.6	49.5
13.0	73.8	56.8	51.1	50.0	50.9	53.3	57.8	64.1	73.5
14.0	104.1	77.6	71.1	70.7	73.1	77.7	84.8	94.5	109.6
15.0	139.9	107.0	100.1	100.9	105.7	113.7	125.0	140.9	164.4

MEWMA ATFS FOR $p = 8$

λ	0.1	0.2	0.3	0.4	0.5	0.6	0.7	0.8	0.9
h									
1.0	2.2	1.6	1.4	1.3	1.2	1.2	1.2	1.2	1.2
2.0	3.6	2.4	2.0	1.7	1.6	1.6	1.5	1.5	1.5
3.0	5.1	3.3	2.7	2.3	2.1	2.0	1.9	1.8	1.9
4.0	6.9	4.4	3.5	3.0	2.7	2.5	2.4	2.4	2.4
5.0	8.8	5.6	4.5	3.9	3.5	3.3	3.2	3.2	3.2
6.0	11.1	7.1	5.7	5.0	4.6	4.3	4.2	4.2	4.3
7.0	14.0	9.0	7.3	6.4	5.9	5.7	5.6	5.7	6.0
8.0	17.5	11.4	9.3	8.3	7.8	7.5	7.5	7.8	8.3
9.0	21.8	14.4	11.9	10.7	10.3	10.1	10.3	10.8	11.7
10.0	27.4	18.4	15.4	14.2	13.7	13.6	14.2	15.0	16.7
11.0	34.6	23.8	20.2	18.9	18.4	18.7	19.6	21.3	23.8
12.0	44.1	30.6	26.5	25.3	25.3	26.0	27.8	30.4	34.3
13.0	56.3	40.2	35.7	34.5	34.8	36.6	39.3	43.4	49.9
14.0	72.9	53.3	48.4	47.5	48.7	51.6	56.3	63.3	73.0
15.0	95.7	71.4	66.2	66.0	69.0	73.9	81.6	91.8	107.7

MEWMA ATFS FOR $p = 9$

λ \ h	0.1	0.2	0.3	0.4	0.5	0.6	0.7	0.8	0.9
1.0	2.0	1.5	1.3	1.2	1.2	1.2	1.1	1.1	1.1
2.0	3.3	2.2	1.8	1.6	1.4	1.4	1.4	1.4	1.4
3.0	4.5	3.0	2.4	2.0	1.9	1.8	1.7	1.7	1.6
4.0	6.0	3.9	3.1	2.6	2.4	2.2	2.1	2.1	2.1
5.0	7.7	4.9	3.9	3.3	3.0	2.8	2.7	2.7	2.7
6.0	9.6	6.1	4.9	4.2	3.8	3.6	3.5	3.5	3.6
7.0	11.9	7.6	6.1	5.3	4.9	4.7	4.6	4.6	4.8
8.0	14.6	9.4	7.6	6.7	6.3	6.0	6.0	6.2	6.5
9.0	18.1	11.8	9.6	8.6	8.1	7.9	8.0	8.3	8.9
10.0	22.2	14.7	12.1	11.1	10.6	10.5	10.7	11.3	12.3
11.0	27.4	18.5	15.4	14.4	14.0	14.1	14.6	15.7	17.3
12.0	34.0	23.3	20.1	18.8	18.6	19.1	20.1	21.8	24.7
13.0	42.7	30.0	26.1	25.0	25.0	26.3	27.8	30.8	35.2
14.0	54.1	38.8	34.8	33.7	34.3	36.1	39.2	43.8	50.6
15.0	68.9	50.9	46.3	45.7	47.3	50.7	55.5	62.6	73.3

MEWMA ATFS FOR $p = 10$

λ \ h	0.1	0.2	0.3	0.4	0.5	0.6	0.7	0.8	0.9
1.0	1.9	1.4	1.2	1.1	1.1	1.1	1.1	1.1	1.1
2.0	3.0	2.0	1.6	1.4	1.4	1.3	1.3	1.2	1.3
3.0	4.1	2.7	2.1	1.9	1.7	1.6	1.5	1.5	1.5
4.0	5.4	3.5	2.7	2.3	2.1	2.0	1.9	1.9	1.8
5.0	6.8	4.3	3.4	2.9	2.7	2.5	2.4	2.3	2.3
6.0	8.4	5.4	4.2	3.7	3.3	3.1	3.0	3.0	3.0
7.0	10.3	6.7	5.2	4.6	4.2	3.9	3.8	3.8	3.9
8.0	12.5	8.0	6.4	5.7	5.2	5.0	4.9	5.0	5.2
9.0	15.2	9.8	8.0	7.1	6.6	6.4	6.4	6.7	7.0
10.0	18.4	12.1	9.9	8.9	8.5	8.3	8.5	8.9	9.6
11.0	22.4	14.9	12.4	11.4	10.9	10.9	11.2	11.9	13.3
12.0	27.3	18.5	15.7	14.6	14.2	14.5	15.2	16.4	18.5
13.0	33.6	23.2	20.0	18.9	18.8	19.4	20.6	22.6	25.8
14.0	41.6	29.5	25.9	24.9	25.2	26.2	28.5	31.5	36.4
15.0	52.2	37.7	33.8	33.1	33.9	36.0	39.5	44.3	51.8

Appendix C: Tables

MEWMA ATFS FOR $p = 15$

λ	0.1	0.2	0.3	0.4	0.5	0.6	0.7	0.8	0.9
h									
1.0	1.4	1.1	1.1	1.0	1.0	1.0	1.0	1.0	1.0
2.0	2.1	1.4	1.3	1.2	1.1	1.1	1.1	1.1	1.1
3.0	2.9	1.9	1.5	1.3	1.3	1.2	1.2	1.2	1.1
4.0	3.6	2.3	1.8	1.6	1.5	1.4	1.3	1.3	1.3
5.0	4.4	2.8	2.2	1.9	1.7	1.6	1.5	1.5	1.5
6.0	5.3	3.4	2.6	2.2	2.0	1.9	1.8	1.7	1.7
7.0	6.2	3.9	3.1	2.6	2.4	2.2	2.1	2.0	2.0
8.0	7.3	4.6	3.6	3.1	2.8	2.6	2.5	2.5	2.5
9.0	8.4	5.3	4.2	3.7	3.3	3.1	3.0	3.0	3.1
10.0	9.8	6.2	5.0	4.3	3.9	3.7	3.6	3.7	3.9
11.0	11.4	7.2	5.8	5.1	4.7	4.5	4.5	4.5	4.8
12.0	13.2	8.3	6.8	6.1	5.8	5.5	5.5	5.7	6.2
13.0	15.1	9.8	8.1	7.3	6.9	6.8	6.9	7.4	8.0
14.0	17.5	11.7	9.6	8.7	8.4	8.4	8.7	9.4	10.4
15.0	20.4	13.9	11.5	10.6	10.4	10.5	11.1	12.1	13.7

MEWMA ATFS FOR $p = 20$

λ	0.1	0.2	0.3	0.4	0.5	0.6	0.7	0.8	0.9
h									
1.0	1.2	1.0	1.0	1.0	1.0	1.0	1.0	1.0	1.0
2.0	1.7	1.2	1.1	1.0	1.0	1.0	1.0	1.0	1.0
3.0	2.2	1.5	1.2	1.1	1.1	1.1	1.1	1.1	1.0
4.0	2.8	1.8	1.4	1.3	1.2	1.1	1.1	1.1	1.1
5.0	3.3	2.2	1.7	1.4	1.3	1.3	1.2	1.2	1.2
6.0	3.9	2.5	2.0	1.7	1.5	1.4	1.3	1.3	1.3
7.0	4.5	2.9	2.3	1.9	1.7	1.6	1.5	1.5	1.4
8.0	5.2	3.3	2.6	2.2	1.9	1.8	1.7	1.6	1.6
9.0	5.9	3.7	2.9	2.5	2.2	2.1	1.9	1.9	1.9
10.0	6.7	4.2	3.3	2.8	2.5	2.3	2.2	2.2	2.2
11.0	7.5	4.7	3.7	3.2	2.9	2.7	2.6	2.5	2.6
12.0	8.4	5.3	4.3	3.7	3.3	3.2	3.0	3.0	3.1
13.0	9.5	6.0	4.8	4.2	3.9	3.6	3.5	3.6	3.8
14.0	10.7	6.8	5.5	4.8	4.4	4.3	4.2	4.4	4.6
15.0	11.8	7.7	6.3	5.6	5.2	5.1	5.0	5.3	5.7

Multivariate Cumulative Sum Detection Method Tables

The following tables provide estimated thresholds to achieve various ATFS as a function of k and h for the MCUSUM detection method for dimensions $p = 3, 4, \ldots, 10, 15$, and 20. See Table 8.3 on page 234 for $p = 2$. As with the other methods, the thresholds in these tables are for data distributed $N_p(\mathbf{0}, \mathbf{I})$.

To use the tables, read down the chosen k column until an ATFS value close to that desired is reached. Then read across to the left to find the threshold h. The thresholds achieve the specified ATFS values with standard errors of less than 0.1. Blank cells indicate combinations of h and k that result in AFTS values in excess of 365 (i.e., average times between false signal greater than 365 days or less than one false signal per year for a daily monitoring scheme).

MCUSUM ATFS FOR $p = 3$

k	0.2	0.4	0.6	0.8	1.0	1.2	1.4	1.6	1.8	2.0
h										
1.0	2.3	2.8	3.5	4.5	6.3	9.2	14.3	23.2	39.5	71.0
2.0	4.9	6.6	9.7	15.5	27.4	53.7	115.1	246.8		
3.0	9.0	13.9	24.6	50.7	124.4					
4.0	14.9	26.7	59.2	168.9						
5.0	23.1	49.0	143.9							
6.0	34.0	88.2								
7.0	48.6	158.3								
8.0	68.4	248.4								
9.0	94.3									
10.0	128.6									
11.0	173.6									
12.0	233.2									
13.0	312.0									
14.0										
15.0										

MCUSUM ATFS FOR $p = 4$

k	0.2	0.4	0.6	0.8	1.0	1.2	1.4	1.6	1.8	2.0
h										
1.0	1.8	2.1	2.5	3.1	4.0	5.5	7.9	12.1	19.6	33.2
2.0	3.7	4.7	6.3	9.2	14.6	25.6	50.0	106.7	244.3	
3.0	6.6	9.3	14.6	26.1	54.4	134.7				
4.0	10.7	16.9	31.5	73.5	217.9					
5.0	16.1	29.0	67.7	218.3						
6.0	23.2	48.8	148.2							
7.0	32.3	80.7	332.5							
8.0	43.9	133.8								
9.0	59.0	223.0								
10.0	77.7									
11.0	101.5									
12.0	131.8									
13.0	170.0									
14.0	219.1									
15.0	281.5									

MCUSUM ATFS FOR $p = 5$

k	0.2	0.4	0.6	0.8	1.0	1.2	1.4	1.6	1.8	2.0
h										
1.0	1.6	1.7	2.0	2.4	2.9	3.8	5.1	7.3	11.2	18.0
2.0	3.0	3.2	4.7	6.4	9.3	14.8	26.2	50.8	108.4	249.0
3.0	5.3	7.0	10.0	16.0	29.5	63.3	159.1			
4.0	8.4	12.1	19.9	39.9	99.2	308.3				
5.0	12.3	19.8	39.3	103.1	366.8					
6.0	17.4	31.7	77.9	282.1						
7.0	23.8	49.6	157.5							
8.0	31.9	77.4	328.9							
9.0	41.7	121.1								
10.0	54.1	190.5								
11.0	69.0	303.5								
12.0	87.5									
13.0	110.3									
14.0	138.1									
15.0	172.6									

MCUSUM ATFS FOR $p = 6$

k	0.2	0.4	0.6	0.8	1.0	1.2	1.4	1.6	1.8	2.0
h										
1.0	1.4	1.5	1.7	1.9	2.3	2.8	3.7	5.0	7.1	10.8
2.0	2.6	3.0	3.7	4.5	6.5	9.7	15.6	27.8	54.9	118.0
3.0	4.4	5.6	7.5	11.1	18.3	34.9	77.8			
4.0	6.9	9.4	14.2	24.9	53.5	142.3				
5.0	10.1	14.9	26.1	57.8	170.6					
6.0	14.0	22.9	47.8	140.2						
7.0	18.9	34.5	88.7							
8.0	24.9	51.3	169.2							
9.0	32.2	76.4	334.0							
10.0	41.0	114.1								
11.0	51.5	171.5								
12.0	64.1	260.7								
13.0	79.4									
14.0	97.7									
15.0	119.4									

MCUSUM ATFS FOR $p = 7$

k	0.2	0.4	0.6	0.8	1.0	1.2	1.4	1.6	1.8	2.0
h										
1.0	1.3	1.4	1.5	1.7	1.9	2.3	2.8	3.6	4.9	7.2
2.0	2.3	2.6	3.1	3.8	5.0	6.9	10.4	17.1	30.7	62.1
3.0	3.8	4.7	6.0	8.3	12.7	21.8	43.3	100.3	268.3	
4.0	5.9	7.7	10.9	17.4	32.7	76.1	218.2			
5.0	8.5	11.9	18.9	36.6	91.9	306.8				
6.0	11.8	17.8	32.5	80.3	283.8					
7.0	15.7	25.9	56.7	186.3						
8.0	20.4	37.6	100.3							
9.0	26.1	53.6	182.6							
10.0	32.7	76.8								
11.0	40.8	110.0								
12.0	50.2	159.5								
13.0	61.5	233.3								
14.0	74.5									
15.0	89.9									

MCUSUM ATFS FOR $p = 8$

k	0.2	0.4	0.6	0.8	1.0	1.2	1.4	1.6	1.8	2.0
h										
1.0	1.2	1.3	1.4	1.5	1.7	1.9	2.3	2.8	3.7	5.1
2.0	2.0	2.3	2.7	3.2	4.0	5.3	7.5	11.5	19.2	35.7
3.0	3.4	4.1	5.0	6.6	9.4	14.9	26.9	56.0	135.5	
4.0	5.2	6.5	8.8	13.1	22.3	45.7	114.7			
5.0	7.4	9.9	14.7	25.6	55.7	159.0				
6.0	10.1	14.5	24.2	51.5	152.2					
7.0	13.4	20.7	39.8	108.8						
8.0	17.3	29.1	66.1	243.7						
9.0	21.9	40.6	112.8							
10.0	27.4	56.0	197.6							
11.0	33.8	77.6								
12.0	41.1	108.0								
13.0	49.6	151.8								
14.0	59.7	214.8								
15.0	71.1	308.5								

MCUSUM ATFS FOR $p = 9$

k	0.2	0.4	0.6	0.8	1.0	1.2	1.4	1.6	1.8	2.0
h										
1.0	1.1	1.2	1.3	1.4	1.5	1.7	1.9	2.3	2.9	3.8
2.0	1.9	2.1	2.4	2.8	3.4	4.8	5.7	8.3	12.9	22.4
3.0	3.1	3.6	4.3	5.5	7.4	11.0	18.2	34.4	75.5	191.3
4.0	4.6	5.7	7.4	10.4	16.2	30.0	66.9	182.5		
5.0	6.5	8.5	11.9	19.1	36.9	91.7	297.5			
6.0	8.9	12.2	18.9	35.9	90.8	323.8				
7.0	11.7	17.1	29.7	69.9	245.6					
8.0	15.1	23.6	47.4	143.9						
9.0	18.9	32.1	76.2	314.3						
10.0	23.4	43.5	125.5							
11.0	28.7	58.5	213.5							
12.0	34.9	79.1	375.3							
13.0	41.7	103.2								
14.0	49.6	146.4								
15.0	58.9	202.0								

MCUSUM ATFS FOR $p = 10$

k	0.2	0.4	0.6	0.8	1.0	1.2	1.4	1.6	1.8	2.0
h										
1.0	1.1	1.1	1.2	1.3	1.3	1.5	1.7	2.0	2.4	3.0
2.0	1.7	1.9	2.1	2.5	2.9	3.6	4.6	6.3	9.3	15.0
3.0	2.8	3.2	3.8	4.7	6.1	8.5	13.2	22.9	45.9	105.8
4.0	4.2	5.0	6.3	8.5	12.5	21.2	42.4	103.2	307.0	
5.0	5.9	7.4	10.0	15.1	26.5	58.0	164.1			
6.0	7.9	10.5	15.5	26.7	59.1	180.7				
7.0	10.4	14.5	23.6	48.7	144.5					
8.0	13.3	19.7	35.8	92.8						
9.0	16.7	26.5	55.4	186.9						
10.0	20.6	35.1	86.7							
11.0	25.0	46.4	139.1							
12.0	30.1	61.2	230.4							
13.0	35.9	80.9								
14.0	42.5	107.1								
15.0	50.0	143.2								

MCUSUM ATFS FOR $p = 15$

k	0.2	0.4	0.6	0.8	1.0	1.2	1.4	1.6	1.8	2.0
h										
1.0	1.0	1.0	1.0	1.1	1.1	1.1	1.2	1.2	1.4	1.5
2.0	1.2	1.4	1.5	1.6	1.8	2.0	2.3	2.7	3.4	4.3
3.0	2.0	2.2	2.5	2.8	3.3	3.9	4.9	6.5	9.3	14.8
4.0	2.9	3.3	3.8	4.5	5.6	7.3	10.5	16.7	30.8	67.7
5.0	4.0	4.7	5.6	7.0	9.4	14.0	24.1	50.3	132.1	
6.0	5.4	6.4	8.0	10.7	16.0	28.3	63.1	188.3		
7.0	6.9	8.5	11.1	16.2	27.7	62.0	194.9			
8.0	8.6	11.0	15.2	24.5	50.7	152.7				
9.0	10.6	14.0	20.8	37.9	98.6					
10.0	12.8	17.6	28.1	59.9	208.6					
11.0	15.4	22.0	38.3	98.5						
12.0	18.2	27.2	52.3	169.4						
13.0	21.3	33.4	72.7							
14.0	24.7	41.1	102.1							
15.0	28.6	50.1	146.5							

MCUSUM ATFS FOR $p = 20$

k	0.2	0.4	0.6	0.8	1.0	1.2	1.4	1.6	1.8	2.0
h										
1.0	1.0	1.0	1.0	1.0	1.0	1.0	1.0	1.1	1.1	1.1
2.0	1.1	1.2	1.2	1.3	1.3	1.5	1.6	1.8	2.0	2.3
3.0	1.6	1.7	1.9	2.1	2.3	2.6	3.0	3.5	4.3	5.6
4.0	2.3	2.6	2.9	3.2	3.6	4.3	5.3	6.9	9.8	15.3
5.0	3.2	3.5	4.0	4.6	5.6	7.1	9.6	14.4	25.2	52.8
6.0	4.1	4.7	5.5	6.6	8.2	11.7	18.2	33.7	80.3	248.2
7.0	5.2	6.1	7.3	9.2	12.7	19.8	31.5	94.2		
8.0	6.5	7.7	9.6	12.8	19.3	35.2	87.4			
9.0	7.9	9.6	12.4	17.7	30.0	68.1	236.0			
10.0	9.5	11.8	16.0	24.5	48.3	144.2				
11.0	11.2	14.4	20.3	34.5	82.0					
12.0	13.2	17.4	25.8	48.9	148.1					
13.0	15.2	20.8	32.9	71.5	287.9					
14.0	17.6	24.6	41.8	107.3						
15.0	20.1	29.2	53.4	167.8						

References

Ackelsberg, J., Balter, S., Bornschelgel, K., Carubis, E., Cherry, C., Das, D., Fine, A., Karpati, A., Layton, M., Mostashari, F., Nivin, B., Reddy, V., Weiss, D., Hutwagner, L., Seeman, G.M., McQuiston, J., Treadwell, T., & Rhodes, J. 2002. Syndromic Surveillance for Bioterrorism Following the Attacks on the World Trade Center – New York City, 2001. *Morbidity and Mortality Weekly Report*, **51 (Special Issue)**, 13–15.

Andridge, R.R., & Little, R.J.A. 2010. A Review of Hot Deck Imputation for Survey Non-response. *International Statistical Review*, **78**(1), 40–64.

Bolstad, C.A., Cuevas, H.M., Wand-Costello, J., Endsley, M.R., Page, W.J., & KassHout, T.A. 2011. Integrating Human Capabilities into Biosurveillance Systems: A Study of Biosurveillance and Situation Awareness. *Pages 79–94 of:* Kass-Hout, T.A., & Zhang, X. (eds), *Biosurveillance: Methods and Case Studies*. CRC Press.

Borror, C.M., Champ, C.W., & Rigdon, S.E. 1998. Poisson EWMA Control Charts. *Journal of Quality Technology*, **30**(4), 352–361.

Borror, C.M., Montgomery, D.C., & Runger, G.C. 1999. Robustness of the EWMA Control Chart to Non-normality. *Journal of Quality Technology*, **31**(3), 309–316.

Box, G.E.P., Jenkins, G.M., & Reinsel, G.C. (eds). 2008. *Time Series Analysis: Forecasting and Control*. 4 edn. Wiley.

Bravata, D.M., McDonald, K.M., Smithe, W.M., Rydzak, C., Szeto, H., Buckeridge, D.L., Haberland, C., & Owens, D.K. 2004. Systematic review: Surveillance Systems for Early Detection of Bioterrorism-Related Diseases. *Annals of Internal Medicine*, **140**(11), 910–922.

Brockwell, P.J., & Davis, R.A. 2002. *Introduction to Time Series and Forecasting*. Springer.

Brook, D., & Evans, D.A. 1972. An Approach to the Probability Distribution of CUSUM Run Length. *Biometrika*, **59**, 539–549.

Brookmeyer, R., & Stroup, D.F. (eds). 2004. *Monitoring the Health of Populations: Statistical Principles and Methods for Public Health Surveillance*. Oxford University Press.

Brown, R.G. 1959. *Statistical Forecasting for Inventory Control*. McGraw-Hill.

Brown, R.G. 1963. *Smoothing Forecasting and Prediction of Discrete Time Series*. Prentice-Hall.

Brownstein, J.S., Freifeld, C.C., Reis, B.Y., & Mandl, K.D. 2008. Surveillance Sans Frontières: Internet-Based Emerging Infectious Disease Intelligence and the HealthMap Project. *PLoS Medicine*, **5**(7), 1019–1024.

Buckeridge, D.L., Burkom, H.S., Moore, A., Pavlin, J., Cutchis, P., & Moore, A.W. 2004. Evaluation of Syndromic Surveillance Systems – Design of an Epidemic Simulation Model. *Morbidity and Mortality Weekly Report*, **53 (Supplement)**, 137–143.

Buckeridge, D.L., Burkom, H.S., Campbell, M., Hogan, W.R., & Moore, A.W. 2005. Algorithms for Rapid Outbreak Detection: A Research Synthesis. *Journal of Biomedical Informatics*, 99–113.

Buckeridge, D.L., Owens, D.K., Switzer, P., Frank, J., & Musen, M.A. 2006. Evaluating Detection of an Inhalational Anthrax Outbreak. *Emerging Infectious Diseases*, **12**(12), 1942–1949.

Buehler, J.W., Sonricker, A., Paladini, M., Soper, P., & Mostashari, F. 2008. Syndromic Surveillance Practice in the United States: Findings from a Survey of State, Territorial, and Selected Local Health Departments. *Advances in Disease Surveillance*, **6**(3), 1–20.

Burkom, H.S. 2006. Personal communication, December 22, 2006.

Burkom, H.S., Murphy, S.P., & Shmueli, G. 2006. Automated Time Series Forecasting for Biosurveillance. *Statistics in Medicine*, 26, 4202–4218.

California Department of Public Health. 2010. Accessed at http://www.cdph.ca.gov/programs/vrdl/Pages/CaliforniaSentinelProviderProgram.aspx, on December 3, 2010.

CDC. 2003. *Syndrome Definitions for Diseases Associated with Critical Bioterrorism-associated Agents Dated October 23, 2003*. Accessed at http://www.bt.cdc.gov/surveillance/syndromedef/ on November 21, 2006.

CDC. 2006a. Accessed at www.cdc.gov/biosense/publichealth.htm on November 16, 2006.

CDC. 2006b. *Annotated Bibliography for Syndromic Surveillance*. Accessed at http://www.cdc.gov/EPO/dphsi/syndromic/evaluation.htm on November 28, 2006.

CDC. 2006c. *BioSense*. Accessed at www.cdc.gov/biosense/ on November 27, 2006.

CDC. 2006d. *BioSense User Guide, Version 2.0*. Accessed at http://0-www.cdc.gov.mill1.sjlibrary.org/biosense/files/CDC_BioSense_User_Guide_v2.0.pdf on November 28, 2006.

CDC. 2006e. *EARS V4.5 User's Guide*. September 19.

CDC. 2007. *Early Aberration Reporting System*. Accessed at http://www.bt.cdc.gov/surveillance/ears on April 30, 2007.

CDC. 2008. Accessed at http://www.cdc.gov/BioSense/publichealth.htm on October 11, 2008.

CDC. 2009. Notifiable Diseases/Deaths in Selected Cities Weekly Information. *Morbidity and Mortality Weekly Report*, **58**(46), 1304–1315.

CDC. 2010a (February). *National Biosurveillance Strategy for Human Health, Version 2.0*. Accessed at http://www.cdc.gov/osels/pdf/NBSHH_V2_FINAL.PDF on July 13, 2012.

CDC. 2010b. *NETSS website*. Accessed at http://www.cdc.gov/ncphi/disss/nndss/netss.htm on June 5, 2010.

CDC. 2010c. *NNDSS website*. Accessed at http://www.cdc.gov/ncphi/disss/nndss/nndsshis.htm on June 5, 2010.

CDC. 2012a. *BioSense*. Accessed at http://www.cdc.gov/biosense/ on June 23, 2012.

CDC. 2012b (April). *BioSense 2.0 Analytics: Aberration Detection Algorithms*. Accessed at https://sites.google.com/site/biosenseredesign/file-cabinet on July 14, 2012.

Chang, J.T., & Fricker, R.D., Jr. 1999. Detecting When a Monotonically Increasing Mean Has Crossed a Threshold. *Journal of Quality Technology*, **31**, 217–233.

Clarke, T.L., Liberman, A., Wang, M., Nieves, K., Cattani, J., & Summer, J. 2007. Epidemic Simulation for Syndromic Surveillance. *The Health Care Manager*, **26**, 297–302.

Cleveland, W.S. 1993. *Visualizing Data*. 1 edn. Hobart Press.

Cleveland, W.S. 1997. Robust Locally Weighted Regression and Smoothing Scatterplots. *Journal of the American Statistical Association*, **368**, 829–836.

Cleveland, W.S., & McGill, M.E. 1988. *Dynamic Graphics for Statistics*. Wadsworth & Brooks/Cole.

Coberly, J.S., Murphy, S.P., Babin, S.M., Burkom, H.S., Feighner, B., Lin, J., & Lombardo, J. 2006. The Development of Virtual Data for Syndromic Surveillance Exercises. *Advances in Disease Surveillance*, **1**, 15.

Cody, R. 2008. *Cody's Data Cleaning Techniques Using SAS*. 2 edn. SAS Institute.

Cook, D., & Swayne, D.F. 2007. *Interactive and Dynamic Graphics for Data Analysis with R and Ggobi*. Springer.

Cooper, D.L. 2006. Can Syndromic Surveillance Data Detect Local Outbreaks of Communicable Disease? A Model Using a Historical Cryptosporidiosis Outbreak. *Epidemiology and Infection*, **134**, 13–20.

Cowling, B.J., Wong, I.O.L., Ho, L., Riley, S., & Leung, G.M. 2006. Methods for Monitoring Influenza Surveillance Data. *International Journal of Epidemiology*, **35**, 1314–1321.

Crosier, R.B. 1988. Multivariate Generalizations of Cumulative Sum Quality Control Schemes. *Technometrics*, **30**, 291–303.

Crowder, S.V. 1989. Design of Exponentially Weighted Moving Average Schemes. *Journal of Quality Technology*, **21**, 155–162.

Crowder, S.V., & Hamilton, M.D. 1992. An EWMA for Monitoring a Process Standard Deviation. *Journal of Quality Technology*, **24**, 12–21.

Diggle, P.J., Knorr-Held, L., Rowlingsos, B., Su, T., Hawin, P., & Bryant, T.N. 2004a. On-line Monitoring of Public Health Surveillance Data. *Pages 233–266 of:* Brookmeyer, R., & Stroup, D.F. (eds), *Monitoring the Health of Populations: Statistical Principles & Methods for Public Health Surveillance*. Oxford University Press.

Diggle, P.J., Rowlingsos, B., & Su, T. 2004b. *Point Process Methodology for On-line Spatiotemporal Disease Surveillance*. Tech. Rept. 37. Johns Hopkins University. Department of Biostatistics Working Papers.

DoD. 2006. Accessed at http://www.geis.fhp.osd.mil/GEIS/SurveillanceActivities/ESSENCE/ESSENCE.asp on November 27, 2006.

Doyle, A.C. 1890. *The Sign of Four*. The works of Sir Arthur Conan Doyle: Complete and unabridged edn. Kingsport Press. Published in 1981.

Dunfee, D.A., & Hegler, B.L. 2007. *Biological Terrorism Preparedness: Evaluating the Performance of the Early Aberration Reporting System (EARS) Syndromic Surveillance Algorithms*. Naval Postgraduate School. Master's thesis.

Endsley, M.R. 1995. Toward a Theory of Situation Awareness in Dynamic Systems. *Human Factors*, **37**, 32–64.

Endsley, M.R. 2001. *Designing for Situation Awareness in Complex Systems*. Proceedings of the Second International Workshop on Symbiosis of Humans, Artifacts, and Environment. Kyoto, Japan.

Endsley, M.R., & Garland, D.J. 2000. *Situation Awareness: Analysis and Measurement*. Lawrence Erlbaum Associates.

Endsley, M.R., Bolte, B., & Jones, D.G. 2003. *Designing for Situation Awareness: An Approach for Human-centered Design*. Taylor & Francis.

Ewan, W.D. 1963. When and How to Use Cu-Sum Charts. *Technometrics*, **5**, 1–22.

Farrington, C.P., Andrews, N.J., Beale, A.D., & Catchpole, M.A. 1996. A Statistical Algorithm for the Early Detection of Outbreaks of Infectious Disease. *Journal of the Royal Statistical Society, Series A (Statistics in Society)*, **159**, 547–563.

Follmann, D. 1996. A Simple Multivariate Test for One-Sided Alternatives. *Journal of the American Statistical Association*, **91**, 854–861.

Forsberg, L., Jeffery, C., Ozonoff, A., & Pagano, M. 2006. A Spatiotemporal Analysis of Syndromic Data for Biosurveillance. *Pages 173–191 of:* Wilson, A., Wilson, G., & Olwell, D.H. (eds), *Statistical Methods in Counterterrorism: Game Theory, Modeling, Syndromic Surveillance, and Biometric Authentication*. Springer.

Fraker, S.E., Woodall, W.H., & Mousavi, S. 2008. Performance Metrics for Surveillance Schemes. *Quality Engineering*, **20**, 451–464.

Freedman, D., Pisani, R., & Purves, R. 1998. *Statistics*. Third edn. W.W. Norton & Company.

Fricker, R.D., Jr. 2007. Directionally Sensitive Multivariate Statistical Process Control Methods with Application to Syndromic Surveillance. *Advances in Disease Surveillance*, 3(1). Available at http://www.isdsjournal.org.

Fricker, R.D., Jr. 2010. Methodological Issues in Biosurveillance. *Statistics in Medicine*, **30**, 403–441.

Fricker, R.D., Jr., & Chang, J.T. 2008. A Spatio-temporal Methodology for Real-time Biosurveillance. *Quality Engineering*, **20**, 465–477.

Fricker, R.D., Jr., & Hanni, K. 2010. *Biosurveillance: Detecting, Tracking, and Mitigating the Effects of Natural Disease and Bioterrorism*. Online presentation, Military Operations Research Society, Monterey, CA, February 10, 2010. Available at http://faculty.nps.edu/rdfricke/frickerpr.htm.

Fricker, R.D., Jr., & Rolka, H.R. 2006. Protecting Against Biological Terrorism: Statistical Issues in Electronic Biosurveillance. *Chance*, **19**, 4–13.

Fricker, R.D., Jr., Hegler, B.L., & Dunfee, D.A. 2008a. Comparing Biosurveillance Detection Methods: EARS Versus a CUSUM-based Methodology. *Statistics in Medicine*, **27**, 3407–3429.

Fricker, R.D., Jr., Knitt, M.C., & Hu, C.X. 2008b. Directionally Sensitive MCUSUM and MEWMA Procedures with Application to Biosurveillance. *Quality Engineering*, **20**, 478–494.

Frisen, M., & Sonesson, C. 2005. Optimal Surveillance. *Pages 31–52 of:* Lawson, A.B., & Kleinman, K. (eds), *Spatial & Syndromic Surveillance for Public Health*. John Wiley & Sons.

Gan, F.F. 1991. An Optimal Design of CUSUM Quality Control Charts. *Journal of Quality Technology*, **23**, 279–286.

GAO. 2009 (December). *BIOSURVEILLANCE: Developing a Collaboration Strategy Is Essential to Fostering Interagency Data and Resource Sharing*. Tech. rept. GAO-10-171. U.S. Government Accountability Office.

GAO. 2010 (June). *BIOSURVEILLANCE: Efforts to Develop a National Biosurveillance Capability Need a National Strategy and a Designated Leader*. Tech. Rept. GAO-10-645. U.S. Government Accountability Office.

GAO. 2011 (October). *BIOSURVEILLANCE: Nonfederal Capabilities Should Be Considered in Creating a National Biosurveillance Strategy*. Tech. Rept. GAO-12-55. U.S. Government Accountability Office.

Gerstman, B.B. (ed). 2003. *Epidemiology Kept Simple: An Introduction to Classic and Modern Epidemiology*. Wiley-Liss.

Ginsberg, J., Mohebbi, M.H., Patel, R.S., Brammer, L., Smolinski, M.S., & Brilliant, L. 2009. Detecting Influenza Epidemics Using Search Engine Query Data. *Nature*, **457**, 1012–1014.

Goldenberg, A., Shmueli, G., Caruana, R.A., & Fienberg, S.E. 2002. Early Statistical Detection of Anthrax Outbreaks by Tracking Over-the-counter Medication Sales. *Proceedings of the National Academy of Sciences*, **99**, 5237–5240.

Gomes, I.C., Mingoti, S.A., & Oliveira, C.D. 2011. A Novel Experience in the Use of Control Charts for the Detection of Nosocomial Infection Outbreaks. *Clinics*, **66**, 1681–1689.

Gonick, L. and W. Smith, 2009. *The Cartoon Guide to Statistics*. Harper Perrenial.

Google. 2012. *Flu Trends*. Accessed at http://www.google.org/flutrends/about/how.html on May 21, 2012.

Green, M. 2008. *Syndromic Surveillance for Detecting Bioterrorist Events – The Right Answer to the Wrong Question?* Presentation given at the Naval Postgraduate School, June 9, 2008.

Grey, M.R., & Spaeth, K.R. (eds). 2006. *The Bioterrorism Sourcebook*. McGraw-Hill.

Hagen, K.S., R.D. Fricker, Jr., Hanni, K., Barnes, S., & Michie, K. 2011. Assessing the Early Aberration Reporting System's Ability to Locally Detect the 2009 Influenza Pandemic. *Statistics, Politics, and Policy*, **2**.

Han, S.W., Tsui, K., Ariyajunya, B., & Kim, S.B. 2009. A Comparison of CUSUM, EWMA, and Scan Statistics for Detection of Increases in Poisson Rates. *Quality and Reliability Engineering International*, **26**, 279–289.

Hanni, K.D. 2011. Comments on "Some Methodological Issues in Biosurveillance." *Statistics in Medicine*, **30**, 423–425.

Hawkins, D.M., & Olwell, D.H. 1998. *Cumulative Sum Charts and Charting for Quality Improvement*. Springer.

HealthMap. 2012. *About HealthMap*. Accessed at http://www.healthmap.org/about/ on April 12, 2012.

Healy, J.D. 1987. A Note on Multivariate CUSUM Procedures. *Technometrics*, **29**, 409–412.

Henning, K.J. 2004. Overview of Syndromic Surveillance: What Is Syndromic Surveillance? *Morbidity and Mortality Weekly Report*, **53 (Supplement)**, 5–11.

Holt, C.C. 1957. *Forecasting Trends and Seasonal by Exponentially Weighted Averages*. Tech. Rept. 57. Office of Naval Research Memorandum.

Hotelling, H. 1947. Multivariate Quality Control – Illustrated by the Air Testing of Sample Bombsights. *Pages 409–412 of:* Eisenhart, C., Hastay, M.W., & Wallis, W.A. (eds), *Techniques of Statistical Analysis*. McGraw-Hill.

Hutwagner, L., Thompson, W., Seeman, G.M., & Treadwell, T. 2003a. The Bioterrorism Preparedness and Response Early Aberration Reporting System (EARS). *Journal of Urban Health: Bulletin of the New York Academy of Medicine*, **80**(2 (**Supplement 1**)), 89i–96i.

Hutwagner, L., Thompson, W., Seeman, G.M., & Treadwell, T. 2003b. The Bioterrorism Preparedness and Response Early Aberration Reporting System (EARS). *Journal of Urban Health: Bulletin of the New York Academy of Medicine*, **80**, 89i–96i.

Hutwagner, L.C., Browne, T., Seeman, G.M., & Fleischauer, A.T. 2005. Comparing Aberration Detection Methods with Simulated Data. *Emerging Infectious Diseases*, **11**, 314–316.

Jackson, J.E. 1972. All Count Distributions Are Not Alike. *Journal of Quality Technology*, **4**, 86–92.

Joner, M.D., Jr., Woodall, W.H., & Reynolds, M.R., Jr. 2008a. Detecting a Rate Increase Using a Bernoulli Scan Statistic. *Statistics in Medicine*, **27**, 2555–2575.

Joner, M.D., Jr., Woodall, W.H., Reynolds, M.R., Jr., & Fricker, R.D., Jr. 2008b. A One-Sided MEWMA Chart for Health Surveillance. *Quality and Reliability Engineering International*, **24**, 503–519.

Kass-Hout, T.A. 2012a. Personal communication, June 26, 2012.

Kass-Hout, T.A. 2012b. https://sites.google.com/site/changepointanalysis/ accessed on July 8, 2012.

Kass-Hout, T.A., & Zhang, X. (eds). 2011. *Biosurveillance: Methods and Case Studies*. CRC Press.

Kass-Hout, T.A., Zhiheng, X., McMurray, P., Park, S., Buckeridge, D.L., Brownstein, J.S., Finelli, L., & Groseclose, S.L. 2012. Application of Change Point Analysis to Daily Influenza-like Illness Emergency Department Visits. *Journal of the American Medical Informatics Association*.

Kay, A. 1984. Computer Software. *Scientific American*, **251**, 53–59.

Kleinman, K. 2005. Generalized Linear Models and Generalized Linear Mixed Models for Small Area Surveillance. *Pages 77–94 of:* Lawson, A.B., & Kleinman, K. (eds), *Spatial & Syndromic Surveillance*. John Wiley & Sons.

Kleinman, K., & Abrams, A. 2006. Assessing Surveillance Using Sensitivity, Specificity, and Timeliness. *Statistical Methods in Medical Research*, **15**, 445–464.

Kleinman, K., Lazarus, R., & Platt, R. 2004. A Generalized Linear Mixed Models Approach for Detecting Incident Clusters of Disease in Small Areas, with an Application to Biological Terrorism. *American Journal of Epidemiology*, **159**, 217–224.

Kleinman, K., Abrams, A., Mandl, K., & Platt, R. 2005. Simulation for Assessing Statistical Methods of Biologic Terrorism Surveillance. *Morbidity and Mortality Weekly Report*, **53 (Supplement)**, 101–108.

Knitt, M.C., & Hu, C.X. 2007. *A Comparative Analysis of Multivariate Statistical Detection Methods Applied to Syndromic Surveillance*. Naval Postgraduate School. Master's thesis.

Koetsier, A., de Keizer, N.F., de Jonge, E., Cook, D.A., & Peek, N. 2012. Performance of Risk-Adjusted Control Charts to Monitor In-Hospital Mortality of Intensive Care Unit Patients: A Simulation Study. *Critical Care Medicine*, **40**, 1799–1807.

Kudô, A. 1963. A Multivariate Analogue of the One-Sided Test. *Biometrika*, **50**, 403–418.

Kulldorff, M. 1997. A Spatial Scan Statistic. *Communications in Statistics, Theory and Methods*, **26**, 1481–1496.

Kulldorff, M. 2001. Prospective Time Periodic Geographical Disease Surveillance Using a Scan Statistic. *Journal of the Royal Statistical Society, Series A (Statistics in Society)*, **164**, 61–72.

Lawson, A.B. 2004. Some Considerations in Spatial-Temporal Analysis of Public Health Surveillance Data. *Pages 289–314 of:* Brookmeyer, R., & Stroup, D.F. (eds), *Monitoring the Health of Populations: Statistical Principles & Methods for Public Health Surveillance*. Oxford University Press.

Lawson, A.B., & Kleinman, K. (eds). 2005. *Spatial & Syndromic Surveillance for Public Health*. John Wiley & Sons.

Lazarus, R., Kleinman, K., Dashevsky, I., Adams, C., Kludt, P., A. DeMaria, Jr., & Platt, R. 2002. Use of Automated Ambulatory-Care Encounter Records for Detection of Acute Illness Clusters, Including Potential Bioterrorism Events. *Emerging Infectious Diseases*, **8**, 753–760.

Le Strat, Y., & Carrat, F. 1999. Monitoring Epidemiologic Surveillance Data Using Hidden Markov Models. *Statistics in Medicine*, **18**, 3463–3478.

Lombardo, J.S., & Buckeridge, D.L. (eds). 2007. *Disease Surveillance: A Public Health Informatics Approach*. John Wiley & Sons.

Lombardo, J.S., Burkom, H.S., & Pavlin, J. 2004. ESSENCE II and the Framework for Evaluating Syndromic Surveillance Systems. *Morbidity and Mortality Weekly Report*, **53 (Supplement)**, 159–165.

Lorden, G. 1971. Procedures for Reacting to a Change in Distribution. *Annals of Mathematical Statistics*, **42**, 1897–1908.

Lotze, T., Shmueli, G., & Yahav, I. 2007. *Simulating Multivariate Syndromic Time Series and Outbreak Signatures*. Working Paper RHS-06-054. University of Maryland. Available at http://ssrn.com/abstract=990020.

Lotze, T., Murphy, S. P., & Shmueli, G. 2008. Implementation and Comparison of Preprocessing Methods for Biosurveillance. *Advances in Disease Surveillance*, **6**, 1–14.

Lowry, C.A., & Montgomery, D.C. 1995. A Review of Multivariate Control Charts. *IIE Transactions*, **27**, 800–810.

Lowry, C.A., Woodall, W.H., Champ, C.W., & Rigdon, S.E. 1992. A Multivariate Exponentially Weighted Moving Average Control Chart. *Technometrics*, **34**, 46–53.

Lucas, J.M., & Saccucci, M.S. 1990. Exponentially Weighted Moving Average Control Schemes: Properties and Enhancements. *Technometrics*, **32**, 1–12.

Maciejewski, R., Hafen, R., Rudolph, S., Tebbetts, G., Cleveland, W.S., & Ebert, D.S. 2009. Generating Synthetic-Syndromic Data for Evaluatinig Visual-Analytics Techniques. *IEEE Computer Graphics and Applications*, **29**, 18–28.

Mandl, K.D., Overhage, J.M., Wagner, M.M., Lober, W.B., Sebastiani, P., Mostashari, F., Pavlin, J.A., Gesteland, P.H., Treadwell, T., Koski, E., Hutwagner, L., Buckeridge, D.L., Aller, R.D., & Grannis, S. 2004. Implementing Syndromic Surveillance: A Practical Guide Informed by the Early Experience. *The Journal of the American Medical Informatics Association*, **11**, 141–150.

McKnight, P.E., McKnight, K.M., Sidani, S., & Figueredo, A.J. 2007. *Missing Data: A Gentle Introduction*. The Guilford Press.

Mei, Y. 2010. Scalable Robust Schemes for Monitoring Multiple Data Streams. *Biometrica*.

M'ikanatha, N.M., Lynfield, R., Van Beneden, C.A., & de Valk, H. (eds). 2007. *Infectious Disease Surveillance*. 1 edn. Blackwell.

Montes de Oca, V., Jeske, D.R., Zhang, Q., Rendon, C., & Marvasti, M. 2010. A CUSUM Change-point Detection Algorithm for Non-stationary Sequences with Application to Data Network Surveillance. *Journal of Systems and Software*, **83**, 1288–1297.

Montgomery, D.C. 2004. *Introduction to Statistical Quality Control*. 5 edn. John Wiley & Sons.

Montgomery, D.C., Jennings, C.L., & Kulachi, M. 2008. *Introduction to Time Series Analysis and Forecasting*. 1 edn. John Wiley & Sons.

Montgomery, D.C., Peck, E.A., & Vining, G.G. 2012. *Introduction to Linear Regression Analysis*. 5 edn. John Wiley & Sons.

Morton, A.P., Whitby, M., McLaws, M.L., Dobson, A., McElwain, S., Looke, D., Stackelroth, J., & Sartor, A. 2001. The application of statistical process control charts to the detection and monitoring of hospital-acquired infections. *Journal of Quality in Clinical Practice*, **21**, 112–117.

Moustakides, G.V. 1986. Optimal Stopping Times for Detecting a Change in Distribution. *Technometrics*, **14**, 1379–1388.

Nau, R.F. 2012. *Decision 411 Forecasting website: Averaging and Exponential Smoothing Models*. Accessed at http://www.duke.edu/ rnau/411avg.htm on June 21, 2012.

NIST. 2012. *NIST website: What is EDA?* Accessed at http://www.itl.nist.gov/div898/handbook/eda/section1/eda11.htm on June 13, 2012.

Olson, K.L., Bonetti, M., Pagano, M., & Mandl, K.D. 2005. Real Time Spatial Cluster Detection Using Interpoint Distances Among Precise Patient Locations. *BMC Medical Informatics and Decision Making*, **5**.

OSD. 2005. *ESSENCE IV Improves Nation's Bio-Surveillance Capability*. Accessed at http://deploymentlink.osd.mil/news/jan05/news_20050125_001.shtml on November 27, 2006.

Ostrom, C.W. 1990. *Time Series Analysis: Regression Techniques*. Sage Publications, Inc.

Page, E.S. 1954. Continuous Inspection Schemes. *Biometrika*, **41**, 100–115.

Paterson, B., Caddis, R., & Durrheim, D. 2011. *Use of Workplace Absenteeism Surveillance Data for Outbreak Detection [letter]*. Accessed at http://wwwnc.cdc.gov/eid/article/17/10/11-0202_article.htm#mainbody.

Perlman, M.D. 1969. One-Sided Testing Problems in Multivariate Analysis. *The Annals of Mathematical Statistics*, **40**, 549–567.

Pignatiello, J.J., Jr., & Runger, G.C. 1990. Comparisons of Multivariate CUSUM Charts. *Journal of Quality Technology*, **3**, 173–186.

Pirsig, R.M. 1999. *Zen and the Art of Motorcycle Maintenance: An Inquiry Into Values*. William Morrow & Company, Inc.

Reingold, A. 2003. If Syndromic Surveillance Is the Answer, What Is the Question? *Biosecurity and Bioterrorism: Biodefense Strategy, Practice, and Science*, **1**, 1–5.

Reis, B.Y., & Mandl, K.D. 2003. Time Series Modeling for Syndromic Surveillance. *BMC Medical Informatics for Decision Making*, **3**.

Reis, B.Y., Pagano, M., & Mandl, K.D. 2003. Using Temporal Context to Improve Biosurveillance. *Proceedings of the National Academy of Sciences of the United States of America*, **100**, 1961–1965.

Rice, J.A. 2006. *Mathematical Statistics and Data Analysis*. 3 edn. Duxbury Press.

Ritov, Y. 1990. Decision Theoretic Optimality of the CUSUM procedure. *The Annals of Statistics*, **18**, 1464–1469.

Roberts, S.W. 1959. Control Chart Tests based on Geometric Moving Averages. *Technometrics*, **1**, 239–250.

RODS. 2010. *RODS Laboratory website*. Accessed at https://www.rods.pitt.edu/site/ on June 5, 2010.

Rogerson, P.A., & Yamada, I. 2004a. Approaches to Syndromic Surveillance When Data Consist of Small Regional Counts. *Morbidity and Mortality Weekly Report*, **53**, 79–84.

Rogerson, P.A., & Yamada, I. 2004b. Monitoring Change in Spatial Patterns of Disease: Comparing Univariate and Multivariate Cumulative Sum Approaches. *Statistics in Medicine*, **23**, 2195–2214.

Rolka, H.R. 2006. Data Analysis Research Issues and Emerging Public Health Biosurveillance Directions. *Pages 101–107 of:* Wilson, A., Wilson, G., & Olwell, D.H. (eds). *Statistical Methods in Counterterrorism: Game Theory, Modeling, Syndromic Surveillance, and Biometric Authentication*. Springer.

Rolka, H.R., & O'Connor, J.C. 2010. Real-Time Public Health Biosurveillance: Systems and Policy Considerations. *In: Infectious Disease Informatics and Biosurveillance: Research, Systems and Case Studies*. Springer.

Rolka, H.R., Bracy, D., Russell, C., Fram, D., & Ball, R. 2005. Using Simulation to Assess the Sensitivity and Specificity of a Signal Detection Tool for Multidimensional Public Health Surveillance Data. *Statistics in Medicine*, **24**, 551–562.

Rolka, H.R., Burkom, H.S., Cooper, G.F., Kulldorff, M., Madigan, D., & Wong, W. 2007. Issues in Applied Statistics for Public Health Bioterrorism Surveillance Using Multiple Data Streams: Research Needs. *Statistics in Medicine*, **26**, 1834–1856.

Rolka, H.R., O'Connor, J.C., & Walker, D. 2008. Public Health Information Fusion for Situation Awareness. *Pages 1–9 of:* Zeng, D., Chen, H., Rolka, H., & Lober, B. (eds). *Biosurveillance and Biosecurity*. Lecture Notes in Computer Science, vol. 5354. Springer, Berlin/Heidelberg.

Schaeffer, R.L. and L. Young, 2009. *Introduction to Probability and Its Applications*. Duxbury Press.

Sebastiani, P., Mandl, K.D., Szolovits, P., Kohane, I.S., & Ramoni, M.F. 2006. A Bayesian Dynamic Model for Influenza (with discussion). *Statistics in Medicine*, **25**, 1803–1825.

Shattuck, L.G., & Miller, N.L. 2006. Extending Naturalistic Decision Making to Complex Organizations: A Dynamic Model of Situated Cognition. *Organization Studies*, **27**, 989–1009.

Shewhart, W.A. 1931. *Economic Control of Quality of Manufactured Product*. D. van Nostrand Company, Inc.

Shmueli, G. 2005. *Wavelet-Based Monitoring for Modern Biosurveillance*. University of Maryland, Robert H. Smith School of Business. Technical Report RHS-06-002.

Shmueli, G., & Burkom, H.S. 2010. Statistical Challenges Facing Early Outbreak Detection in Biosurveillance. *Technometrics*, **52**, 39–51.

Siegmund, D. 1985. *Sequential Analysis, Tests and Confidence Intervals*. Springer-Verlag.

Smolinski, M.S., Hamburg, M.A., & Lederberg, J. (eds). 2003. *Microbial Threats to Health: Emergence, Detection, and Response*. National Academies Press.

Sonesson, C. 2007. A CUSUM Framework for Detection of Space-Time Disease Clusters using Scan Statistics. *Statistics in Medicine*, **26**, 4770–4789.

Sonesson, C., & Bock, D. 2003. A Review and Discussion of Prospective Statistical Surveillance in Public Health. *Journal of the Royal Statistical Society, Series A*, **166**, 5–21.

Sosin, D.M. 2003. Syndromic Surveillance: The Case for Skillful Investment View. *Biosecurity and Bioterrorism: Biodefense Strategy, Practice, and Science*, **1**, 247–253.

Stoto, M.A. 2006. *Syndromic Surveillance in Public Health Practice*. Presentation to Institute of Medicine Forum on Microbial Threats, December 12, 2006.

Stoto, M.A., Schonlau, M., & Mariano, L.T. 2004. Syndromic Surveillance: Is It Worth the Effort? *Chance*, **17**, 19–24.

Stoto, M.A., Fricker, R.D., Jr., Jain, A., Diamond, A., Davies-Cole, J.O., Glymph, C., Kidane, G., Lum, G., Jones, L., Dehan, K., & Yuan, C. 2006. Evaluating Statistical Methods for Syndromic Surveillance. *Pages 141–172 of:* Wilson, A., Wilson, G., & Olwell, D.H. (eds), *Statistical Methods in Counterterrorism: Game Theory, Modeling, Syndromic Surveillance, and Biometric Authentication*. Springer.

Stroup, D.F., Williamson, G.D., Herndon, J.L., & Karon, J.M. 1989. Detection of Aberrations in the Occurrence of Notifiable Dieseases Surveillance Data. *Statistics in Medicine*, **8**, 323–329.

Stroup, D.F., Wharton, M., Kafadar, K., & Dean, A.G. 1993. Evaluation of a Method for Detecting Aberrations in Public Health Surveillance Data. *American Journal of Epidemiology*, **137**(3), 373–380.

Szarka, J.L., III, Gan, L., & Woodall, W.H. 2011. Comparison of the Early Abberation Reporting System (EARS) W2 Methods to an Adaptive Threshold Method. *Statistics in Medicine*, **30**, 489–504.

Taylor, W.A. 2012a. *Change-Point Analysis: A Powerful New Tool for Detecting Changes*. Accessed at http://www.variation.com/cpa/tech/changepoint.html on July 2, 2012.

Taylor, W.A. 2012b. *Change-Point Analyzer Software*. Accessed at http://www.variation.com/cpa/index.html on July 3, 2012.

Testik, M.C., & Runger, G.C. 2006. Multivariate One-Sided Control Charts. *IIE Transactions*, **30**, 635–645.

Thacker, S.B. 2000. Historical Development. *Pages 1–16 of:* Teutsh, S.M., & Churchill, R.E. (eds), *Principles and Practices of Public Health Surveillance*. Oxford University Press.

Tokars, J. 2006. *The BioSense Application*. Presentation at the 2006 PHIN Conference, Atlanta, GA. Accessed at http://0-www.cdc.gov.mill1.sjlibrary.org/biosense/files/Jerry_Tokars.ppt#387,1,The BioSense Application on November 27, 2006.

Toner, E.S. 2009. *Creating Situational Awareness: A Systems Approach*. Accessed at http://www.upmc-biosecurity.org/website/resources/ publications/2009/2009-06-10-SituationalAwarenessSystemsApproach on May 24, 2012.

Toprani, A., Ratard, R., Straif-Bourgeois, S., Sokol, T., Averhoff, F., Brady, J., Staten, D., Sullivan, M., Brooks, J.T., Rowe, A.K., Johnson, K., Vranken, P., & Sergienko, E. 2006. Surveillance in Hurricane Evacuation Centers – Louisiana. *Morbidity and Mortality Weekly Report*, **55**, 32–35.

Tufte, E.R. 1990. *Envisioning Information*. Graphics Press.

Tufte, E.R. 2001. *The Visual Display of Quantitative Information*. 2 edn. Graphics Press.

Tukey, J.W. (ed). 1977. *Exploratory Data Analysis*. Addison Wesley.

US Government. 2007. *Homeland Security Presidential Directive 21: Public Health and Medical Preparedness*. Accessed at http://www.fas.org/irp/offdocs/ nspd/hspd-21.htm on September 29, 2009.

Uscher-Pines, L., Farrell, C.L., Babin, S.M., Cattani, J., Gaydos, C.A., Hsieh, Y., Moskal, M.D., & Rothman, R.E. 2009. Framework for the Development of Response Protocols for Public Health Syndromic Surveillance Systems: Case Studies of 8 US States. *Disaster Medicine and Public Health Preparedness*, **3 (Supplement)**, S29–S36.

Verzani, J. 2005. *Using R for Introductory Statistics*. Hungry Minds, Inc.

Voelker, D.H., Orton, P.Z., & Adams, S.V. 2001. *Statistics*. Hungry Minds, Inc.

Wackerly, D., Mendenhall, W., and R.L. Scheaffer. 2007. *Mathematical Statistics with Applications*. Duxbury Press.

Wagner, M.M., Robinson, J.M., Tsui, F-C., Espino, J.U., & Hogan, W.R. 2003. Design of a National Retail Data Monitor for Public Health Surveillance. *Journal of the American Medical Informatics Association*, **10**, 409–418.

Wagner, M.M., Moore, A.W., & Aryel, R.M. (eds). 2006. *Handbook of Biosurveillance*. Elsevier Academic Press.

Wald, A. 1947. *Sequential Analysis*. John Wiley & Sons.

Waller, L.A. 2004a. Detecting Disease Clustering in Time or Space. *Pages 167–202 of:* Brookmeyer, R., & Stroup, D.F. (eds). *Monitoring the Health of Populations: Statistical Principles & Methods for Public Health Surveillance*. Oxford University Press.

Waller, L.A. 2004b. Invited Commentary: Syndromic Surveillance – Some Statistical Comments. *American Journal of Epidemiology*, **159**, 225–227.

Waller, L.A., & Gotway, C.A. (eds). 2004. *Applied Spatial Statistics for Public Health Data*. John Wiley & Sons.

Winters, P.R. 1960. Forecasting Sales by Exponentially Weighted Moving Averages. *Management Science*, **6**, 324–342.

Wong, D.M. 2010. *The Wall Street Journal Guide to Information Graphics: The Dos and Don'ts of Presenting Data, Facts, and Figures*. W.W. Norton & Company.

Wong, W., Moore, A., Cooper, G., & Wagner, M. 2003. WSARE: What's Strange About Recent Events? *Journal of Urban Health: Bulletin of the New York Academy of Medicine*, **80 (Supplement)**, 66i–75i.

Wong, W., Cooper, G., Dash, D., Levander, J., Dowling, J., Hogan, W., & Wagner, M. 2005. Use of Multiple Data Streams to Conduct Bayesian Biologic Surveillance. *Morbidity and Mortality Weekly Report*, **54 (Supplement)**, 63–69.

Woodall, W.H. 2006. The Use of Control Charts in Health-Care and Public-Health Surveillance. *Journal of Quality Technology*, **38**, 1–16.

Woodall, W.H., & Adams, B.M. 1993. The Statistical Design of CUSUM Charts. *Quality Engineering*, **5**, 559–570.

Woodall, W.H., & Ncube, M.M. 1985. Multivariate CUSUM Quality Control Procedures. *Technometrics*, **27**, 285–292.

Woodall, W.H., Marshall, B., Joner, M.D., Fraker, S.E., & Abdel-Salam, A.G. 2008. On the Use and Evaluation of Scan Methods for Health-related Surveillance. *Journal of the Royal Statistical Society: Series A (Statistics in Society)*, **171**, 223–237.

Young, F.W., Valero-Mora, P.M., & Friendly, M. (eds). 2006. *Visual Statistics: Seeing Data with Dynamic Interactive Graphics*. Wiley-Interscience.

Zhang, J., Tsui, F., Wagner, M., & Hogan, W. 2003. Detection of Outbreaks from Time Series Data Using Wavelet Transform. *AMIA Annual Symposium Proceedings*, 748–752.

Zhu, Y., Wang, W., Atrubin, D., & Wu, Y. 2005. Initial Evaluation of the Early Aberration Reporting System – Florida. *Morbidity and Mortality Weekly Report*, **54 (Supplement)**, 123–130.

Zubay, G. (ed). 2005. *Agents of Bioterrorism: Pathogens and Their Weaponization*. Columbia University Press.

Author Index

Subject Index